T0321969

Pattern and Data Analysis in Healthcare Settings

Vivek Tiwari
Maulana Azad National Institute of Technology, India

Basant Tiwari
Devi Ahilya University, India

Ramjeevan Singh Thakur
Maulana Azad National Institute of Technology, India

Shailendra Gupta
AISECT University, India

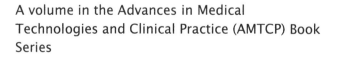

A volume in the Advances in Medical Technologies and Clinical Practice (AMTCP) Book Series

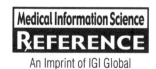

Medical Information Science
REFERENCE
An Imprint of IGI Global

Published in the United States of America by
    Medical Information Science Reference (an imprint of IGI Global)
    701 E. Chocolate Avenue
    Hershey PA, USA 17033
    Tel: 717-533-8845
    Fax: 717-533-8661
    E-mail: cust@igi-global.com
    Web site: http://www.igi-global.com

Library of Congress Cataloging-in-Publication Data

Names: Tiwari, Vivek, 1982- editor. I Tiwari, Basant, 1975- editor. I Thakur,
    Ramjeevan Singh, 1974- editor. I Gupta, Shailendra, editor.
Title: Pattern and data analysis in healthcare settings / Vivek Tiwari,
    Basant Tiwari, Ramjeevan Singh Thakur, and Shailendra Gupta, editors.
Description: Hershey, PA : Medical Information Science Reference, [2017] I
    Includes bibliographical references and index.
Identifiers: LCCN 2016017556I ISBN 9781522505365 (hardcover) I ISBN
    9781522505372 (ebook)
Subjects: I MESH: Medical Informatics
Classification: LCC R858 I NLM W 26.5 I DDC 610.285--dc23 LC record available at https://lccn.loc.gov/2016017556

This book is published in the IGI Global book series Advances in Medical Technologies and Clinical Practice (AMTCP) (ISSN: 2327-9354; eISSN: 2327-9370)

British Cataloguing in Publication Data
A Cataloguing in Publication record for this book is available from the British Library.

For electronic access to this publication, please contact: eresources@igi-global.com.

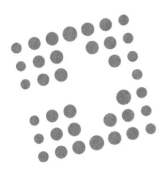

Advances in Medical Technologies and Clinical Practice (AMTCP) Book Series

Srikanta Patnaik
SOA University, India
Priti Das
S.C.B. Medical College, India

ISSN: 2327-9354
EISSN: 2327-9370

MISSION

Medical technological innovation continues to provide avenues of research for faster and safer diagnosis and treatments for patients. Practitioners must stay up to date with these latest advancements to provide the best care for nursing and clinical practices.

The **Advances in Medical Technologies and Clinical Practice (AMTCP) Book Series** brings together the most recent research on the latest technology used in areas of nursing informatics, clinical technology, biomedicine, diagnostic technologies, and more. Researchers, students, and practitioners in this field will benefit from this fundamental coverage on the use of technology in clinical practices.

COVERAGE

- Medical Imaging
- Patient-Centered Care
- Clinical Nutrition
- Biomedical Applications
- E-Health
- Neural Engineering
- Clinical Data Mining
- Clinical Studies
- Diagnostic Technologies
- Telemedicine

IGI Global is currently accepting manuscripts for publication within this series. To submit a proposal for a volume in this series, please contact our Acquisition Editors at Acquisitions@igi-global.com or visit: http://www.igi-global.com/publish/.

Titles in this Series

For a list of additional titles in this series, please visit: www.igi-global.com

Emerging Research in the Analysis and Modeling of Gene Regulatory Networks
Ivan V. Ivanov (Texas A&M University, USA) Xiaoning Qian (Texas A&M University, USA) and Ranadip Pal (Texas Tech University, USA)
Medical Information Science Reference • copyright 2016 • 418pp • H/C (ISBN: 9781522503538) • US $195.00 (our price)

Applied Case Studies and Solutions in Molecular Docking-Based Drug Design
Siavoush Dastmalchi (Tabriz University of Medical Sciences, Iran) Maryam Hamzeh-Mivehroud (Tabriz University of Medical Sciences, Iran) and Babak Sokouti (Tabriz University of Medical Sciences, Iran)
Medical Information Science Reference • copyright 2016 • 367pp • H/C (ISBN: 9781522503620) • US $225.00 (our price)

Methods and Algorithms for Molecular Docking-Based Drug Design and Discovery
Siavoush Dastmalchi (Tabriz University of Medical Sciences, Iran) Maryam Hamzeh-Mivehroud (Tabriz University of Medical Sciences, Iran) and Babak Sokouti (Tabriz University of Medical Sciences, Iran)
Medical Information Science Reference • copyright 2016 • 456pp • H/C (ISBN: 9781522501152) • US $235.00 (our price)

Advancing Pharmaceutical Processes and Tools for Improved Health Outcomes
Tagelsir Mohamed Gasmelseid (International University of Africa, Sudan)
Medical Information Science Reference • copyright 2016 • 388pp • H/C (ISBN: 9781522502487) • US $185.00 (our price)

Classification and Clustering in Biomedical Signal Processing
Nilanjan Dey (Techno India College of Technology, India) and Amira Ashour (Tanta University, Egypt)
Medical Information Science Reference • copyright 2016 • 463pp • H/C (ISBN: 9781522501404) • US $225.00 (our price)

Virtual Reality Enhanced Robotic Systems for Disability Rehabilitation
Fei Hu (University of Alabama, USA) Jiang Lu (University of Houston -Clear Lake, USA) and Ting Zhang (University of Alabama, USA)
Medical Information Science Reference • copyright 2016 • 383pp • H/C (ISBN: 9781466697409) • US $210.00 (our price)

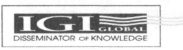

www.igi-global.com

701 E. Chocolate Ave., Hershey, PA 17033
Order online at www.igi-global.com or call 717-533-8845 x100
To place a standing order for titles released in this series, contact: cust@igi-global.com
Mon-Fri 8:00 am - 5:00 pm (est) or fax 24 hours a day 717-533-8661

Table of Contents

Section 2
Knowledge Visualization and Big Data

Section 3
Data Mining: Utilization and Application

Detailed Table of Contents

Section 1
Healthcare Settings and Security

Chapter 1

Agnieszka Dardzinska, Bialystok University of Technology, Poland

Action rule is an implication rule that shows the expected change in a decision value of an object as a result of changes made to some of its conditional values. An example of an action rule is 'patients are expected to control their health regularly if they receive an information about free medical tests once a year'. In this case, the decision value is the health status, and the condition value is whether the information is sent to the patient. Because of some complex medical problems this paper discusses a strategy which generates action rules to using new knowledge base consisting of classification rules. As one of the testing domains for our research, we take new system for gathering and processing clinical data on patients with throat disorders, and mining action rules will suggest in simply way how to construct the decision support module for easier given diagnosis for patients.

Chapter 2

Grasha Jacob, Rani Anna Govt. College, Tirunelveli
Murugan Annamalai, Dr. Ambedkar Govt. Arts College, India

Telemedicine has become a common method for transmission of medical images and patient data across long distances. With the growth of computer networks and the latest advances in digital technologies, large amount of digital data gets exchanged over various types of insecure networks - wired or wireless. Modern Healthcare Management Systems need to change to accommodate these new advances. There is an urgent need to protect the confidentiality of health care records that are stored in common databases and transmitted over public insecure channels. This chapter outlines DNA sequence based cryptography which is easy to implement and is robust against cryptanalytic attack as there is insignificant correlation between the original record and the encrypted image for the secure storage and transmission of health records.

Chapter 3

Ramgopal Kashyap, AISECT University, India
Pratima Gautam, AISECT University, India

Medical applications became a boon to the healthcare industry. It needs correct and fast segmentation associated with medical images for correct diagnosis. This assures high quality segmentation of medical images victimization. The Level Set Method (LSM) is a capable technique, however the quick process using correct segments remains difficult. The region based models like Active Contours, Globally Optimal Geodesic Active Contours (GOGAC) performs inadequately for intensity irregularity images. During this cardstock, we have a new tendency to propose an improved region based level set model motivated by the geodesic active contour models as well as the Mumford-Shah model. So that you can eliminate the re-initialization process of ancient level set model and removes the will need of computationally high priced re-initialization. Compared using ancient models, our model are sturdier against images using weak edge and intensity irregularity.

Chapter 4

Shaligram Prajapat, Maulana Azad National Institute of Technology, India & Devi Ahilya University, India
Ramjeevan Singh Thakur, Maulana Azad National Institute of Technology, India

"Key" plays a vital role in every symmetric key cryptosystem. The obvious way of enhancing security of any cryptosystem is to keep the key as large as possible. But it may not be suitable for low power devices since higher computation will be done for longer keys and that will increase the power requirement which decreases the device's performance. In order to resolve the former specified problem an alternative approach can be used in which the length of key is fixed and its value varies in every session. This is Time Variant Key approach or Automatic Variable Key (AVK) approach. The Security of AVK based cryptosystem is enhanced by exchanging some parameters instead of keys between the communicating parties, then these parameters will be used to generate required keys at the receiver end. This chapter presents implementation of the above specified Mechanism. A model has been demonstrated with parameterized scheme and issues in AVK approach. Further, it has been analyzed from different users' perspectives. This chapter also highlights the benefits of AVK model to ensure two levels of security with characterization of methods for AVK and Estimation of key computation based on parameters only. The characteristic components of recent styles of key design with consideration of key size, life time of key and breaking threshold has also been pointed out. These characteristics are essential in the design of efficient symmetric key cryptosystem. The novel approach of AVK based cryptosystem is suitable for low power devices and useful for exchanging very large objects or files. This scheme has been demonstrated with Fibonacci-Q matrix and sparse matrix based diffused key information exchange procedures. These models have been further tested from perspective of hackers and cryptanalyst, to exploit any weakness with fixed size dynamic keys.

Chapter 5

Aditi Nema, BIRT, India

The detection portion of Intrusion Detection System is the most complicated. The IDS goal is to make the network more secure, and the prevention portion of the IDS must accomplish that effort. After malicious or unwanted traffic is identified, using prevention techniques can stop it. When an IDS is placed in an inline configuration, all traffic must travel through an IDS sensor. In this paper the reduced the features and perform layered architecture for identify various attack (DoS, R2L, U2R, Probe) and show accuracy using SVM with genetic approach.

Section 2
Knowledge Visualization and Big Data

Chapter 6

Ram Kumar, Barkatullah University, India
Shailesh Jaloree, SATI, India
R. S. Thakur, MANIT, India

Knowledge-based systems have become widespread in modern years. Knowledge-base developers need to be able to share and reuse knowledge bases that they build. As a result, interoperability among different knowledge-representation systems is essential. Domain ontology seeks to reduce conceptual and terminological confusion among users who need to share various kind of information. This paper shows how these structures make it possible to bridge the gap between standard objects and Knowledge-based Systems.

Chapter 7

Monica Sankat, Barkatullah University, India
R. S. Thakur, MANIT, India
Shailesh Jaloree, SATI, India

In this paper, we present a (semi) automatic framework that aims to produce a domain concept from text and to derive domain ontology from this concept. This paper details the steps that transform textual resources (and particularly textual learning objects) into a domain concept and explains how this abstract structure is transformed into more formal domain ontology. This methodology targets particularly the educational field because of the need of such structures (Ontologies and Knowledge Management). The paper also shows how these structures make it possible to bridge the gap between core concepts and Formal ontology.

Chapter 8

Girraj Prasad Rathor, AISECT University, India
Sanjeev Kumar Gupta, AISECT University, India

Image fusion based on different wavelet transform is the most commonly used image fusion method, which fuses the source pictures data in wavelet space as per some fusion rules. But, because of the uncertainties of the source images contributions to the fused image, to design a good fusion rule to incorporate however much data as could reasonably be expected into the fused picture turns into the most vital issue. On the other hand, adaptive fuzzy logic is the ideal approach to determine uncertain issues, yet it has not been utilized as a part of the outline of fusion rule. A new fusion technique based on wavelet transform and adaptive fuzzy logic is introduced in this chapter. After doing wavelet transform to source images, it computes the weight of each source images coefficients through adaptive fuzzy logic and then fuses the coefficients through weighted averaging with the processed weights to acquire a combined picture: Mutual Information, Peak Signal to Noise Ratio, and Mean Square Error as criterion.

Chapter 9

Vinod Kumar, Maulana Azad National Institute of Technology, India
Ramjeevan Singh Thakur, Maulana Azad National Institute of Technology, India

With every passing day, data generation is increasing exponentially, its volume, variety, velocity are making it quite challenging to analyze, interpret, visualize for gaining the greater insights from the available data. Billions of networked sensors are being embedded in devices such as smart phones, automobiles, social media sites, laptop, PC's and industrial machines etc. that operates, generate and communicate data. Thus, the data obtained from various resources exists in structured, semi-structured and unstructured form. The traditional database system is not suitable to handle these data formats. Therefore, new tools and techniques are developed to work with these data. NoSQL is one of them. Currently, many NoSQL database are available in the market, each one of them specially designed to solve specific type of data handling problems, most of the NoSQL databases are developed with special attention to problem of business organizations and enterprises. The chapter focuses various aspects of NoSQL as tool for handling the big data.

Section 3
Data Mining: Utilization and Application

Chapter 10

Sachin Kamley, SATI, India
Shailesh Jaloree, SATI, India
R. S. Thakur, MANIT, India

Stock market nature is considered to be dynamic and susceptible to quick changes because it depends on various factors like share price, fundamental variables like P/E ratio, dividend yield etc. election results, rumors etc. Now a day's prediction is an important process which determines the future worth of a company. The successful prediction brings motivation and awareness in stock community as well as economic growth of the country. In past various theories and methods like Efficient Market Hypothesis (EMH), Random Walk Theory, fundamental and technical analyses have been proposed. These methods or combination of methods have not got as much success even yet because these methods are very complex and time consuming and performed well on short data. These days stock market users mostly rely on intelligent trading system which would be help them to predict share prices based on various situations and conditions. Data mining is a broad area and also supports various business intelligence techniques. It has mastery to raise various financial issues like buying/selling security, bond analysis, contract analyses etc. in this study various prediction techniques like linear regression, multiple regression, association rule mining, clustering, neural network have been proposed and their significant performances will be compared by Bombay Stock Exchange (BSE) data.

Chapter 11

Vivek Badhe, MANIT, India
R. S. Thakur, MANIT, India
G. S. Thakur, MANIT, India

Problem of decision making is a crucial task in every business. Profit Pattern Mining hit the target by minimizes the gap between statistical based pattern generation and value base decision making. But this job is found very difficult when it depends on the large, imprecise and vague environment, which is frequent in recent years. The concept of soft computing with data mining is novel way to address this difficulty. The general approaches to association rule mining focus on inducting rule by using correlation among data and finding frequent occurring patterns. The major technique uses support and confidence measures for generating rules which is not adequate nowadays as a measure of interest, since the data have become more multifaceted these days, it's a necessary to find solution that deals with such problems and uses some new measures like profit, significance etc. In this chapter, authors apply concept of pattern mining with vague set theory, Genetic algorithm theory and related properties to the commercial management to deal with business decision making problem.

Chapter 12

Suraj Kumar Nayak, National Institute of Technology Rourkela, India
Utkarsh Srivastava, National Institute of Technology Rourkela, India
D. N. Tibarewala, Jadavpur University, India
Goutam Thakur, Manipal Institute of Technology, India
Biswajit Mohapatra, Vesaj Patel Hospital, India
Kunal Pal, National Institute of Technology Rourkela, India

The current study delineates the effect of Odia and Tamil music on the Autonomic Nervous System (ANS) and cardiac conduction pathway of Odia volunteers. The analysis of the ECG signals using Analysis of Variance (ANOVA) showed that the features obtained from the HRV domain, time-domain and wavelet transform domain were statistically insignificant. But non-linear classifiers like Classification and Regression Tree (CART), Boosted Tree (BT) and Random Forest (RF) indicated the presence of important features. A classification efficiency of more than 85% was achieved when the important features, obtained from the non-linear classifiers, were used. The results suggested that there is an increase in the parasympathetic activity when music is heard in the mother tongue. If a person is made to listen to music in the language with which he is not conversant, an increase in the sympathetic activity is observed. It is also expected that there might be a difference in the cardiac conduction pathway.

As we know use of Internet flourishes with its full velocity and in all dimensions. Enormous availability of Text documents in digital form (email, web pages, blog post, news articles, ebooks and other text files) on internet challenges technology to appropriate retrieval of document as a response for any search query. As a result there has been an eruption of interest in people to mine these vast resources and classify them properly. It invigorates researchers and developers to work on numerous approaches of document clustering. Researchers got keen interest in this problem of text mining. The aim of this chapter is to summarised different document clustering algorithms used by researchers.

Analyzing clustering of mixed data set is a complex problem. Very useful clustering algorithms like k-means, fuzzy c-means, hierarchical methods etc. developed to extract hidden groups from numeric data. In this paper, the mixed data is converted into pure numeric with a conversion method, the various algorithm of numeric data has been applied on various well known mixed datasets, to exploit the inherent structure of the mixed data. Experimental results shows how smoothly the mixed data is giving better results on universally applicable clustering algorithms for numeric data.

Foreword

The fields of computer science have given us much to think and work with. Data analysis and Mining might not have satisfied all its buildup, but rather it had an exceptionally solid role in stimulating thought about what knowledge can and cannot be demonstrated.

The whole book dedicated to data analysis, pattern and their utility. Data analysis is not just about having more insight into the data, but far more. There are various aspects and dimensions to see the same data and the utility of the outcome depends on this. I think, the medical sector is one of the most promising and challenging dimensions of data analysis. It is promising because having direct impact on our society and livelihood and challenging because of having complex data, variety of formats, data confidentiality, and many more. I think, this book provides enough information and necessary components for aforesaid issues.

Reviewing the contents of this book, I am struck by the different and diverse nature of the field as well as how much convergence and coherence has emerged in such a short time. This book figures out with every aspect of the field without turning into an immense awkward black box of a thing concentrated on data, information, knowledge and everything else under the sun. It is interesting to see just how much agreement there exists among researchers and practitioners as to what data analysis, security and mining are. This book is a decent stride in that heading.

R.K. Pateriya
Maulana Azad National Institute of Technology (MA-NIT), India

Preface

Nowadays, many applications are generating huge quantities of data (medical, clinical, reports, stock, logs, etc.) and it becomes difficult to manage efficiently. Instant and correct decisions are always key factors in business and health care industries. However, there are numbers of approaches have been discovered such as data warehousing, databases, Bigdata, cloud, etc., but, all are concentrating on only data management and it can be viewed as two ways, daily transaction data management and historical data management. Transaction data are managed and maintained by operational database which is also known as Database Management Systems (DBMS). Historical data are managed by data warehouses and it is used for analysis and decision making. These both approaches are the best for data management, but they do not allow to facilitate *knowledge on–demand*. Noteworthy, Users have to do analysis repeatedly whenever the need arises. Nowadays, databases are huge and dynamic because it comes from various application domains and a variety of patterns can be extracted. It is clear that business users do not have an interest in data, but they are striving for trends hidden within the data. So, more elaborated and advanced techniques are needed to be investigated to mine the hidden trends and let them available for further analysis. Many techniques are developed to extract patterns, especially in the context of data mining and the results of such techniques are abstract and compact representations of the original data. The data processing methods such as data mining produce the results such as clusters, association rules, decision trees and others. The output of all the data mining and knowledge discovery techniques represent big portions of the raw data by a few number of knowledge-carrying representatives, which call *patterns*. The pattern is useful because it describes a recurrent behavior and trends. The pattern is a compact representation of raw data, but, usually, in a form that cannot lead us significant meaning directly to real life use. The volume of extracting patterns from various knowledge discovery applications is increasing exponentially, so there requires an effective pattern analysis system that will permit us to compare, query and store the patterns.

The beginning of 90s, it was considered that huge amount of data is available and data warehousing was getting tremendous success as a central data repository system. The working of a data warehouse is represented as multiple layers of data and their processing unit, where, data move from one layer to another. A data warehouse is a central data repository system where data are integrated from external data sources. Basically, data coming from external source are heterogeneous in nature. Often, external data sources are transaction and production system so data are frequently changed. Moreover, these systems may suffer with one major problem of schema changes. So, there is need a system that works as a facilitator for data analysis. Data warehouses can be considered as a separate and dedicated repository of historical data. Furthermore, data warehouse provides a basic framework for analytical processing, decision making, and data mining applications. Several benefits exist when data warehouses are used together with Electronic Healthcare Record (EHRs). First, data warehouses combine data from many disparate sources—including legacy and retired systems—obviating the need for time-consuming manual extraction and assimilation of data from multiple systems. Furthermore, as data are combined, they are often standardized to allow comparisons to be made (e.g. gender of "male," "M," and "1" might be converted into a uniform value). Second, the integration with tools to perform data mining and statistical analyses allows a wide variety of exploratory analyses to be rapidly performed. Third, because data warehouses are separate from the primary systems that hold the source data, performing analyses does not result in additional load and a concomitant reduction in response time to the "live" EHR system used in clinical practice. Finally, unlike EHRs that typically store data in a patient-centric manner, data warehouses store data in a format that easily allows cross patient searches (e.g. "find all patients with systolic blood pressure greater than 140").

Basically, data mining is able to extract the knowledge from a variety of data. Furthermore, underlying methods and algorithms may differ with the view of different types of data. Data mining techniques should be able to handle the challenges carried by data due to their diversity. All pattern generating methods produce knowledge in the form of patterns and most importantly, these patterns are not persistent by nature. Means, the pattern gets lost when it goes out of memory inspite of having long and complex process behind the pattern generation and It is time and resource consuming as well. The major drawbacks with these pattern generating methods are:

1. Patterns are not persistent, i.e. each time when patterns are in need, it is necessary to execute pattern generating method again and again.
2. Patterns have become stale when data source is updated i.e., as source of data or data warehouse is updated then the same pattern extracting method may give different patterns as compared to earlier.
3. In some cases patterns are huge itself and it is hard to manage in main memory because the algorithm which generates patterns itself resides in memory and occupy major portion. This situation makes the whole process slow.
4. In some cases, the data warehouse is not maintained by the organizations, i.e. data need to be accessed from various locations on-demand. It may face some authentication and authorization issues because there is a need to make connection with various data sources on the fly and even this complex process is required to be repeated again and again to get the patterns on different moments.
5. The process of collecting the data every time is not a single issue, but further preprocessing of data (cleaning, transformation, etc.) is required to make it suitable for analysis.

Due to all above said issues data management through data warehousing and pattern generation through data mining is still suffering from many problems. So, this kind of data management and decision making process is not full proof, suitable in critical business application and health care decision making.

This book aims to investigate all the approaches which help with efficient and flexible data analysis specially in medical and bioinformatics domain. Through this book, we are looking forward new approaches or existing methods which can modify to accommodate in on-demand bioinformatics knowledge retrieval concept. There is found little investigation on pattern management for business and health care industries. Healthcare practices have been enhanced through the use of information technologies and analytical methods. Nowadays, there is a need to optimize health care data or trends management through knowledge on-demand concept. This book investigates the incorporation of pattern management into business technologies and health care for the decision making and prediction process. This book brings together the common issues of business and health care pattern management. These two areas have not been tackled collectively till date. This book tries to uncover the various strategies, techniques and approaches which may improve the organization's pattern management power and helps for quick and efficient decision making. Instant and correct decisions are always key factors in business and health care industries. There need a separate system which helps to organize, store, manipulate and retrieval of patterns. This book will spread an awareness about bioinformatics pattern management, its need and applications. We are looking forward attention on business applications health care data management, but is not limited to.

So as to give the most thorough, in-depth, and current scope of every single related subject and their applications, and also to offer a solitary reference source on all conceptual, methodological and technical, We are satisfied to offer a rich collection on this quickly developing discipline. This collection intends to enable specialists, researchers, understudies, and professionals by encouraging their extensive comprehension of the most basic data analysis in medical territories inside this field of study. This collection, entitled '*Pattern and data analysis in healthcare settings*' is organized into three distinct sections, which are as follows: (1) Healthcare settings and security (2) Knowledge visualization and Big data (3) Data Mining: Utilization and Application. The following paragraphs provide a summary of what is covered in each chapter.

Chapter 1 (*Association Action Rules Mining in Laryngological Disorders*): These days we can watch extremely dynamic development in the field of computer based medical systems. It is the consequence of perceptible enhancements in medical care. Finding valuable rules of the medical data is a critical assignment of a knowledge discovery process. However, in the meantime, individuals are overpowered by countless rules. In this way, a requirement for new techniques with the capacity to help clients in breaking down an extensive number of rules. An action rule is a rule extracted from a decision system that describes a possible reclassification of objects from one state to another. Mining action rules can propose how to develop the decision support module for better patients' diagnosis. This chapter built a system to support flat feet treatment. The model suggested that the arch height correction is increased by age and place of living, and decreased as body mass increased.

Chapter 2 (*Secure Storage and Transmission of Health Care Records*): Electronic Health Record (EHR) is a step by step being executed in numerous nations. It is the need of great importance since it enhances the nature of medical services and is additionally financially savvy. In this perspective, Telemedicine has turned into a typical technique for transmission of medical pictures and patient information crosswise over long separations over different sorts of unstable systems - wired or remote. There is an earnest need to ensure the confidentiality of health care records that are put away in like manner databases and transmitted over open unstable channels. This chapter plots DNA grouping based cryptography, which is easy to implement but difficult to execute and is robust against cryptanalytic attack as there is an insignificant correlation between the original record and the encrypted image for the secure storage and transmission of health records.

Chapter 3 (*Fast Medical Image Segmentation Using Energy-Based Method*): Medical applications turned into a shelter to the healthcare industry. It needs right and quick segmentation connected with medicinal pictures for right finding. This guarantees high quality segmentation of medical images exploitation. The level set method (LSM) is a proficient system, however the brisk procedure utilizing correct segments stays troublesome. The region based models like Active Contours, Globally Optimal Geodesic Active Contours (GOGAC) performs inadequately for intensity irregularity images. This chapter objective is to discover 'under segmented' spots in GOGAC and enhance it by outskirt extension technique. We have utilized the Globally Optimal Geodesic Active Contours based division calculation.

Chapter 4 (*Towards Parameterized Shared Key for AVK Approach*): "Information security is the sole target of each communication system significantly in critical medical record exchange. "Key" assumes an indispensable part in each symmetric key cryptosystem and for upgrading security of any cryptosystem is to keep the key as large as would be prudent. However, it may not be appropriate for low power gadgets since higher calculation will be ruined longer keys. An alternative methodology can be utilized as a part of which the length of the key is settled and its value fluctuates in each session. This is Time Variant Key approach or Automatic Variable Key (AVK) approach. The Security of AVK based cryptosystem is enhanced by exchanging some parameters instead of keys between the communicating parties.

Chapter 5 (*Innovative Approach for Improving Intrusion Detection Using Genetic Algorithm with Layered Approach*): The detection portion of Intrusion Detection System (IDS) is the most complicated. The IDS goal is to make the network more secure, and the prevention portion of the IDS must accomplish that effort. After malicious or unwanted traffic is identified, using prevention techniques can stop it. When an IDS is placed in an inline configuration, all traffic must travel through an IDS sensor. In this chapter, the reduced the features and perform layered architecture for identifying various attacks (DoS, R2L, U2R, Probe) and show accuracy using SVM with genetic approach.

Chapter 6 (*Knowledge Extraction from Domain-Specific Documents*): Knowledge-based systems have become widespread in present day years. Knowledge-base developers should have the capacity to share and reuse knowledge bases that they build. As a result, interoperability among different knowledge-representation systems is essential. Domain ontology seeks to reduce conceptual and terminological confusion among users who need to share various kinds of information. This chapter shows how these structures make it possible to bridge the gap between standard objects and Knowledge-based Systems.

Chapter 7 (*Semi-Automatic Ontology Design for Educational Purposes*): Ontology characterizes a common vocabulary for researchers who need to share information in a domain. Ontology can be dealt with as set of themes connected with different types of relations. Development of such ontology from a given corpus can be an exceptionally tedious assignment for the user. This chapter presents a (semi) automatic framework that aims to produce a domain concept from the text and to derive a domain ontology from this concept. This chapter details the steps that transform textual resources (and particularly textual learning objects) into a domain concept and explains how this abstract structure is transformed into more formal domain ontology.

Chapter 8 (*Improving Multimodality Image Fusion through Integrate AFL and Wavelet Transform*): Multimodalities data fusion has turned a discipline to which more and more general formal solutions to a number of application cases are required. A few circumstances (i.e. Medical diagnosis) in image processing, simultaneously require high spatial and high spectral information in a single composite image. In this view, The integration of 2D DWT image fusion with adaptive fuzzy logic in the broader framework of 2D DWT image processing and visualization is the definitive objective of this chapter. Chapter 9 (*Big Data: Techniques, Tools, and Technologies – NoSQL Database*): Today, the world is suffocating in data however starving for information. With each passing day, data generation is expanding exponentially in its volume, variety, velocity, variability, and complexity is making it quite challenging to analyze, interpret, visualize for gaining the greater insights from the available data. Here, in chapter, a brief introduction of architecture and working of NoSQL Database with MapReduce is discussed. Furthermore, a summarized difference between NoSQL Database and Traditional database is likewise discussed.

Chapter 10 (*Bombay Stock Exchange of India: Patterns and Trends Prediction Using Data Mining Techniques*): Stock market nature is considered to be dynamic and susceptible to speedy changes since it relies on upon different variables. Presently a day's, forecast is a vital process which determines the future worth of an organization. Data mining is a broad area and also supports various business intelligence techniques. It has the mastery to raise various financial issues like buying/selling security, bond analysis, contract analyses etc. In this study, various prediction techniques like linear regression, multiple regression, association rule mining, clustering, neural network have been proposed and their significant performances will be compared with Bombay Stock Exchange (BSE) data.

Chapter 11 (*Profit Pattern Mining Using Soft Computing for Decision Making: Pattern Mining Using Vague Set and Genetic Algorithm*): In this chapter, a method is planned for decision making by joining vague set theory as a tool in association rule mining. The rules generated by conventional Apriori are compared with the rules generated by our algorithm that finds vague rules. The Apriori algorithm is implemented and the dataset is fed to find the rules. The presented algorithm uses vague set theory concepts to find rules in the datasets. For that, there is give few propositions and definitions regarding the vague terminology of the database, such as, vague percentage, true vague support, and true vague confidence.

Chapter 12 (*Effect of Odia and Tamil Music on the ANS and the Conduction Pathway of Heart of Odia Volunteers*): The present study depicts the effect of Odia and Tamil music on the Autonomic Nervous System (ANS) and cardiac conduction pathway of Odia volunteers. The analysis of the ECG signals using Analysis of Variance (ANOVA) showed that the features obtained from the HRV domain, time-domain and wavelet transform domain were statistically insignificant. But non-linear classifiers like Classification and Regression Tree (CART), Boosted Tree (BT) and Random Forest (RF) indicated the presence of important features. The outcomes suggested that there is an expansion in the parasympathetic activity when music is heard in the mother tongue. If a person is made to listen to music in the language with which he is not conversant, an increase in the sympathetic activity is observed.

Chapter 13 (*Document Clustering: A Summarized Survey*): Nowaday, internet thrives with its full velocity and in all dimensions. Enormous availability of Text documents in digital form (email, web pages, blog post, news articles, ebooks and other text files) on internet challenges technology to appropriate retrieval of document as a reaction for any search query. Subsequently, there has been an emission of enthusiasm for individuals to mine these vast resources and classify them appropriately. It empowers researchers and designers to work on numerous approaches of document clustering. The aim of this chapter is to summarize different document clustering algorithms used by researchers.

Chapter 14 (*Cluster Analysis with Various Algorithms for Mixed Data*): Investigating clustering of a mixed data set is a mind boggling issue. Extremely valuable clustering algorithms like k-means, fuzzy c-means, hierarchical methods, etc. developed to extract hidden groups from numeric data. In this chapter, the mixed data is changed over into pure numeric with a conversion method, the various algorithms of numeric data has been applied to various well known mixed datasets, to exploit the inherent structure of the mixed data. Experimental results demonstrate how easily the mixed data are giving better results on universally applicable clustering algorithms for numeric data.

TARGET AUDIENCE

By focusing on concepts such as pattern management, conceptual modeling, logical modeling, access control, quality issues, security, clustering, fusion, knowledge retrieval, knowledge updating, pattern comparison, data filtering, this book is a comprehensive reference source for policy makers, academicians, researchers, students, technology developers, and professionals interested in the development of pattern management system for business application health care decision making. This book brings attention of researchers/professionals who are working in the area of Data management, Data mining, Data warehousing, Knowledge, management, Information Retrieval, Business decision maker, Health care data manager, Big data worker.

Vivek Tiwari
Maulana Azad National Institute of Technology, India

Basant Tiwari
Devi Ahilya University, India

Ramjeevan Singh Thakur
Maulana Azad National Institute of Technology, India

Shailendra Gupta
AISECT University, India

Acknowledgment

The editors would like to express appreciation to the numerous individuals who saw us through this book; for all those who provided support, talked things over, read, composed, offered remarks, allowed us to cite their comments and assisted in the editing, proofreading and design. Without their support, this book would not have become a reality.

I believe that the team of authors provides the perfect blend of knowledge and skills that went into composing this book. I thank each of the authors for devoting their time and effort towards this book; I believe that it will be a great asset to the community! Much obliged for everything, I look forward to writing the second edition soon! The editors wish to acknowledge the significant commitments of the reviewers regarding the improvement of quality, coherence, and content presentation of chapters. Some of the authors also served as referees; we highly appreciate their twofold undertaking.

We would like to thank to our mentor Dr. Kamal Raj Pardasani, Dr. R.K. Pateriya, Dr. Kanak Saxena, Dr. Millie Pant, Dr. D.K. Mishra, Dr. Shailendra Singh, Dr. D.K. Rajoriya, Dr. A.K. Sachan, Dr. Manish Billore, Dr. Jagdish Chand Bansal. They have been our inspiration and motivation for continuing to improve our knowledge and experience. We are likewise exceptionally appreciative of Mr. Pawan Grover for providing all support and faith when required.

Last and not least: I beg forgiveness of all those who have been with me over the course of the years and whose names I have failed to mention.

Vivek Tiwari
Maulana Azad National Institute of Technology, India

Ramjeevan Singh Thakur
Maulana Azad National Institute of Technology, India

Basant Tiwari
Devi Ahilya University, India

Shailendra Gupta
AISECT University, India

Section 1
Healthcare Settings and Security

Chapter 1
Action Rules Mining in Hoarseness Disease

Agnieszka Dardzinska
Bialystok University of Technology, Poland

ABSTRACT

Action rule is an implication rule that shows the expected change in a decision value of an object as a result of changes made to some of its conditional values. An example of an action rule is 'patients are expected to control their health regularly if they receive an information about free medical tests once a year'. In this case, the decision value is the health status, and the condition value is whether the information is sent to the patient. Because of some complex medical problems this paper discusses a strategy which generates action rules to using new knowledge base consisting of classification rules. As one of the testing domains for our research, we take new system for gathering and processing clinical data on patients with throat disorders, and mining action rules will suggest in simply way how to construct the decision support module for easier given diagnosis for patients.

INTRODUCTION

Support of decision making plays an extremely wide role in many fields, especially medicine. In medical databases many attributes can be misunderstood, unclear or missing. It could be very complicated for medical staff, because of luck of full information which can be useful in patient's diagnosis and treatment. Each medical database stores information about patient's age, gender, diagnosis, treatments, etc. It uses attributes suitable for locally collected information. Values of attributes can be disease code, treatment code, patient category, etc. One coded attribute can be replaced by several others with a small numbers of values and clear meaning. For instance, a code for broken bone indicates broken bone, the location, the type of fracture, etc. There have been a lot of methods to extract rules from complete information system in the literature, while it is much more difficult to extract rules from incomplete information system. When we look into laryngological diseases, the main symptom in almost all kind of diseases is hoarseness. Therefore it is possible to make a fast and incorrect diagnosis, which leads to treatment that means waste of time and sometimes even human life. Our proposed new method analyzes different

DOI: 10.4018/978-1-5225-0536-5.ch001

symptoms for different patients and suggests actions which can be made to improve medical treatment for their faster recovery. The primary purpose of this approach is to improve diagnostic accuracy, reduce inappropriate antibiotic or steroid use, inappropriate use of antireflux medications, radiographic imaging, and promote appropriate use of laryngoscopy, voice therapy, and surgery (Traister, 2014). Evaluation of a patient with hoarseness includes very careful history of illness, physical examination, and in many cases, also laryngoscopy (Feierabend, 2009; Mau, 2010).

BACKGROUND

Finding useful rules is an important task of a knowledge discovery process. Most researchers mainly focus on techniques for generating classification rules. A need for new methods with the ability to assist users in analyzing a large number of rules for a useful knowledge (Dardzinska, 2013) is still seeking. All patients, called objects, together with many symptoms and laboratory results, called attributes, form so called information When additional attributes, describing e.g. the situation of a patient are given, this system is called a decision information system. In such case, each object can be classified into one of the several given groups. An action rule is a rule extracted from a decision system, which gives suggestions helpful in reclassification process of objects in given information system from one state to another with respect to a distinguished attribute called a decision attribute (Ras, 2006). We assume that attributes are partitioned into stable (they cannot be changed, e.g. sex, name, height) and flexible (they can change, e.g. blood pressure, level of hoarseness). In paper (Ras,2008,2009) a new subclass of attributes called semistable attributes was introduced. They are typically a function of time, and undergo deterministic changes. It was shown in (Ras, 2008; Dardzinska, 2013) that some semistable attributes can be treated the same way as flexible attributes.

MAIN FOCUS OF THE CHAPTER

Issues, Controversies, Problems

While working on real medical data, it is easy to notice that correct diagnosis under given assumptions is not easy at all and accuracy in such data can be rather low. It is caused by several problems, which can be connected with the nature of kinds of diseases. In case of larynx problems, many conditions can cause e.g. hoarseness. Evaluation of a patient with hoarseness is time consuming task. Therefore we can propose a strategy which is helpful in faster and more accurate diagnosis of patients. Under some circumstances we are also able to suggest what changes in patient's behaviour should be made to reclassify him. It can be done using action rules.

Action rules mining initially was based on comparing profiles of two groups of targeted objects (Dardzinska, 2013,2006; Ras, 2008). An action rule was defined as a term $r = \left[\omega * \left(\alpha \to \beta \right) \right] \to \left(\varphi \to \psi \right)]$, where $\omega, \alpha, \beta, \varphi$ and ψ are descriptions of objects, in our case seen as patients. The term r states that when a fixed condition ω is satisfied and the changeable behavior $\left(\alpha \to \beta \right)$ occurs in patients registered in a database so we obtian the suggestion to move object from one state φ to anoter $\psi : \left(\varphi \to \psi \right)$. We propose a method for constructing action rules directly from single classification rules. It has been implemented as one of the modules in new computer aided support system, which consists of a medical database and a set of tests and procedures, facilitating decision-making process for patients with throat and larynx disorders.

An information system (Dardzinska, 2013; Pawlak, 1991) can be seen as a triple $S = (X, A, V)$, where:

1. X is a nonempty, finite set of objects,
2. A is a nonempty, finite set of attributes,
3. V is a set of values of attributes i.e. $a : X \rightarrow V_a \, for \, a \in A$,

where V_a is called the domain of attribute a. Information systems can be seen as decision tables. Formally, by a decision table we mean an information system $S = (X, A_{St} \cup A_{Fl} \cup D_i)$, where D_i, $i \in 1, \ldots, k$ is a set of k decisions, and $. d \in D_i .$, $d \notin A_{St} \cup A_{Fl}$ is a distinguished attribute called the decision. The elements of A_{St} are called stable conditions, whereas the elements of $A_{Fl} \cup D_i$ are called flexible ones. Our goal is to change values of attributes in A_{Fl} for some objects in X, so the values of the decision attribute d from D_i for these objects may also change. Relationships between attributes from $A_{St} \cup A_{Fl}$ and the attribute d have to be discovered first. By $(a, v \rightarrow w)$ we denote the fact that the value of attribute a changed from v to w. The notion $(a, v \rightarrow v)$ means, that the value of attribute a, which is v, did not change.

Solutions and Recommendations

For the purpose of suggested method we can build a simple decision acion tree. It is built on the base of extracted rules, forming knowledge base for the information system. The algorithm starts at the root node of the tree representing all classification rules extracted from S (which gives primary knowledge base) (Dardzinska, 2013). A stable attribute is the one which divide these rules. For each value of that attribute an outgoing edge from the root node is created, and the corresponding subset of rules that have the attribute value assigned to that edge is moved to the child node. This process is repeated recursively for each child node. When we are done with all stable attributes, the last split is based on a decision attribute for each current leaf of action tree. Every path to the decision attribute node, represents a subset of the extracted classification rules when the stable attributes have the same value. Each leaf node represents a set of rules, which do not contradict on stable attributes and also define decision value d_i.

NEW COMPUTER SUPPORTED DIAGNOSIS SYSTEM

First steps and ideas in constructing this system were created in collaboration between the Department of Mechanics and Computer Science at Bialystok University of Technology and physicians at the Department of Clinical Phonoaudiology and Logopedics at Medical University of Bialystok, and Laryngologic Medical Centre. The collaboration between these two instistutions allows easily for systematic collection and processing of clinical data of hoarseness patients diagnosed and treated in the medical centre. The proposed system is equipped with a smart diagnostic module built around several statistical and KDD methods that have been found useful during the whole process of diagnosis. The current database contains approximately 1000 patients. Each case is described by over 30 different medical findings, such as patient self-reported data, results of physical examination, laboratory tests and finally a histopatologically verified diagnosis. The patients from this database have been classified by clinicians into five adequate throat and larynx diseases: A – normal (healthy), B - vocal cord polyps, C1 - voice nodules, C2 - voice nodules and reflux disease, D -functional dysphonia, E-larynx-cancer. A medical treatment is naturally associated with reclassification of patients from one decision class into another one. We are especially interested in objects reclassification from more serious treatment class to another, which includes objects with lighter diseases. In our research we are mainly interested in reclassification of patients from the class C2 into class C1 and from class C1 to class A. The description of attributes (tests) listed in rules is given below:

$$R = \left\{ a, g, ii, sa, ya, is, h, sp, hh, bi, vi, ad, ph, vw, sd \right\},$$

where . a .–age, g –gender, ii –inhalation injuries, sa –seasonal allergy, ya –year-round allergy, is –irritating substances, h –hoarseness, sp – surgeries in the past (stable) hh – history of hospitalization (stable), bi – bacterial infection, vi – viral infection, ad – autoimmune diseases, ph – ph level, vw – voice work, sd – special diet.

Many action rules have discovered. Two of them, quite interesting, for men and women separately with high confidence (close to 90) are given below:

$$\left[(hh,1) \cdot (g,2) \cdot (h,1) \right] \cdot (sd, 2 \rightarrow 1) \cdot (ph, 2 \rightarrow 1) \Rightarrow (d, C2 \rightarrow C1) \cdot$$

This first rule is applicable to women with a history of hospitalization. It says that if we change the diet into special one, and we change the level of ph ., then we should be able to reclassify such patients from the category C2 to C1.

$$\left[(hh,1) \cdot (g,1) \right] \cdot (vw, 2 \rightarrow 1) \cdot (sa, 2 \rightarrow 1) \Rightarrow (dd, C1 \rightarrow A1) \cdot$$

The second rule is applicable to men with history of hospitalization. It says that if we minimize seasonal allergy and we minimize voice expose then we should be able to reclassify such patients from the category C1 to A1.

FUTURE RESEARCH DIRECTIONS

In future the authors will construct a flexible temporal feature retrieval system based on grouping patients of similar visiting frequencies with connection to an action-rules engine, which consists of four modules: a data grouping device, a temporal feature extraction engine, a decision tree classification device, and an action rules generation device. The data grouping device is to filter out less relevant records in terms of visiting duration patterns measured from the initial visits. The temporal feature extraction engine is to project temporal information into patient-based records for classic classifiers to learn effects of treatment upon patients. The action rules generation device is to build action rules from certain pairs of classification rules.

CONCLUSION

Action rules mining can be successfully applied in other medical databases. We initially tested flat feet and orthopedic databases (Dardzinska, 2013). We already developed a flexible temporal feature retrieval system based on grouping plano-valgus patients of similar visiting frequencies with connection to an action-rules engine, which consists of four modules: a data grouping device, a temporal feature extraction engine, a decision tree classification device, and an action rules generation device. There exist also initial studies on pancreas database. Based on the research we can conclude that the occurrence of chronic pancreatitis can affect reception of the non-steroidal anti-inflammatory drugs. Patients who do not take these drugs suffer from chronic pancreatitis. In addition, we can notice a strong relationship between the intake of aspirin and to the occurrence of chronic pancreatitis. With the learned rules shows that patients who were not taking aspirin (in excess of two tablets per week) suffered from chronic pancreatitis. Therefore the results seem to be also very promising.

REFERENCES

Dardzinska, A. (2013). *Action Rules Mining, Studies in Computational Intelligence* (Vol. 468). Springer. doi:10.1007/978-3-642-35650-6

Dardzinska, A., & Ras, Z. (2006). *Extracting rules from incomplete decision systems. In Foundations and Novel Approaches in Data Mining, Studies in Computational Intelligence* (pp. 143–154). Springer.

Feierabend, R., & Shahram, M. (2009). Hoarseness in adults. *American Family Physician, 80*(4), 363–370.

Kosztyła-Hojna, B. (2013). Ocena przydatności metody szybkiego filmu highspeed imaging (HSI) w diagnostyce zaburzeń jakości głosu. *Annals of the Rheumatic Diseases, 72*(suppl. 3), 837–840. doi:10.1136/annrheumdis-2013-eular.2491

Kosztyła-Hojna, B. et al.. (2007). Usefulness of some diagnostic methods in differential diagnosis of occupational voice disorders. *Polish Journal of Environmental Studies, 16*(no 1A), 23–29.

Kosztyła-Hojna B., Moskal, D., Kuryliszyn-Moskal, A., & Rutkowski, R. (2013). The innovative method of visualization of vocal folds vibrations in the chosen cases of occupational dysphonia. *Otorynolaryngologia - Przegląd Kliniczny*, 23-28.

Mau, T. (2010). Diagnostic evaluation and management of hoarseness. *The Medical Clinics of North America, 94*(5), 945–960. doi:10.1016/j.mcna.2010.05.010

Pawlak, Z. (1991). Information systems - theoretical foundations. *Information Systems Journal, 6*(3), 205–218. doi:10.1016/0306-4379(81)90023-5

Ras, Z., & Dardzinska, A. (2006). Action rules discovery, a new simplified strategy. *Foundations of Intelligent Systems, Proceedings of ISMIS'06 Symposium* (LNAI) (vol. 4203, pp. 445-453). Springer.

Ras, Z., & Dardzinska, A. (2008). Action rules discovery without pre-existing classification rules. *Proceedings of the International Conference on Rough Sets and Current Trends in Computing* (LNAI), (vol. 5306, pp. 181-190). Springer.

Ras, Z., & Wieczorkowska, A. (2000). Action-Rules: How to increase profit of a company. *Proceedings of PKDD 2000* (LNAI), (vol. 1910, pp. 587-592). Springer.

Rubin J., Sataloff, R.T., & Korovin, G.S. (2006). *Diagnosis and treatment of voice disorders*. Plural Publishing Inc.

Schwartz, S. R., Cohen, S. M., Dailey, S. H., Rosenfield, R. M., Deutsch, E. S., Gillepsie, M. B., & Patel, M. M. et al. (2009). Clinical practice guideline: Hoarseness (dysphonia). *Otolaryngology - Head and Neck Surgery, 141*(3Suppl 2), S1–S31. doi:10.1016/j.otohns.2009.06.744

Skrodzka D., et al. (2006). Powikłania laryngologiczne choroby refluksowej przełyku. *Prz. Lek. 2006, 63*(9), 752-755. (in Polish)

Traister, R. S., Fajt, M. L., Landsittl, D., & Petrov, A. A. (2014). A novel scoring system to distinguish vocal cord dysfunction from asthma. *Journal of Allergy Clinical Immunology Practice, 2*(10), 65–69. doi:10.1016/j.jaip.2013.09.002

KEY TERMS AND DEFINITIONS

Action Rule: Rule extracted from an information system that describes a possible transition of objects from one state to another with respect to a distinguished attribute called a decision attribute.

Decision System: Information system, which additional attribute – decision.

Flexible Attribute: Attribute, which value can be changed.

Incomplete Information System: Information system, where some of the values of attributes remain unknown.

Information System: System, which contains set of objects, set of attributes, set of values of attributes.

Stable Attribute: Attribute, which value cannot be changed.

Chapter 2
Secure Storage and Transmission of Healthcare Records

Grasha Jacob
Rani Anna Govt. College, Tirunelveli

Murugan Annamalai
Dr. Ambedkar Govt. Arts College, India

ABSTRACT

Telemedicine has become a common method for transmission of medical images and patient data across long distances. With the growth of computer networks and the latest advances in digital technologies, large amount of digital data gets exchanged over various types of insecure networks - wired or wireless. Modern Healthcare Management Systems need to change to accommodate these new advances. There is an urgent need to protect the confidentiality of health care records that are stored in common databases and transmitted over public insecure channels. This chapter outlines DNA sequence based cryptography which is easy to implement and is robust against cryptanalytic attack as there is insignificant correlation between the original record and the encrypted image for the secure storage and transmission of health records.

INTRODUCTION

India is providing quality health care of international standards at a relatively low cost and has attracted the patients from across the globe. India is now one of the favorite destinations for the health care services. With the advances in technology that is witnessed each passing day, there is not a dimension of development that can sustain unless technology is embraced by it. Information Technology receives a benevolent face when it delivers value addition to medical field. It ranges from processing of patient data to computer aided drug discovery. One of the greatest challenges facing mankind in the 21st century is to make high-quality health care available to all. Such a vision has been expressed by the World Health Organization (WHO) in its health-for-all strategy in the 21st century. A Health Telematics Policy, a

DOI: 10.4018/978-1-5225-0536-5.ch002

document from World Health Organization states telemedicine motivation as - "…integrate the appropriate use of health telematics in the overall policy and strategy for the attainment of health for all in the 21st century, thus fulfilling the vision of the world in which benefits of science, technology and public health development are made equitable available to all people everywhere". Telemedicine is defined as, "the delivery of health care and the exchange of health information across distances including all medical activities: making diagnosis, treatment, prevention, education and research" (Wootton & Craig, 1999). Telemedicine is connecting remote locations and helps in addressing the inadequacies associated with health care. Telemedicine can improve equity of access to health care in the rural and urban areas. Widespread adoption of telemedicine would permit decentralization and could potentially have the greatest effect, allowing underserved people to benefit from a greatly improved standard of health care. In remote or rural areas, telemedicine could have a great impact, permitting better diagnostic and therapeutic services, faster and easier access to medical knowledge, obviating the need for patients and health-care workers to travel. Even in urban areas, however, telemedicine can improve access to health services and to information. A health record may contain patient information along with a scanned image. According to Norcen et al (2003), "The organization of today's health systems often suffers from the fact that different doctors do not have access to each other's patient data. The enormous waste of resources for multiple examinations, analyses, and medical check-ups is an immediate consequence. In particular, multiple acquisitions of almost identical medical image data and loss of former data of this type have to be avoided to save resources and to provide a time-contiguous medical report for each patient. A solution to these problems is to create a distributed database infrastructure where each doctor has electronic access to all existing medical data related to a patient, in particular to all medical image data acquired over the years. When such an infrastructure is established, it is possible to give precise, advanced, and entire information about patients at the time of care, permit speedy access to patient records for more synchronized and well organized care and distribute digital information to patients and other clinicians Additionally, many medical professionals are convinced that the future of health care will be shaped by tele-radiology, tele-cardiology and technologies such as telemedicine in general. Telemedicine is of most use to the remote and disconnected areas which do not have access to best of medical care, both infrastructural and human resource. With advancement in mobile technologies, mobile apps can be developed which can work in synchronization with the ERP system at the hospital. Thus, Telemedicine reaches wider audience through the outreach of smartphones. Remote prescription, drug administration, oversight etc. can be managed remotely and thus reducing the travel, nursing and hospital admitting costs. In the fields like psychiatry, telemedicine is the most effective way, as videoconferencing is required. Post-surgical monitoring can also be done remotely as patient may be allowed to recover in congenial homely environment. Shortage of physicians and paramedical persons can be addressed with initial investment in telemedicine technology. Though there are several advantages of Tele-medicine, several threats like accidental disclosure, insider curiosity, insider subordination, uncontrolled secondary usage and outsider intrusion exist to patient information confidentiality. Accidental disclosure occurs when medical personnel make innocent mistakes during multiple electronic transfers of data to various entities, medical personnel and cause disclosure of data. Insider curiosity is the result of misusing their access rights to patient information out of curiosity. Insider subordination results when medical personnel leak out personal medical information for spite, profit, revenge, or other purposes. Uncontrolled secondary usage occurs when those who are granted access to patient information solely for the purpose of supporting primary care can exploit that permission for reasons not listed in the contract, such as research. Outsider intrusion occurs when former employees, network intruders, hackers, or others may access information, damage systems or disrupt operations. All electronic health information must be encrypted and decrypted as necessary according to user defined preferences in accordance with the best available encryption key strength. During data exchange all electronic health information must be suitably encrypted and decrypted when exchanged in accordance with an encrypted and integrity protected link. All actions related to electronic health information must be recorded with the date, time, patient identification, and user identification whenever any electronic health information is created, modified, deleted, or printed; and an indication of which action(s) took place must also be recorded. As health care records contain health information which is protected under legislation, image encryption schemes for health care records have been increasingly studied to meet the demand for real-time secure storage and transmission over the Internet.

BACKGROUND

In the past, the medical record was a warehouse of information in papers that was reviewed or used for clinical, research, administrative, and financial purposes. It was strictly restricted in terms of accessibility, available to only one user at a time. The paper-based record sometimes had bad handwritten information written by physicians which could not be read or understood and was updated manually, resulting in delays for record completion that persisted from 1 to 6 months or more. Most medical record departments were housed in institutions' basements because the weight of the paper precluded other locations. The physician was in control of the care and documentation processes and authorized the release of information. Patients rarely viewed their medical records. Another limitation of the paper-based medical record was the lack of security. Right to use was controlled by doors, locks, identification cards, and tedious sign-out procedures for authorized users. Unauthorized access to patient information triggered no warnings, nor was it known what information had been observed. It is "the right of individuals to keep information about themselves from being disclosed to others; the claim of individuals to be let alone, from surveillance or interference from other individuals, organizations or the government". The information that is shared as a result of a clinical relationship is considered confidential and must be secure. The information can take several forms (including identification data, diagnoses, treatment and progress notes, and laboratory results) and can be stored in numerous ways. Patient information should be released to others only with the patient's permission or as allowed by law. This is not, however, to say that physicians cannot gain access to patient information. Information can be released for treatment, payment, or administrative purposes without a patient's authorization. The patient, too, has federal, state, and legal rights to view, obtain a copy of, and amend information in his or her health record. The key to preserving confidentiality is making sure that only authorized individuals have the right to use the information. The process of controlling the access - restricting who can see what—begins with authorizing users. In the case of health record access, the practice administrator identifies the users, determines what level of information is needed by whom and for what purpose it is needed, and assigns usernames and passwords. Basic standards for passwords include requiring that they be changed at set intervals, setting a minimum number of characters, and prohibiting the reuse of passwords. The user's access is based on pre-established, role-based privileges. A physician, a nurse and a receptionist have very different tasks and responsibilities; therefore, they do not have access to the same information. Hence, designating user privileges is a critical aspect of medical record security: all users who have access to the information have to realize their roles and responsibilities, and must know that they are accountable for use or misuse of the information they view and change.

SECURE STORAGE OF HEALTH RECORDS

Telemedicine is good for every nation for the betterment of Medicare services and for developed nations, it is even more necessary to setup and generate immediate and expert medical care. Government and healthcare people are converting the paper-based health records into electronic health records in order to reduce the healthcare cost, improving the patient care and decreasing the medical faults. A health care record may include medical history, notes, and other information about health including the symptoms, diagnoses, medications, lab results, vital signs, immunizations, and reports from diagnostic tests such as x-rays and scans. Health records aim to store a patients' health information in one place, providing quick access when required. Telemedicine improves efficiency and coordination of the administration of hospitals. Telemedicine reduces the communication distance between experts and consultants, as the sharing of reports of patient and discussion over the treatment becomes online. But there are lots of research issues in storing and transmitting electronic health records which require an optimal solution. These facts show very clearly that there is an urgent need to provide and protect the confidentiality of patient related medical image data when stored in databases or cloud and transmitted over networks of any kind" (Norcen et. al, 2003). Measures that can be built in to such systems may include: "Access control" tools like passwords and PIN numbers, to help limit access to your information to authorized individuals, "Encrypting" the stored information - health information is unintelligible except by those using a system that can "decrypt" it with a "key" and an "audit trail" feature, which records the details such as who accessed your information, what changes were made and when. When a message is generated by the user and transmitted by the application software, until it is received by an authorised recipient the data is subject to a range of security risks. These risks are inclusive of standard security protections relating to hardware, software, human interventions, natural disasters, network issues and logical problems. Clinical information must be transferred securely and like other types of secure transmission must include identification, authorization, authentication, confidentiality, integrity and nonrepudiation. Protecting the data in transit is subject to the same security threats as required for other sensitive data; data may be subject to loss, late delivery, damage, or attack. All information in a patient's health care record is confidential and subject to the prevailing privacy laws and policies. Like all computerized systems, electronic records are vulnerable to crashes. Back-ups should be taken now and then and should be stored in two or more databases or multi-cloud to prevent loss of information.

Secure Transmission of Health Records

An electronic health record (EHR) is a record of a patient's medical details (including history, physical examination, investigations and treatment) in digital format. Physicians and hospitals are implementing EHRs because they offer several advantages over paper records. They increase access to health care, improve the quality of care and decrease costs. However, ethical issues related to EHRs confront health personnel. Telemedicine can make health care more efficient and less expensive, and improve the quality of care by making patients' medical history easily accessible to all who treat them. But as health care providers adopt electronic records, the challenges have proved daunting, with a potential for mix-ups and confusion that can be frustrating, costly and even dangerous. The medical record, either paper-based or electronic, is a communication tool that supports clinical decision making, coordination of services, evaluation of the quality and efficacy of care, research, legal protection, education, and accreditation and regulatory processes. The way to keep the information in these exchanges secure is a major concern. There is no way to control what information is being transmitted, the level of detail, whether communications are being intercepted by others, what images are being shared, or whether the mobile device is encrypted or secure. Mobile devices are largely designed for individual use and were not intended for centralized management by an information technology (IT) department. Computer workstations are rarely lost, but mobile devices can easily be misplaced, damaged, or stolen. Encrypting mobile devices that are used to transmit confidential information is of the utmost importance. Another potential threat is that data can be hacked, manipulated, or destroyed by internal or external users, so security measures and on-going educational programs must include all users. Some security measures that protect data integrity include firewalls, antivirus software, and intrusion detection software. Regardless of the type of measure used, a full security program must be in place to maintain the integrity of the data, and a system of audit trails must be operational. Providers and organizations must formally designate a security officer to work with a team of health information technology experts who can inventory the system's users, and technologies; identify the security weaknesses and threats; assign a risk or likelihood of security concerns in the organization; and address them. The responsibilities for privacy and security can be assigned to a member of the physician office staff or can be outsourced. With the advent of audit trail programs, organizations can precisely monitor who has had access to patient information. Audit trails track all system activity, generating date and time stamps for entries; detailed listings of what was viewed, for how long, and by whom; and logs of all modifications to electronic health records. Administrators can even detail what reports were printed, the number of screen shots taken, or the exact location and computer used to submit a request. Alerts are often set to flag suspicious or unusual activity, such as reviewing information on a patient one is not treating or attempting to access information one is not authorized to view, and administrators have the ability to pull reports on specific users or user groups to review and chronicle their activity. Software companies are developing programs that automate this process. End users should be mindful that, unlike paper record activity, all EHR activity can be traced based on the login credentials. Audit trails do not prevent unintentional access or disclosure of information but can be used as a deterrent to ward off would-be violators. To prevent intentional and unauthorized access, encryption renders a helping hand.

MAIN FOCUS OF THE CHAPTER

From time immemorial, the art of communicating secretly has been imperative. German's Enigma machine and American Indian Language Navajo used during World War II are concrete examples to explain everything about cryptographic techniques. A cryptosystem is a system that allows two parties to communicate secretly by transforming an intelligible message into unintelligible form and then retransforming that back to its original form. The main objective of cryptography is confidentiality. The usefulness of developing techniques of DNA computing and ultimately developing working DNA computers can be described as falling into one of the following three general categories:

1. Applications making use of "classic" DNA computing schemes where the use of massive parallelism holds an advantage over traditional computing schemes, including potential polynomial time solutions to hard computational problems;
2. Applications making use of the "natural" capabilities of DNA, including those that make use of informational storage abilities and those that interact with existing and emerging biotechnology;
3. Contributions to fundamental research within both computer science and the physical sciences especially concerned with exploring the limitations of computability and understanding and manipulating biomolecular chemistry.

DNA Computing is an exciting fast developing interdisciplinary area concerned with the use of DNA molecules and associated quaternary coding for the implementation of computational processes. Adleman's pioneering experimental work in 1994 opened a new world of possibilities in computing. He established the use of nucleic-acid strand interactions for computing and solved the travelling-salesman problem (Hamiltonian Path Problem - to find the shortest route that visits each city exactly once in a given network of connected cities), in a test tube using specially sequenced DNA molecules and standard molecular-biology procedures in a biological laboratory. Although solving such a specific task is a far cry from building a general-purpose computer, this ground-breaking work revealed that information could indeed be processed using interactions between the strands of DNA. Adleman's work urged other researchers to develop DNA-based logic circuits using a variety of approaches. The resulting circuits were able to perform simple mathematical and logical operations, recognize patterns based on incomplete data and play simple games. Molecular circuits even detect and respond to a disease signature inside a living cell and open up the possibility of medical treatments based on man-made molecular software. Lipton extended the work of Adleman and investigated the solution of Satisfiability of Propositional Formula pointing to new opportunities of DNA computing. Research work is being done on DNA Computing either using test tubes (biologically) or simulating the operations of DNA using computers (Pseudo or Virtual DNA computing). L. Kari (1997) gave an insight of the various biological operations concerning DNA.

Taylor et al. (1997) proposed a substitution cipher for plaintext encoding where base triplet was assigned to each letter of the alphabet, numeral and special characters and demonstrated a steganographic approach by hiding secret messages encoded as DNA strands among multitude of random DNA. Decryption was difficult with the use of sub-cloning, sequencing and there was a need of an additional triplet coding table. Gehani et al.(2000) introduced a trial of DNA based Cryptography and proposed two methods: i) a substitution method using libraries of distinct one time pads, each of which defines a specific, randomly generated, pair-wise mapping and ii) an XOR scheme utilizing molecular computation and indexed random key strings were used for encryption. They used the natural DNA sequences to encode the information and encrypted an image by using the XOR logic operation. Such experiments could be done only in a well-equipped lab using modern technology, and it would involve high cost. Leier et al. (2000) also presented two different cryptographic approaches based on DNA binary strands with the idea that a potential interceptor cannot distinguish between dummies and message strand. The first approach hid information in DNA binary strands and the second designed a molecular checksum. Decryption was done easily using PCR and subsequent gel electrophoresis without the use of sub-cloning, sequencing and additional triplet coding table. Although the approach of generating bit strands shown here had advantages such as rapid readout, it also had practical limitations. One of the limitations was the resolution of the used agarose-gels. Chen (2003) presented a novel DNA-based cryptography technique that took advantage of the massive parallel processing capabilities of biomolecular computation. A library of one time pads in the form of DNA strands was assembled. Then, a modulo-2 addition method was employed for encryption whereby a large number of short message sequences could be encrypted using one time pads. A novel public-key system using DNA was developed by Kazuo et al. (2005) based on the one-way function. The message-encoded DNA hidden in dummies could be restored by PCR amplification, followed by sequencing.The YAEADNA algorithm (Sherif et al., 2006) used a search technique in order to locate and return the position of quadruple DNA nucleotide sequence representing the binary octets of plain text characters. Plain text character and a random binary file were given as input and the output PTR was a pointer to the location of the found quadruple DNA nucleotide sequence representing the binary octet. The encryption process was tested on images to show how random the selection of DNA octet's locations is on the encrypting sequence. Cui et al. (2008) designed an encryption scheme by using the technologies of DNA synthesis, PCR amplification, DNA digital coding and the theory of traditional cryptography. The data was first pre-processed to get completely different ciphertext to prevent attack from a possible word as PCR primers. Then, the DNA digital encoding technique was applied to the ciphertext. After coding sender synthesizes the secret-message DNA sequence which was flanked by forward and reverse PCR primers, each 20-mer oligo nucleotides long. Thus, the secret-message DNA sequence was prepared and at last sender generated a certain number of dummies and put the sequence among them. Once the data in encrypted form reached the receiver's side the reverse procedure was followed to decrypt it. Biological difficult issues and cryptography computing difficulties provided a double security safeguard for the scheme. The intended PCR two primer pairs used as the key of this scheme was designed by the complete cooperation of sender and receiver to increase the security of this encryption scheme. Ning (2009) explained the pseudo encryption methodology based upon the work of Gehani. The plain text was converted to DNA sequences and these sequences were converted to the spliced form of data and protein form of data by cutting the introns according to the specified pattern and it was translated to mRNA form of data and mRNA was converted into protein form of data. The protein form of data was sent through the secure channel. The method did not really use DNA sequences, but only the mechanisms of the DNA function; therefore, the method was a kind of pseudo DNA cryptography methods. The method only simulates the transcription, splicing, and translation process of the central dogma; thus, it was a pseudo DNA cryptography method.

Sadeg et al. (2010) proposed a symmetric key block cipher algorithm which included a step that simulated ideas from the processes of transcription (transfer from DNA to mRNA) and translation (from mRNA into amino acids). Though the encryption algorithm (OTP) proposed was theoretically unbreakable, it experienced some disadvantages in its algorithm. These drawbacks had prevented the common use of its scheme in modern cryptosystems. In 2010, Qinghai had also proposed a method to protect information, including representing information using biological alphabets to enhance the security of traditional encryption, using DNA primer for secure communication and key distribution, and using the chemical information of DNA bases for steganography. Alice and Bob share a secret DNA sequence codebook. Alice can design a sequence that can maximally match one of the sequences in the codebook and then send the designed sequence to Bob through a public channel. When Bob receives the sequence he would use the non-matching letters in the private sequence as the encryption key. Knowing the public string only, an attacker cannot decrypt the transmitted information. L.Xuejia et al. (2010) also proposed an asymmetric encryption and signature cryptosystem by combining the technologies of genetic engineering and cryptology. It was an exploratory research of biological cryptology. DNA-PKC uses two pairs of keys for encryption and signature, respectively. Using the public encryption key, everyone can send encrypted message to a specified user, only the owner of the private decryption key can decrypt the ciphertext and recover the message; in the signature scheme, the owner of the private signing key can generate a signature that can be verified by other users with the public verification key, but no else can forge the signature. DNA-PKC differs from the conventional cryptology in that the keys and the cipher texts are all biological molecules. The security of DNA-PKC relies on difficult biological problems instead of computational problems; thus DNA-PKC is immune from known attacks, especially the quantum computing based attacks. In the image encryption algorithm based on DNA sequence addition operation combined with logistic chaotic map to scramble the location and value of pixel of an image presented by Qiang et al., (2010) a DNA sequence matrix was obtained by encoding the original image and it was divided into some equal blocks and two logistic maps. DNA complementarity and DNA sequence addition operations were utilized to add these blocks. DNA sequence matrix was decoded to get the encrypted image. The experimental results and security analysis showed that the proposed algorithm had larger key space and resisted exhaustive, statistical and differential attacks. In 2012, Qiang et al. presented a novel image encryption algorithm based on DNA subsequence operations that uses the idea of DNA subsequence operations (such as elongation operation, truncation operation, deletion operation, etc.) combining with the logistic chaotic map to scramble the location and the value of pixel points from the image. The experimental results and security analysis showed that the proposed algorithm was easy to be implemented, had good encryption effect and a wide secret key's space, strong sensitivity to secret key, and had the abilities of resisting exhaustive attack and statistic attack but the defect was its weak ability of resisting differential attack. Encryption protects both data at rest and data in transit or transmission. The concept of using DNA computing in the fields of cryptography is studied in order to enhance the security of cryptographic algorithms. Adleman, with his pioneering work set the foundation for the new field of bio-computing research. His main notion was to use actual chemistry to solve problems that were either unsolvable by conventional computers, or required a massive amount of computation. Gehani et al. introduced the first trial of DNA-based cryptography. In this work, the principle ideas of the central dogma of molecular biology are used for computing instead of real biological DNA strands. The method simulates the transcription, splicing, and translation process of the central dogma; thus, it is a virtual DNA cryptographic method.

DNA Coding

An electronic computer needs only two digits, 0 and 1 for coding information. As a single strand of DNA is similar to a string consisting of a combination of four different symbols, A, C, G and T, DNA coding should reflect the biological characteristics of the four nucleotide bases- A, C, G and T along with the Watson-Crick complementary rule (A is complementary to T and C is complementary to G). Out of the twenty four combinations of the four nucleotides, only eight combinations (00 01 10 11 - C T A G, 00 01 10 11 - C A T G, 00 01 10 11 - G T A C, 00 01 10 11 - G A T C, 00 01 10 11 - T C G A, 00 01 10 11- T G C A, 00 01 10 11 - A C G T, 00 01 10 11 - A G C T) satisfy the complementary rule of the nucleotides.

In accordance with the increasing molecular weight of the four nucleotides, (C -111.1 g/mol, T - 126.1133 g/mol, A - 135.13 g/mol and G - 151.13 g/mol) C T A G, is the best coding pattern and is used as DNA Coding. According to DNA Coding Technology, C denotes the binary value 00, T denotes 01, A denotes 10 and G denotes 11 so that Watson-Crick complementary also holds good. Table 1 gives the DNA Coding used in this work. This pattern perfectly reflects the biological characteristics of the four nucleotide bases and has biological significance.

Table 1. DNA Coding

Digital value	DNA base	Molecular weight g/mol
00	C	111.1
01	T	126.11
10	A	135.13
11	G	151.13

Axiomatic Definition of DNA Algebra

DNA algebra is an algebraic structure defined on a set of elements B{C, T, A, G} together with two binary operators '∨' and '∧' provided the following Huntington postulates are satisfied.

1. a. Closure with respect to the operator ∨.
    b. Closure with respect to the operator ∧.
2. a. An identity element with respect to ∨, designated by C:

$$x \vee C = x, \forall x \in B$$

b. An identity element with respect to ∧, designated by G:

$$x \wedge G = x, \forall x \in B$$

3. a. Commutative with respect to ∨.

$$x \vee C = C \vee x, \forall x \in B$$

b. Commutative with respect to ∧.

$$x \wedge G = G \wedge x, \forall x \in B$$

4. a. ∨ is Distributive over ∧.

$$x \vee (y \wedge z) = (x \vee y) \wedge (x \vee z), \forall x, y, z \in B$$

b. ∧ is Distributive over ∨.

$$x \wedge (y \vee z) = (x \wedge y) \vee (x \wedge z), \forall x, y, z \in B$$

5. For every element $x \in B$, there exists an element $x' \in B$ (called the complement of x) such that
    a. $x \vee x' = G$ and

b. $x \wedge x' = C$

6. There exists at least two elements $x, y \in B$, such that $x \neq y$.

The following De' Morgan's laws also hold good.

$$(x \vee y)' = x' \wedge y', \forall x, y \in B$$

$$(x \wedge y)' = x' \vee y', \forall x, y \in B$$

The primitive logic operations AND, OR, XOR, and NOT can be carried out and the results will be obtained as given in the characteristic tables Table 2, Table 3, Table 4 and Table 5.

DNA Sequence Based Image Representation

The term image refers to a two-dimensional light intensity function, denoted by f(x,y), where the value of f at spatial coordinates(x,y) gives the intensity(brightness) of the image at that point. As light is a form of energy f(x,y) must be nonzero and finite, that is f(x) must lie between zero and infinity (0 < f(x,y) < ∞). A digital image is an image f(x,y) that has been discretized both in spatial coordinates and brightness. A digital image can be considered a matrix (two dimensional array) whose row and column indices identify a point in the image and the corresponding matrix element value identifies the gray level at that point. The elements of such a picture array are called pixels. Each pixel of the image consists of 8 bits. Using DNA coding principle, substituting C for 00, A for 01, T for 10 and G for 11, each pixel of the DNA image is represented as a quadruple nucleotide sequence.

Table 2. AND characteristic table

>	C	T	A	G
C	C	C	C	C
T	C	T	C	T
A	C	C	A	A
G	C	T	A	G

Table 3. OR characteristic table

V	C	T	A	G
C	C	T	A	G
T	T	T	G	G
A	A	G	A	G
G	G	G	G	G

Table 4. XOR

⊕	C	T	A	G
C	C	T	A	G
T	T	C	G	A
A	A	G	C	T
G	G	A	T	C

Table 5. Not characteristic table

X	C	T	A	G
~X	G	A	T	C

Arithmetic and Logic Operations on Images

Arithmetic and logic operations between pixels are used extensively in most of the branches of image processing and are generally carried out on images pixel by pixel. The principle use of image addition is for image averaging - to reduce noise. Image addition is mainly done using XOR operation for brightening the image and for image security applications. Image subtraction is a basic tool in medical imaging where it is used to remove static background information. Image multiplication or division is used to correct gray level shading resulting from non-uniformities in illumination or in the sensor used to acquire the image. Arithmetic operations can be done "in place" such that the result of performing an operation can be stored in that location in one of the existing images. With DNA computing, two DNA images can be added using parallel addition of the rows of the two images.

DEFINITIONS FOR THE PROPOSED SYSTEM

Cryptosystem

A cryptosystem is a five tuple $(M, C, \kappa, \varepsilon, D)$, where the following conditions are satisfied.

1. M is a finite set of possible plain-text (images).
2. C is a finite set of possible cipher-text.
3. κ is a finite set of possible keys.
4. E is a finite set of encryption rules indexed by K, such that for each $K \in \kappa$, there is a function E_K: $M \to C$.
5. D is a finite set of encryption rules indexed by K, such that for each $K \in \kappa$, there is a function D_K: $C \to M$.
6. For each $K \in \kappa$, $D_K(E_K(x)) = x$, for every plain-text $x \in M$..

Condition (vi) enables a user to decrypt a received cipher-text, since $D_K(E_K(x)) = x$, for every plain-text $x \in M$.

For unambiguous decryption, it is required that $E_K(x1) \neq E_K(x2)$, if $x_1 \neq x_2$. On the other hand, if $E_K(x_1) = E_K(x_2)$, and $x_1 \neq x_2$ then decryption is not unique and hence it is impossible for a recipient to decide whether the intended plain text was x_1 or x_2 upon receipt of $E_K(x_1) = E_K(x_2)$.

Synthesis

In standard solid phase DNA synthesis, a desired DNA molecule is built up nucleotide by nucleotide on a support particle in sequential coupling steps. For example, the first nucleotide (monomer), say A, is bound to a glass support. A solution containing C is poured in, and the A reacts with the C to form a two-nucleotide (2-mer) chain AC. After washing the excess C solution away, one could have the C from the chain AC coupled with T to form a 3-mer chain (still attached to the surface) and so on.

Creation of DNA sequences for the image data is referred to as Synthesis. DNA sequences are made up of four bases – A, C, T and G. According to the DNA Coding Technology, C denotes 00, T – 01, A

- 10 and G – 11. According to the coding method proposed for each pixel of a digital image by Qiang et al, each pixel of the digital image is converted into its corresponding DNA coded value.

Translation

When the positions of sequences are translated, the sequences are interchanged.
Translation is represented as

$$P_1P_2P_3P_4 \leftrightarrow P_5P_6P_7P_8$$

Substitution

Each quadruple nucleotide sequence is substituted by the value returned by the DNA Sequence Crypt function. Substitution is represented by the following expression.

$$V \leftarrow DNASequenceCryptfn(P_1P_2P_3P_4)$$

Re-Substitution

Each value, V in the encrypted image is replaced by the corresponding quadruple nucleotide sequence from that position in the DNA Sequence File.

$$P_1P_2P_3P_4 \leftarrow V$$

Detect

Detect searches for a quadruple nucleotide sequence of the image starting from a random position in the DNA sequence file and returns true if a match is found and false otherwise.

Re-Synthesis

Re-synthesis is the process of converting each sequence into its digital form.

KEY DEPENDENT DYNAMIC S-BOX FUNCTION

A Key Dependent Dynamic S-Box function is a mapping function,

$$f:\{0,1\}^m \rightarrow \{0,1\}^n,$$

that maps n bit input string X into n bit output string Y based on the codeword and has the following properties:

1. **Bijection**: A bijection (or bijective function or one-to-one correspondence) is a function between the elements of two sets, where every element of one set is paired with exactly one element of the other set, and every element of the other set is paired with exactly one element of the first set. A bijective function f: X → Y is a one to one and onto mapping of a set X to a set Y. A bijection from the set X to the set Y has an inverse function from Y to X.

2. **Strict Avalanche Criterion**: If a one bit change in the input results in at least 50 percent changes in the output bits, then there is Strict Avalanche criteria.

3. **Correlation-Immunity:** If the output bits act independently from each other, then there is Correlation-immunity.

4. **Nonlinearity**: A function with its corresponding vector is said to be highly nonlinear when the resulting vector $_{yi}$ from a function f_i has a high Hamming distance with all the linear vectors in the set of B_n.

5. **Balance**: An S-box with n input bits and m output bits, m ≤ n, is balanced if each output occurs 2^{n-m} times. For the S-box to be balanced it should have the same number of 0's and 1's.

Hamming Distance

Hamming distance between two binary vectors of equal length is the number of places for which the corresponding entries are different.

DNA Sequence Crypt Function

DNA Sequence Crypt function is a function that returns one of the many positions of the quadruple DNA sequence in the key DNA sequence file.

A one to many DNA Sequence Crypt function is a one-to-many function d(x), which has the following three properties:

1. A pointer, h maps an input quadruple nucleotide sequence, x to one of the many positions obtained in random in the key DNA sequence file.

2. Ease of computation: Given d and an input x, d(x) is easy to compute.

3. Resistance to guess: In order to meet the requirements of a cryptographic scheme, the property of resistance to guess is required of a crypt function with input x, x_1 and outputs y, y_1.

As similar quadruple nucleotide sequence that occur in a plain text are mapped to different positions in the DNA nucleotide sequence file(one to many mapping), it is difficult for a recipient to guess the plain-text. The sender and receiver agree on a key DNA sequence file, R which can be freely and easily downloaded from the DNA GenBank®, the NIH genetic sequence database, an annotated collection of all publicly available DNA sequences. GenBank is part of the International Nucleotide Sequence Database Collaboration, which comprises the DNA DataBank of Japan (DDBJ), the European Molecular Biology Laboratory (EMBL), and GenBank at NCBI. These three organizations exchange data on a daily basis. Query sequence(s) to be used for a BLAST search should be pasted in the 'Search' text area. It accepts a number of different types of input and automatically determines the format or the input.

A sequence in FASTA format begins with a single-line description, followed by lines of sequence data. The description line is distinguished from the sequence data by a greater-than (">") symbol at the beginning. It is recommended that all lines of text be shorter than 80 characters in length. In cryptographic applications, long DNA sequences are generally used.

DUAL ENCRYPTION METHOD

The Dual Encryption method consists of two phases. Phase I is the encryption process and Phase II is the decryption process. The decryption is the reverse of the encryption process. In Phase I of the proposed Encryption scheme, a codeword is first generated based upon a 64 bit key. For simplicity, the key is denoted as Hex value in this paper. Once the codeword is generated, based upon the codeword, a Dynamic key-dependent S-Box is generated and a DNA sequence file is selected at run-time. Then the input image (health record) is transformed into a coded image based on the Dynamic key-dependent S-Box. With the key dependent Dynamic S-Box function, it is a single simple function applied over and over again to each byte of the input image, returning a byte. Each of the 256 possible byte values is transformed to another byte value with the key dependent SubBytes (S-Box) transformation, which is a full permutation, meaning that every element gets changed, and all 256 possible elements are represented as the result of a change, so that no two different bytes are changed to the same byte. Figure 1 represents the key dependent Dynamic SBox generated at runtime, when the key is A451B67290F7DE38 (hex representation of the 64 bit key 1010 0100 0101 0001 1011 0110 0111 0010 1001 0000 1111 0111 1101 1110 0011 1000). The coded image is then synthesized - transformed into DNA image. The encrypted image obtained by substituting each quadruple DNA nucleotides sequence of the translated image by one of the many positions of the quadruple nucleotides sequence (which is randomly obtained) in the gene sequence file by applying DNA Sequence Crypt function is sent to the receiver through any channel or stored in a public database in the encrypted form. The sender and the receiver/retriever should agree upon the 64 bit-key that is generated and the receiver/retriever can decrypt the encrypted image.

Figure 1. Dynamic SBox when the key is A451B67290F7DE38

```
36 C7 77 B7 2F B6 F6 5C 03 10 76 B2 EF 7D BA 67
AC 28 9C D7 AF 95 74 0F DA 4D 2A FA C9 4A 27 0C
7B DF 39 62 63 F3 7F CC 43 5A 5E 1F 17 8D 13 51
40 7C 32 3C 81 69 50 A9 70 21 08 2E BE 72 2B 57
90 38 C2 A1 B1 E6 A5 0A 25 B3 6D 3B 92 3E F2 48
35 1D 00 DE 02 CF 1B B5 A6 BC EB 93 A4 C4 85 FC
0D FE AA BF 34 D4 33 58 54 9F 20 F7 05 C3 F9 8A
15 3A 04 F8 29 D9 83 5F CB 6B AD 12 01 FF 3F 2D
DC C0 31 CE F5 79 44 71 4C 7A E7 D3 46 D5 91 37
06 18 F4 CD 22 A2 09 88 64 EE 8B 41 ED E5 B0 BD
0E 23 A3 A0 94 60 42 C5 2C 3D CA 26 19 59 4E 97
7E 8C 73 D6 D8 5D E4 9A C6 65 4F AE 56 A7 EA 80
AB 87 52 E2 C1 6A 4B 6C 8E DD 47 F1 B4 DB B8 A8
07 E3 5B 66 84 30 6F E0 16 53 75 9B 68 1C D1 E9
1E 8F 89 11 96 9D E8 49 B9 E1 78 9E EC 55 82 FD
C8 1A 98 D0 FB 6E 24 86 14 99 D2 F0 0B 45 BB 61
```

In the retrieval phase, the authorized receiver upon receiving the encrypted image converts it into DNA image by mapping the pointers from the encrypted image onto the key DNA sequence file and the decrypted image is then obtained by Re-Synthesis followed by Inverse S-Box substitution.

Algorithm Dynamic_S-Box

```
Input :     codeword cw
Output:     D_ S-Box
Begin
Z = Bin2dec(cw) + 1
Case Z of
  1 - 32      : D_ S-Box = row transformation of AES_S-Box
  33 - 64     : D_ S-Box = column transformation of AES_S-Box
  65 - 96     : D_ S-Box = transpose of results obtained in case 1- 32
  97 - 128    : D_ S-Box = transpose of results obtained in case 33- 64
 129 - 160    : D_ S-Box = nibble exchange of results obtained in case 1- 32
 161 - 192 : D_ S-Box = nibble exchange of results obtained in case 33- 64
193 - 224    : D_ S-Box = transpose of results obtained in case 129- 160
225 -256     : D_ S-Box = transpose of results obtained in case 161- 192
EndCase
Return D_ S-Box
End Dynamic_S-Box
```

Generation of Codeword

The key used for encryption is considered to be 64 bits in length. From the key, a codeword of 8 bits $(C_8 C_7 C_6 C_5 C_4 C_3 C_2 C_1)$ is generated at run-time based upon the Hamming Distance and Hamming Weight. The key-dependent S-box generated at runtime based upon the codeword is non-linear in nature. The codeword is also used to randomly select a DNA sequence file. For generating the codeword from the 64 bit key, the following two assumptions are considered.

1. Each bit of the codeword calculates the parity (Hamming weight) for certain bits in the key.
2. A parity bit is set to 1 if the total number of ones in the positions it checks is odd or 0 otherwise.

Algorithm Codeword_Generator

```
Input :     64 bit key K
Output:     codeword cw
Begin
C_8 = (check all the bits of the key(1-64)) ? 1 : 0
C_7 = (check 1 bit, skip 1 bit, check 1 bit  etc. (1,3,5,7,9,11,13,15,...)) ?
1 : 0
C_6 = (check 2 bits, skip 2 bits, check 2 bits etc. (2,3,6,7,10,11,14,15,...))
? 1 : 0
```

```
C₅ =   (check 4 bits, skip 4 bits, check 4 bits etc. (4,5,6,7,12,13,14,15,...))
? 1 : 0
C₄ =   (check 8 bits, skip 8 bits, check 8 bits etc. (8-15,24-31,40-47,...)) ? 1
: 0
C₃ =   (check 16 bits, skip 16 bits, check 16 bits etc. (16-31,48-56)) ? 1 : 0
C₂ =   (check 32 bits, skip 32 bits, check 32 bits etc. (32-63)) ? 1 : 0
C₁ =   (check bit 1 and bit 64) ? 1 : 0
cw = C₈C₇C₆C₅C₄C₃C₂C₁Return cw
End Codeword_Generator
```

The codeword for the key A451 B672 90F7 DE38 and A451 B672 90F7 DE39 are 10111001 and 00111000, respectively.

Algorithm CodeImage

```
Input :  Input image X, codeword cw
Output:  Coded image  C
Begin
DS ← Dynamic_S-Box(cw)
C  ← SubByte Transformation of  X based on DS
Return C
End CodeImage
SubByte Transformation
```

With the Dynamic S-Box function, the SubByte transformation is a single simple function applied over and over again to each byte of the input image. In the SubByte transformation, each of the 256 possible byte values is treated independently and transformed to another byte value based on the Dynamic S-Box, which is a full permutation, meaning that every element gets changed, and all 256 possible elements are represented as the result of a change, so that no two different bytes are changed to the same byte.

The SubByte transformation is pictorially represented in Figure 2. To substitute a byte, the byte is interpreted as two hexadecimal digits. The left digit defines the row and the right digit defines the column of the substitution table. The two hexadecimal digits at the junction of the row and the column is the new byte.

Figure 3 is an illustration of a SubByte transformation of an image of size 4 x 4, when the key is {**F95BBAF3656EFB64**}.

The coded image obtained in the encryption phase is then encrypted based upon the reference DNA Sequence file using the encryption algorithm. The encrypted image thus obtained is sent to the receiver. The sender and the receiver should agree upon the 64 bit-key that is used for encryption. Phase I and II of the proposed scheme can be pictorially represented as shown in Figure 4.

Algorithms EncryptImage, DNASequenceCrypt, Detect and DNA are given below.

Figure 2. SubByte transformation

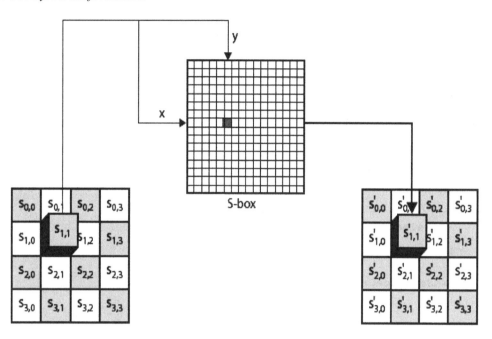

Figure 3. SubByte transformation when the key is {F95BBAF3656EFB64}

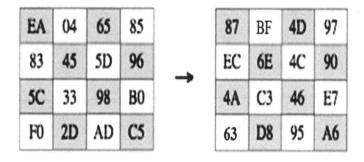

Figure 4. Encryption and decryption phase

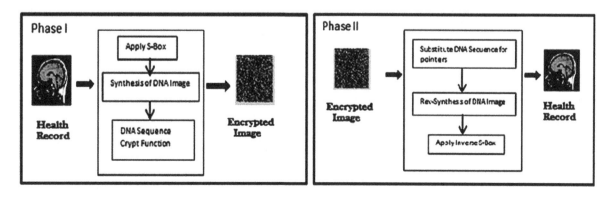

Algorithm EncryptImage

```
Input :      64 bit key, image to be encrypted  Y
Output:      Encrypted image E
Begin
Image X, codedimage C
DNA Sequence file R
Integer I
1.          cw ← Codeword_Generator(key)
2.          C ← CodeImage(Y, cw)
3.          Synthesis
 X ← DNA(Y)    // Convert the coded image into a DNA image
4.          R ← Select a  DNA Sequence file at runtime based on the Codeword
5.          Detection and Substitution
   For each quadruple DNA nucleotide sequence in X
       E(I)←DNASequenceCrypt(R, X(P₁P₂P₃P₄))
       I = I + 1
   End_For
6.          Return E
End EncryptImage
```

Algorithm DNASequenceCrypt

```
Input :  DNA Sequence file R, quadruple nucleotide sequence x(P₁P₂P₃P₄)
Output:  index in DNA Sequence file h
Begin
Integer i, J
J = rnd(30000)
repeat
   rn = rnd(J)
   for  i = rn to length(R) - 4
       if Detect(i, R, x)
           h = i
           Return h
       endif
   end for
     J = J - 100
until J > 5
End DNASequenceCrypt
Algorithm Detect
Input :    search index rn, DNA Sequence file R,
                quadruple nucleotide sequence x(P₁P₂P₃P₄)
Output:    Boolean T
Begin
```

```
Strings, Integeri
    i = rn
    s = R(i)+R(i+1)+R(i+2)+R(i+3)
    if (s = x)
         T ← true
    else
         T ← false
    end if
    return T
End Detect
```

Algorithm DNA

```
Input :   image X
Output:   DNA image Y
Integer i, j, m, n, k
Begin
  m = w(Image) // width of image
  n = h(Image) // height of image
  for i = 1 to h
    k = 1
   for j = 1 to w-1
      if (X(i, j) = 0 and (X(i, j) = 0) then Y(i,k) = 'C'
      if (X(i, j) = 0 and (X(i, j) = 1) then Y(i,k) = 'T'
      if (X(i, j) = 1 and (X(i, j) = 0) then Y(i,k) = 'A'
      if (X(i, j) = 1 and (X(i, j) = 1) then Y(i,k) = 'G'
     k = k + 1
   end  // end for i
   end // end for j
   Return Y
End DNA
```

Decryption Phase

The decryption is just the reverse of the encryption process. In the decryption phase, the received encrypted image (2D array) is actually pointers (index) to the DNA sequence file. The indices are therefore substituted by the quadruple nucleotide sequence starting from that index and the corresponding DNA image in encrypted form is obtained. The encrypted DNA image is converted to binary form and the Inverse SubByte transformation is performed on each byte of the resultant image to get the original image that was transmitted in the encrypted form. The inverse SubByte transformation is the inverse of the SubByte transformation and is obtained from Inverse Dynamic S_Box.

The algorithm for Inverse Dynamic S_Box is given as follows:

Algorithm Inv_Dynamic_S-Box

```
Input :   codeword cw
Output:   Inv_D_SBox
Begin
        Inv_D_SBox  ←Dynamic_S_Box(cw) ⁻¹Return  Inv_D_SBox
End Inv_Dynamic_S-Box
        The Decryption algorithm is given below:
```

Algorithm DecryptImage

```
Input : Encrypted Image E, Codeword cw
Output:Decrypted Image X
Begin
1.        Select the DNA Sequence file based on the Codeword
2.        Re-Substitution
   Convert E into DNA sequence
              F     ←      E
3.        Re-Synthesis
   Convert F into its binary equivalent
4.        Substitution
                X  ←  Apply Inv_Dynamic_S-Box(cw) on F
5.        Return X
End DecryptImage
```

Experimental Results and Analysis

To prove the validity of the proposed scheme, experiments were performed on different images of varied sizes using Matlab 2009a on DELL Inspiron ACPIx64 based notebook PC. Table 2 gives the encoded values of a health care record of size 8 x 8. Figure 5 is an example of an original image and its corresponding encrypted and decrypted images and shows that the encrypted image reveals no information to the invader. The experimental results and security analysis reveal that the proposed algorithm has strong sensitivity to the key and DNA sequence file used. The level of security that the proposed encryption algorithm offers is double-fold – Dynamic S Box and DNA Sequence based.

Security analysis is defined as the technique of finding the weakness of a cryptographic scheme and retrieving whole or a part of the encrypted image without knowing the decryption key or the algorithm. For an encryption scheme to be good, it should be robust against statistical, brute-force and differential attacks, and therefore the proposed method was examined for these attacks.

Statistical Attack

The stability of the proposed method is examined via statistical attacks - correlation between adjacent pixels and the histogram. The encrypted image should not have any statistical likeness (similarity) with the original image to prevent the leakage of information.

Figure 5. Original, encrypted and decrypted images

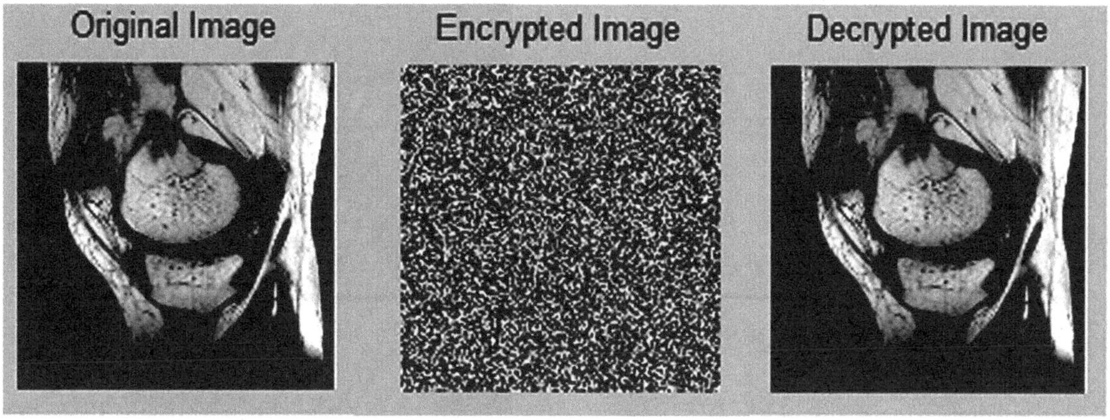

Correlation Coefficient Analysis

In most of the plaintext-images, there exists high correlation among adjacent pixels, while there is little correlation between neighboring pixels in the encrypted image. It is the main task of an efficient image encryption algorithm to eliminate the correlation of pixels. Two highly uncorrelated sequences have approximately zero correlation coefficient and two strongly correlated sequences have a correlation coefficient nearly equal to one. Scatter graphs are drawn taking pixel value at location (x, y) on the x-axis and pixel value at location (x, y+1) on the y-axis for both the original and encrypted images.

The Pearson's Correlation Coefficient is determined using the formula:

$$\gamma = \frac{n \sum xy - (\sum x)(\sum y)}{\sqrt{n(\sum x^2)(\sum x)^2} \sqrt{n(\sum y^2)(\sum y)^2}} \tag{1}$$

where x and y are the grey-scale values of two neighboring pixels in the image and n is the total number of pixels selected from the image for the calculation is used to investigate the correlation between adjacent pixels.

Table 6 tabulates the correlation coefficient between adjacent pixels of the original and encrypted images. If there is insignificant correlation, correlation coefficient is close to 0. It is clear from Table 6 that there is negligible correlation between the two adjacent pixels in the encrypted image and gives no information to the invader regarding the nature of the original image that is being transmitted. However, the two adjacent pixels in the original image are highly correlated. Figure 6 reveals that the correlation of the encrypted images is unvaryingly distributed and reveals no information to the attacker.

Histogram Analysis

The histograms present the statistical characteristics of an image. If the histograms of the original image and encrypted image are different, then the encryption algorithm has good performance. An attacker cannot extract the pixels' statistical nature of the original image from the encrypted image and the algo-

Figure 6. (a) to (f) represent the correlation between the adjacent pixels of the original and encrypted images column-wise, row-wise and diagonal-wise.

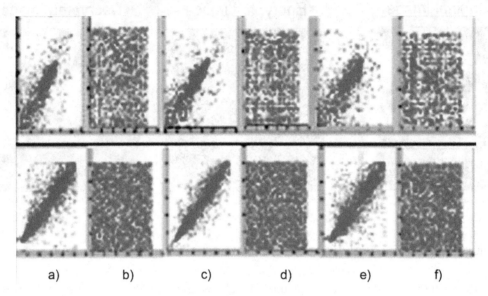

a)   b)   c)   d)   e)   f)

Table 6. Encoded values of a health record of size 8 x 8

10454	57803	33952	33493	62362	70194	37655	43645
8200	1769	37656	35110	53348	42641	71593	77842
53016	18200	40047	4689	66314	4047	57830	66341
49	16522	48211	53335	26241	41520	59784	69671
3	15694	80186	1991	35188	33691	30117	30694
12	13848	3765	67898	76356	2061	15059	44617
261	22420	42508	39119	1820	1796	5334	744
883	31999	78981	43153	14211	50947	23941	14628

rithm can resist a chosen plain image or known plain image attack. Figure 8 reveals that the histograms of the encrypted images are fairly uniform and significantly different from the original image. It is also observed that the histograms of the encrypted images look quite similar (though the original images are different) and are completely different from that of the histograms of the original images and do not provide any information regarding the distribution of gray values to the attacker; As the encrypted image does not provide any information regarding the distribution of gray values to the attacker, the proposed algorithm can resist any type of histogram based attacks and strengthens the security of the encrypted images significantly.

Brute Force Attack

A Brute Force Attack is an approach that can be used against any encrypted data by an intruder who is incapable to take benefit of any weakness in an encryption system that would otherwise make his

Figure 7. Correlation coefficient graph

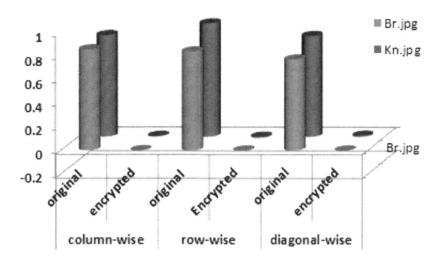

Table 7. Correlation coefficient of original and encrypted images

Image	Correlation Coefficient					
	Column-Wise		Row-Wise		Diagonal-Wise	
	Original	Encrypted	Original	Encrypted	Original	Encrypted
Br.jpg	0.8551	0.0014	0.8371	-0.0037	0.7698	0.00062
Kn.jpg	0.86	0.0062	0.959	-0.0102	0.8539	0.0108

Figure 8. . Histogram of brain and bone image – original and encrypted

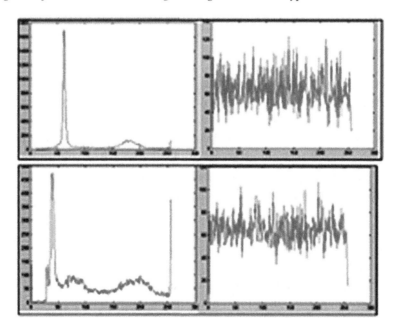

task at ease. It involves methodically examining all probable keys until the right key is established. The encrypted file is principally arbitrarily generated pointers to the DNA sequence file and rarely there is a prospect of more than one quadruple nucleotide sequence pointing to the same position in the DNA sequence file. Moreover, the feature of bio-molecular setting is tougher to access as it is extremely difficult to recover the DNA digital code without knowing the correct coding technology used. An incorrect coding will cause biological pollution, which would lead to a corrupted image. Since there are many web-sites and roughly 55 million publicly accessible DNA sequences, it is practically impossible to guess the key sequence.

Differential Attack

The aim of differential attack analysis is to determine the sensitivity of encryption algorithm to slight changes. If an attack is made to create a small change in the plain image to observe the results, this influence causes a noteworthy change in the encrypted image and the antagonist will not be able to find a meaningful association between the original and encrypted image with respect to diffusion and confusion. A different sequence used or slight change made to the original plain image will result in a completely different encrypted image proving that the algorithm is highly intricate to small changes.

FUTURE RESEARCH DIRECTIONS

The two major drivers of contemporary telemedicine development are a high volume demand for clinical service, and a high criticality of need for security of health care records. These areas offer promise for further study and enhancement of security in health care management system and have the potential for large-scale deployments internationally, which would contribute significantly to the advancement of healthcare.

CONCLUSION

Electronic health record (EHR) is gradually being implemented in many countries. It is the need of the hour because it improves the quality of health care and is also cost-effective. The convolution and haphazardness of DNA based encryption of health record provides a great ambiguity which makes it better than other mechanism of cryptography and guarantees secure storage and transmission of health records. Integrating DNA based encryption along with Dynamic S-Box substitution helps in a double fold security. The proposed Encryption Scheme is easy to implement and can resist brute-force, statistical and differential attack and is suitable for the secure storage and transmission of health-care records.

REFERENCES

Adleman, L. (1994). Molecular Computation of Solutions to Combinatorial Problems. *Science*, *266*(5187), 1021–1024. doi:10.1126/science.7973651 PMID:7973651

Alvarez, G., Li, S., & Hernandez, L. (2007). Analysis of security problems in a medical image encryption system. *Computers in Biology and Medicine, 37*(3), 424–427. doi:10.1016/j.compbiomed.2006.04.002 PMID:16872592

Amos, M., Paun, G., Rozenberg, G., & Salomaa, A. (2002). Topics in the theory of DNA computing. *Theoretical Computer Science, 287*(1), 3–38. doi:10.1016/S0304-3975(02)00134-2

Chen, J. (2003) A DNA-based biomolecular cryptography design.*IEEE International Symposium on Circuits and Systems*, (pp. 822–825).

Craig, J., & Patterson, V. (2005). Introduction to the practice of Telemedicine. *Journal of Telemedicine and Telecare, 11*(1), 3–9. doi:10.1258/1357633053430494 PMID:15829036

Cui, G. Z., Qin, L. M., Wang, Y. F., & Zhang, X. (2007). Information Security Technology Based on DNA Computing.*IEEE International Workshop on Anti-counterfeiting, Security, Identification*, (pp. 288–291). doi:10.1109/IWASID.2007.373746

Cui, G. Z., Qin, L. M., Wang, Y. F., & Zhang, X. (2008). An Encryption Scheme using DNA Technology. *International Conference on Bio-Inspired Computing: Theories and Applications*, (pp. 37-42).

Gehan, A., LaBean, T., & Reif, J. (2000). DNA Based Cryptography. *DIMACS Series in Discrete Mathematics and Theoretical Computer Science., 54*, 233–249.

Joseph, A. A., Lehmanny, C. U., Green, M. D., Pagano, M. W., Zachary, N. J. P., & Rubin, A. D. (2010). *Self-Protecting Electronic Medical Records Using Attribute-Based Encryption.* Retrieved from: https://eprint.iacr.org/2010/565.pdf

Josh, B., Melissa, C., Horvitz, E., & Lauter, K. (n.d.). *Patient Controlled Encryption: Ensuring Privacy of Electronic Medical Records.* Microsoft Research.

Ning, K. (2009). A pseudo DNA cryptography Method. *CoRR*. Retrieved from http://arxiv.org/abs/0903.2693

Norcen, R., Podesser, M., Pommer, A., Schmidt, H. P., & Uhl, A. (2003). Confidential storage and transmission of medical image data. *Computers in Biology and Medicine, 33*(3), 273–292. doi:10.1016/S0010-4825(02)00094-X PMID:12726806

Qiang, Z., Xue, X., & Wei, X. (2012). A Novel Image Encryption Algorithm based on DNA Subsequence Operation. *TheScientificWorldJournal*.

Reif, J. (1997). Local Parallel Biomolecular Computation.*3rd DIMACS workshop on DNA based computers*, (pp. 243-258).

Richa, H. R., & Phulpagar, B. D. (2013). Review on Multi-Cloud DNA Encryption Model for Cloud Security. *Int. Journal of Engineering Research and Applications, 3*(6), 1625–1628.

Richter, C., Leier, A., Banzhaf, W., & Rauhe, H. (2000). Private and Public Key DNA steganography.*6th DIMACS Workshop on DNA Based Computers*, (pp. 1-10).

Risca, V. I. (2001). DNA-based Steganography. *Cryptologia, Taylor and Francis, 25*(1), 37–49. doi:10.1080/0161-110191889761

Rothemund P W K. (1996). A DNA and restriction enzyme implementation of Turing machines. *DNA Based Computers, 6*, 75-120.

Rothemund, P. W. K., Papadakis, N., & Winfree, E. (2004). Algorithmic self-assembly of DNA Sierpinski triangles. *PLoS Biology, 2*(12), e424. doi:10.1371/journal.pbio.0020424 PMID:15583715

Rozenberg, G., Bäck, T., & Kok, J. (2012). *Handbook of Natural Computing*. Springer. doi:10.1007/978-3-540-92910-9

Rozenberg, G., & Salomaa, A. (2006). DNA computing: New ideas and paradigms. Lecture Notes in Computer Science, 7, 188-200.

Sadeg, S. (2010). An Encryption algorithm inspired from DNA.*IEEE International Conference on Machine and Web Intelligence*, (pp. 344 – 349).

Sakakibara, Y. (2005). Development of a bacteria computer: From in silico finite automata to *in vitro* and *invivo. Bulletin of EATCS, 87*, 165–178.

Sánchez, R., Grau, R., & Morgado, E. (2006). A Novel Lie Algebra of the Genetic Code over the Galois Field of Four DNA Bases. *Mathematical Biosciences, 202*(1), 156–174. doi:10.1016/j.mbs.2006.03.017 PMID:16780898

Shannon, C. E. (1949). Communication theory of secrecy system. *Journal of Bell System Technology, 28*(4), 656–715. doi:10.1002/j.1538-7305.1949.tb00928.x

Sherif, T. A., Magdy, S., & El-Gindi, S. (2006). A DNA based Implementation of YAEA Encryption Algorithm.*IASTED International Conference on Computational Intelligence.*

Siromoney, R., & Bireswar, D. (2003). DNA algorithm for breaking a propositional logic based cryptosystem. *Bulletin of the European Association for Theoretical Computer Science, 79*, 170–177.

Stallings W. (n.d.). *Cryptography and Network Security – Principles and Practice* (5th ed.). Prentice Hall.

Susan, K. L., & Hellman, M. E. (1994). Differential-Linear Cryptanalysis. *LNCS, 839*, 17–25.

Tausif, A., Sanchita, P., & Kumar, S. (2014). Message Transmission Based on DNA Cryptography[Review]. *International Journal of Bio-Science and Bio-Technology, 6*(5), 215–222. doi:10.14257/ijbsbt.2014.6.5.22

Taylor, C., Risca, V., & Bancroft, C. (1999). Hiding messages in DNA Microdots. *Nature, 399*(6736), 533–534. doi:10.1038/21092 PMID:10376592

Terec, R. (2011). DNA Security using Symmetric and Asymmetric Cryptography. *International Journal of New Computer Architectures and Their Applications*, 34-51.

Udo, F., Saghaf, S., Wolfgang, B., & Rauhe, H. (2002). DNA Sequence Generator: A program for the construction of DNA sequences. *DNA Computing*, 23-32.

Vazirani, V. (2004). *Approximation Algorithms*. Berlin: Springer.

Volos, C. K., Kyprianidis, I., & Stouboulos, I. (2013). Image encryption process based on chaotic synchronization phenomena. *Signal Processing, 93*(5), 1328–1340. doi:10.1016/j.sigpro.2012.11.008

Wang, X., & Wang, Q. (2014). A novel Image Encryption Algorithm based on Dynamic S-Boxes constructed by chaos. *Nonlinear Dynamics, 75*(3), 567–576. doi:10.1007/s11071-013-1086-2

Wang, Z., & Yu, Z. (2011). Index-based symmetric DNA encryption algorithm.*Fourth International Congress on Image and Signal Processing*, (pp. 15-17).

Watson, J. D., & Crick, F. H. C. (1953). Molecular structure of nucleic acids: A structure for De-oxy ribose nucleic acid. *Nature, 25*(4356), 737–738. doi:10.1038/171737a0 PMID:13054692

Weichang, C., & Zhihua, C. (2000). Digital Coding of the Genetic Codons and DNA Sequences in High Dimension Space. *Acta Biophysica Sinica, 16*(4), 760–768.

Westlund, B. H. (2002). NIST reports measurable success of Advanced Encryption Standard. *Journal of Research of the National Institute of Standards and Technology.*

Winfree, A. (1980). *The Geometry of Biological Time.* Academic Press.

Winfree, E. (1996) On the Computational Power of DNA Annealing and Ligation.*1st DIMACS Workshop on DNA Based Computers.*

Wootton, R., & Craig, J. (1999). *History of Telemedicine. Introduction to telemedicine.* London: Royal Society of Medical Press.

World Health Organization. (1997). *Health-for-all Policy for the 21st Century, HQ (document EB101/8).* Geneva: WHO.

Wu, Y., Noonan, J. P., & Agaian, S. (2011). NPCR and UACI Randomness Tests for Image Encryption. *Journal of Selected Areas in Telecommunications, 4*, 31–38.

Wu, Y., Zhou, Y., Noonan, J. P., & Agaian, S. (2013). Design of Image Cipher Using Latin Squares. *Information Sciences, 00*, 1–30.

Xiao, G., Lu, M., Qin, L., & Lai, X. (2006). New field of cryptography: DNA cryptography. *Chinese Science Bulletin, 51*, 1139–1144.

Xiao, J. H., Zhang, X. Y., & Xu, J. (2012). A membrane evolutionary algorithm for DNA sequence design in DNA computing. *Chinese Science Bulletin, 57*(2), 698–706. doi:10.1007/s11434-011-4928-7

XueJia, L., MingXin, L., Lei, Q., JunSong, H., & XiWen, F. (2010). Asymmetric Encryption and signature method with DNA technology. *Information Sciences, 53*, 506–514.

Youssef, M. I., Emam, A. E., Saafan, S. M., & Abd Elghany, M. (2013). Secured Image Encryption Scheme Using both Residue Number System and DNA Sequence. *The Online Journal on Electronics and Electrical Engineering, 6*(3), 656–664.

Yunpeng, Z. (2012). *Research on DNA Cryptography.* InTech Press.

Yunpeng, Z., Fu, B., & Zhang, X. (2012). DNA cryptography based on DNA Fragment assembly.*IEEE International Conference Information Science and Digital Content Technology.*

KEY TERMS AND DEFINITIONS

DNA Sequence Based Cryptography: A cryptographic technique based on DNA sequences.

Dynamic S-Box: A S-Box generated at run-time to enhance security.

Health Care Record: A record of a patient's medical details (including history, physical examination, investigations and treatment) in digital format.

Healthcare Management System: A system designed and developed for better understanding of health care information and management.

S-Box: A substitution box used in cryptography to obscure the relationship between the key and the cipher text.

SubByte Transformation: Each byte is transformed to another byte based on Dynamic SBox.

Telemedicine: The use of telecommunication and information technology to provide health care eliminating the barriers of distance.

Chapter 3
Fast Medical Image Segmentation Using Energy–Based Method

Ramgopal Kashyap
AISECT University, India

Pratima Gautam
AISECT University, India

ABSTRACT

Medical applications became a boon to the healthcare industry. It needs correct and fast segmentation associated with medical images for correct diagnosis. This assures high quality segmentation of medical images victimization. The Level Set Method (LSM) is a capable technique, however the quick process using correct segments remains difficult. The region based models like Active Contours, Globally Optimal Geodesic Active Contours (GOGAC) performs inadequately for intensity irregularity images. During this cardstock, we have a new tendency to propose an improved region based level set model motivated by the geodesic active contour models as well as the Mumford-Shah model. So that you can eliminate the re-initialization process of ancient level set model and removes the will need of computationally high priced re-initialization. Compared using ancient models, our model are sturdier against images using weak edge and intensity irregularity.

INTRODUCTION

Image Analysis remains one of the major challenges in image Processing. Numerous segmentation algorithms have been developed for a variety of applications. Disappointing outcome has been stumbled upon in some cases, for several existing segmentation methods. The qualitative analysis proved that the proposed methods are less perceptive with respect to noise. As such, the rate of in proper segmentation, pixel loss and trapped center at local minima problems can be avoided. As we all know Improved GO-GAC performs better than GOGAC, by correctly predicting the pixels and it is much faster than Active Contours method (Gao, Kikinis, Bouix, Shenton & Tannenbaum, 2012).

DOI: 10.4018/978-1-5225-0536-5.ch003

In Bioinformatics one of the major challenges is to get precision within the immense amount of information that results from projects involving the sequencing of the human genome. Initially, this category of sequencing was carrying out solely in the laboratory but with such an enormous level of data production, we now rely on computers to accomplish sequencing goals (Majewski & Rosenblatt, 2012). To actually produce a DNA sequence and then store up and examine it, computers are responsible for much of the work. Though, it is a challenge in Bioinformatics to proficiently and fruitfully store such a large quantity of Image data and to do so in such a way that a scientist can easily access the necessary information as needed. Image Data in itself is almost useless until it is analyzed and properly interpreted (Sun, 2013).

MAIN FOCUS OF CHAPTER

Healthcare images are usually ambiguous. If physical objects of fascination and their boundaries could be located the right way, meaningful aesthetic information will be provided to the physicians, making this analysis much simpler. Within the many image segmentation algorithms, active contour model is widely used with its clear curve with the object (Li, Luo & Zou, 2010).

According to the curve representation, there are generally two main kinds of active contour models: parametric versions and geometric versions. Parametric energetic contour versions use parameterized curves to symbolize the shape. Snake model (Kass, Witkin & Terzopoulos, 1988) has been often a representative and popular one in every of parametric energetic contour versions (Shi, 2006). The model has a constant curve to find the boundary on the image. In early grow older, the parametric energetic contour model is definitely an efficient construction for biometric impression segmentation. Nevertheless, it cannot represent this topology change such as the merging and splitting on the evolving curve (Benninghoff & Garcke, 2014).

The geometric energetic contour design, combining level set procedure and curve evolution principle, allows cusps, edges, and programmed topological changes. It may solve difficulties of curve evolution in parametric energetic contour design and extend the application form region of the active contour model (Xu & Zhang, 2014). For the parametric/geometric energetic contour design propagating toward a local optimum and therefore exhibiting a level of sensitivity to first conditions (Bresson, Esedoğlu, Vandergheynst, Thiran & Osher, 2007) a fresh global optimization method inside. This fast active contour is dependant on the level set procedure, replacing this framework having convex leisure approaches. Therefore, the model does not rely on the initial info with velocity.

According to the energy, you will discover two main families of active contour models: edge-based models (Pratondo, Chui & Ong, 2016) and region-based models (Vard, Jamshidi & Movahhedinia, 2012). Edge-based productive contour models count on the graphic gradient to halt the growing contours about the desired subject boundaries. Intended for images with weak limits, the electricity functional of the edge-based productive contour products will seldom approach zero about the boundaries of the objects and the evolving contour may traverse the true boundaries (Yuasa, 2003). For that reason, the edge-based productive contour products always forget to segment health-related images effectively, as blur as well as weak side usually occurs from the medical pictures, especially within MRI mind images, which normally contain large subject of blur limits between gray matter and white subject (Wang, Li, Sun, Xia & Kao, 2009).In contrast to the edge-based productive contour products, the region-based productive contour models tend not to utilize the actual image gradient; they make use of image statistics inside and away from contours to regulate the development with better performance pertaining to images connected with weak perimeters or without edges. Many regions-based active contour algorithms provide the assumption that the image may be approximated by simply the global intensity (Ye & Zhan, 2009). Chan and Vese offered a renowned Chan-Vese (CV) model deriving some coupled contour evolution equations from your single world-wide cost functional to advertise multiple shape to segment multiple-region image(Liu & Peng, 2012).CV model, also called PC (piecewise constant) model is a simplified Mumford-Shah model. The model utilizes the actual global suggest intensities of the interior and exterior regions of images. As a result, it has good segmentation result with the objects with weak as well as discrete limits, but frequently has mistaken segmentation pertaining to images with intensity inhomogeneity (Zheng, 2012). Even so, due for you to technical limits or artifacts introduced through the object fitting imaged, intensity inhomogeneity frequently occurs in many medical images.

Numerous implementation schemes have been proposed to help break the restrictions of CV model. A pair of similar region-based types are suggested independently. These models derive from a standard piecewise sleek (PS) formulation which is originally suggested by Mumford and Shah and also have been often known as piecewise sleek (PS) model. The PS models can handle segmentation problems which might be caused by intensity inhomogeneity. Lankton and Tannenbaum suggested localizing region-based active contours (LRBAC) throughout, allowing any kind of region-based segmentation energy being reformulated in the local means. The approach they proposed can be utilized with any kind of global region-based lively contour vitality, segmenting items with heterogeneous data (Lankton & Tannenbaum, 2008). However, they're computationally too costly. One strategy to reduce the computational cost being suggested is with a contour close to the object boundaries because initial contour.Local region-based lively contour model are suggested to overcome the issue caused by intensity inhomogeneity. The Local binary fitting (LBF) model in the region-scalable fitting (RSF) model is the favorite models. LBF model utilizes image information throughout local locations (Yuan, 2012). RSF model draws when intensity info in local regions for a controllable size. These models possess similar capability to handle intensity inhomogeneity. Nevertheless, they are also sensitive to help initialization.

To generate the segmentation productive piecewise sleek segmentation help quickly figure out localized data and provide. The model is to cope with spatial perturbations of the image intensity directly and much the same flow depending on the computing geodesic curve inside the space of localized means instead of approximating the piecewise sleek model(Tao & Tai, 2011). The approach can discover object limits accurately as well as reduce dependence on initial curve placement. The hybrid lively contour throughout, incorporates the GAC model, which is usually an edge-based lively contour model, and the CV model, which can be a region-based lively contour model. The brand-new model ended up being called since geodesic intensity fitting (GIF) model. It ended up being, then prolonged to a pair of models: Globally geodesic intensity fitting (GGIF) model and Local geodesic intensity fitting (LGIF) model (Ali, Badshah, Chen & Khan, 2016). The GGIF model is designed for images together with intensity homogeneity. Along with the LGIF model is designed for images together with intensity inhomogeneity (Xu & He, 2013).

Motivated with the work throughout, we plan to propose the model which is based on the region information on the images. While it's fast and not accurate throughout using world wide information and it's also accurate and not fast throughout using local information, the modern function uses both of global as well as local information to attain the appropriate result speedily. a hybrid region-based active contour model is displayed for image segmentation(Chen, 2013). The local information is described by utilizing the composition proposed throughout towards the energy throughout, localizing the force. The weights involving the local as well as global size terms are applied to avoid computationally high priced and flawed segmentation.

Information extraction and segmentation is the major foundation progression of image analysis. The key capability of image segmentation is that, the each spot in the image should be segmented properly; it enables accurate analysis of images (Wang & Liu, 2012). One important emerging area of application for Improved GOGAC is in image segmentation. Improved GOGAC in image analysis are that it requires minimal time for image segmentation as GOGAC, and it performs serial segmentation and produces a closed contour of optimal integrated edge strength. It works on each spot independently. Although GO-GAC has great potential in image segmentation, it is important to realize that it also has major drawbacks that include: improper segmentation of spots, difficulty in identification of the borders of the spots in the images (Zou, 2013). Therefore, how to improve the performance of GOGAC for image segmentation is the question we attempt to solve because, the incorrect segmentation reached by GOGAC is high and it's not good for proficient analysis. In order to extend the applications of GOGAC to the areas with high requirements on both robustness and accuracy, it is a critical task to improve the results of GOGAC by further reducing the incorrect spot segmentation. These challenges are addressed in this dissertation via development and application of appropriate technique based on the thresholding of original image which are Integrated with the results of GOGAC to build a system that we refer to as the Improved GOGAC

Medical Image Segmentation Methods: A Brief Review

Image segmentation algorithms for the delineation associated with anatomical structures and other regions associated with interest have become increasingly important in assisting and automating certain radiological duties. These algorithms play a vital role in various biomedical imaging applications, like quantification associated with tissue sizes, diagnosis in addition to localization associated with pathology, review of bodily structures, therapy planning, in addition to computer-guided surgical procedures (Maciejewski, Surtel, Maciejewska & Małecka-Massalska, 2015).

Meaning of Image Segmentation

Classically, image segmentation is understood to be the partitioning of the image directly into nonoverlapping, constituent regions which are homogeneous regarding some characteristic like intensity as well as texture (Dawoud & Netchaev, 2012).When the domain of the image can be given simply by Ω, then the actual segmentation dilemma is to look for the sets $S_K \subset \Omega$, whose union may be the entire website Ω. Therefore, the sets that make up a segmentation need to satisfy:

$$\Omega = \bigcup_{k=1}^{K} S_K$$

Where by $S_K \bigcap S_{J=\varnothing}$ (a null set) for K≠ J, and each and every S_K can be connected. If at all possible, a segmentation approach finds people sets that match distinct bodily structures or aspects of interest from the image.

Image segmentation, instead of classical segmentation, is usually a desirable aim in professional medical images, particularly when disconnected regions are part of the similar tissue category. When the actual constraint which regions need to be connected is taken out of the traditional segmentation, determining the actual sets, S_K is known as pixel group, and the actual sites themselves are referred to as classes. Determining the overall number associated with classes K, can be described as a difficult dilemma (Abdelsamea, Gnecco & Medhat Gaber, 2015) .Typically, the value of K is assumed for being known structured on prior knowledge of the composition being considered. For illustration, in the actual segmentation associated with cardiac images, we presume that K = 3, related to blood-filled region,myocardium region, and lung region (Drapikowski & Domagała, 2014).

The widely used image segmentation procedures include: thresholding, region growing, classifiers, clustering, Markov random field (MRF) versions, artificial neural networks, deformable model and atlas-guided solutions (Ortiz, Gorriz, Ramirez & Salas-Gonzalez, 2012). Several of those techniques tend to be used along with for dealing with different segmentation difficulties. Other methods are available in the actual surveys associated with image segmentation in literature.

Thresholding and Region Growing

Thresholding strategies segment scalar images by creating a binary dividing of this image intensities. It is just a simple and often effective opportunity for obtaining the segmentation involving images through which different constructions have contrasting intensities. Thresholding is frequently used as a possible initial help a string of image processing operations. Its main constraint is that typically it does not take into account the spatial characteristics of the image. This helps it be sensitive to noise in addition to intensity inhomogeneities, which often occur inside medical images (Kim & Park, 2005). Variations in classical thresholding happen to be proposed to add an information dependant on local intensities in addition to connectivity.

Region growing is usually a technique that extracts hooked up regions depending on certain criteria, for instance image high intensity and/or ends. A seed is needed to be inserted inside the desired region to extract the many connected pixels good criteria. Such as thresholding, the most convenient form involving region growing can be sensitive to noise, and it requires this manual placement of seeds divorce lawyers region to get segmented (Kocher & Leonardi, 1986). Region growing is usually seldom utilized alone, although usually joined with other segmentation techniques to delineate smaller, simple structures, for instance tumors in addition to lesions .

Classifiers and Clustering Strategies

Classifiers in addition to clustering strategies are style recognition techniques that affect image segmentation problems. Classifiers are referred to as supervised strategies because the needed training info, and clustering algorithms usually are termed unsupervised since they conduct classification of the data without the application of training info.Classifier strategies seek to partition an attribute space usually image intensities by using training data (Vlachos & Dermatas, 2013). There are a variety of ways that they the coaching data can be employed. The very popular non parametric classifiers incorporate k-nearest neighbors (kNN) in addition to Parzen screen; a parametric classifier is frequently the maximum-likelihood or even Bayes classifier (Soria, Garibaldi, Ambrogi, Biganzoli & Ellis, 2011).The assumption is that this pixel intensities usually are independent samples from a mixture of probability distributions, usually Gaussian pertaining to CT in addition to MRI images.

The estimation of the means, covariances, and mixing coefficients of the K courses is furthermore needed. Staying non-iterative, classifiers usually are relatively computationally productive,and they might be applied to multichannel images. The disadvantage could be the requirement of guide book interaction to have training info, which can be laborious. If a same pair of training info here for numerous images, biased results might be obtained.

Clustering algorithms, conversely, do not want training info. But to compensate just for this, they iteratively switch between segments this image in addition to characterizing this property of the class. Three very popular clustering algorithms are the K-means, the fuzzy c-means, and this expectation maximization (EM) method (Jung, Kang & Heo, 2014).Classifiers in addition to clustering methods don't directly integrate spatial modeling and can be very sensitive to noise. This insufficient spatial modeling, nevertheless, can provide advantages pertaining to fast computation. The by using MRF versions (Can, Leclercq, Lelong & Botteldooren, 2010) can increase the robustness to noise these algorithms.

Active Contour Models

Active contour models, also called deformable models are physically motivated techniques for segmenting objects using closed parametric curves or surfaces that deform under the influence of internal and external forces (Vard, Monadjemi, Jamshidi & Movahhedinia, 2011).The internal forces provide to demand a smoothing regular. The exterior or image forces press the active contour to maneuver toward salient image features such as lines as well as edges. The closed curve or surface is needed to be placed close to the desired boundary and allowed to endure an iterative peace process for you to delineate the item (Li, Luo & Zou, 2010).

Active shape models are actually widely applied inside segmentation involving medical images, either by itself or incorporated with other image segmentation methods. They are actually used for you to segment cerebral cortex MR images, heart MR images, bone CT images (Petitjean & Dacher, 2011). The main benefit from active shape is his or her ability to add the smoothness of the contours as well as image features at the same time.The internal forces help to make the shape robust for you to noise as well as spurious sides.A significant extension involving active shape models is the usage of implicit level-set representation in lieu of explicit parameterization to be able to handle topology modifications (Fussenegger, Roth, Bischof, Deriche & Pinz, 2009). An overview of geometric level-set analogues regarding parametric affective contours are located in, as well as a general review of deformable versions in medical image analysis has located in.Sooner active shape techniques, mostly used image depth gradient because external force inside segmentation design. This sort of approach usually referred to you to as edge-based or gradient-based approaches (Diop & Burdin, 2013). Another sort of technique employs region statistical information such as mean as well as variance of the intensity involving different regions separated by the active shape, and defines the segmentation simply by seeking a new maximum divorce of particular regional measures. This sort of approach can also be referred to like a region-based approach (Karasulu, 2013).

Microarray Image Segmentation

Due to the complexity involving medical images, a sole segmentation procedure usually may not achieve an excellent result regarding desired segmentation objectives. Thus, a combination of different approaches is usually adopted. There exists a huge literature of various types involving medical applications, and the following we solely list several examples involving combining different methods when it comes to segmentation. Baillard combined Bayesian pixel classification as well as active shape models inside a level established formulation for you to segment head structures coming from MRI images (Chen, Deeley, Niermann, Moretti & Dawant, 2010).

A DNA microarray is an array of DNA spots. One type of DNA microarray is called complementary DNA (cDNA) microarray. It contains a very large number of genes and it can examine the expression of hundreds or thousands of genes at once, it promises to revolutionize the way gene expression is examined and its size is very small. Microarray may be used to assay gene expression within a single sample or to compare gene expression in two different cell types or tissue samples, such as in healthy and diseased tissue and provides solutions to a broad range of problems in medical science, medicine, health and environment, drug development, etc. (Shang, 2010).They are used to identify the genes, which are expressed in a particular cell type or an organism. To understand gene functions it provides biologists a best approach for measuring gene expression levels in changeable situation and it has wide applications in medical sciences. As DNA microarray technology comes forward, it is traditional to simple, yet proficient tools for experimental explorations of genomic structures, gene expression programs, gene functions, and cell and organism biology. It is generally believed that gene expression data contain in sequence that permit us to distinguish higher-order arrangement of organisms and their performance. As well their technical consequence, gene expression data have important applications in clinical research (Li & Weng, 2011). A DNA microarray is a microchip or a glass slide, in which DNA molecules are attached at fixed position called spots, each connected to a single gene or we can say the spots are layered in sub-grids. The segmentation of the image is one of the three significant steps in microarray image processing, together with spot gridding and information extraction (Wee-Chung Liew, Yan & Yang, 2003). As we all know, segmentation is one of the most important steps in microarray image processing, and consists of identifying the pixels that belong to the spot from the pixels of the background and noise. Microarray develop the theory of favored binding of complementary single stranded DNA sequences (cDNA, for short), i.e., complementary single stranded DNA sequences tend to attract each other and the longer the complementary parts, the stronger the attraction (Qin, Rueda, Ali & Ngom, 2005). While multi-channel microchips are currently being devised, today's microarray experiments are used to compare gene expression from two samples, one called experimental and the other called control. The two examples are labeled by synthesizing single stranded cDNA that is complementary to the extracted mRNA. In cDNA microarray DNA strands are fastened at fixed spots on glass or plastic slides or silicon chips. A cDNA microarray is a useful tool for analyzing gene expression based on the samples of genes in the spots aligned in a regular pattern. cDNA microarray provide extensive used technology for doing scientific research simultaneously with thousands of genes or entire genomes. This approach is much more proficient than the traditional experiment method which only focuses on a few genes at one time. A critical part in the genetic analysis process is the usefulness of image segmentation analysis. There are four types of segmentation methods described in fixed circle segmentation (Renka,

Figure 1. Fixed circle segmentation

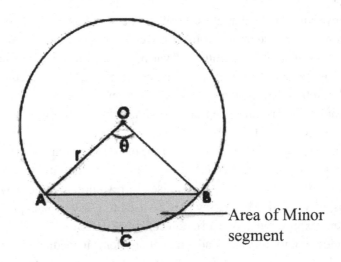

Figure 2. Adaptive circle segmentation

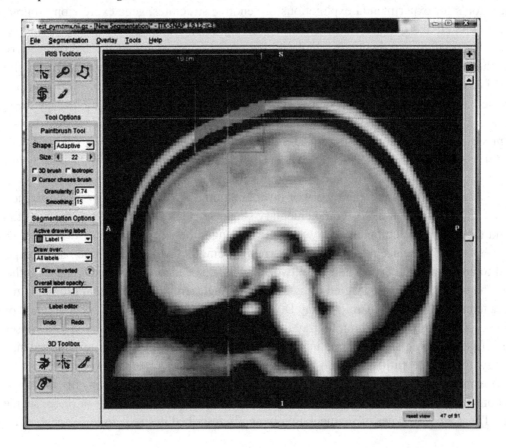

Figure 3. Adaptive shape segmentation

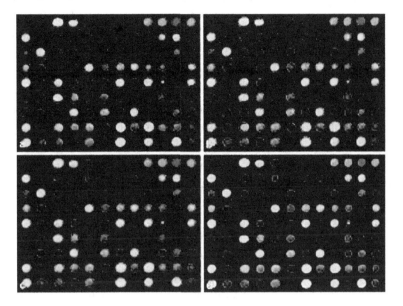

2009), adaptive circle segmentation (Wang & Sun, 2011), adaptive shape segmentation (Wang, Zhang & Ray, 2013) and histogram segmentation (Huang & Pun, 2015). Here we have core diagrams of all above segmentation techniques.

Some cDNA microarray segmentation software has been developed based on several segmentation methods. ScanAlyze developed by Eisen in 1999 is based on the fixed circle segmentation method. This method assumes that the spot has a perfect circle shape and all spots have the similar size (Shao, Li, Zuo, Wu & Liu, 2015).GenePix developed by Axon Instruments Inc. in 1999 uses. Fixed circle segmentation,

Figure 4. Histogram segmentation

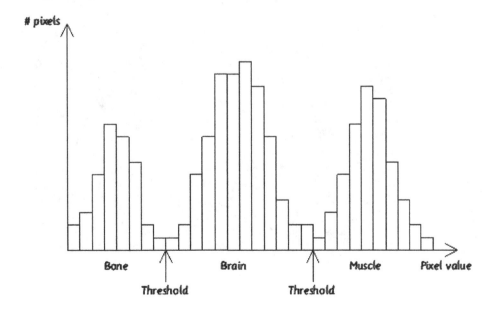

a traditional technique that was first used in ScanAlyze, assigns the same diameter and shape (circle) to all spots. GenePix and ScanArray Express also provide the option for fixed circle method (Jiang & Lin, 2010). A method that was proposed to avoid the drawback of fixed circle is the adaptive circle segmentation technique and can be found in GenePix, ScanAlyze, ScanArray Express, Imagene, and Dapple.

Here diagram shows the imagine adaptive circle segmentation methods below in Figure 5.

Seeded region growing (SRG) has been successfully applied to image segmentation in general, and has recently been introduced in microarray image processing on the other hand, an adaptive circle segmentation method. This method pre supposes as well that the spot has a circular shape, but also allows for adjusting the size of each spot (Chen & Chen, 2009). It provides more precise consequences than the fixed circle method. The method uses a clustering algorithm to partition the pixels based on their pixel intensity values. Most of the histogram segmentation algorithms abandon the spatial information of pixels. Spot Segmentation is the customized method which collective the power of the histogram based and spatial approaches.

Another technique that has been successfully used in microarray image segmentation is the histogram-based approach. Using histograms to classify a pixel into either foreground or background is a simple and intuitive idea. Chen introduced a method that uses a circular target mask to cover all the foreground pixels, and computes a threshold using Mann-Whitney test . Clustering has also been used in microarray image segmentation, showing some advantages when applied to microarray image segmentation, since they are not restricted to a particular shape and size of the spots (Rahman, 2012). Although they produce irregular-shaped spots, clustering-based methods are prone to include noisy pixels in the foreground regions, producing incorrect quantization measures for the spots in such cases.

Figure 5. Genepix software's view

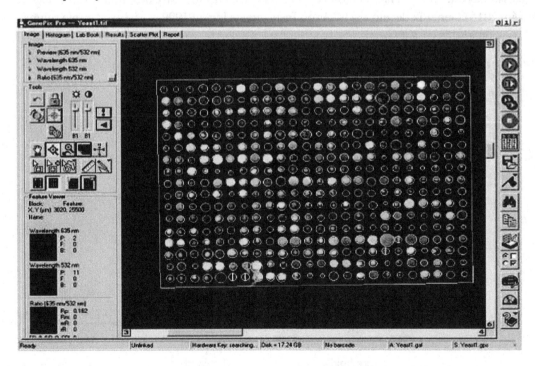

Figure 6. Imagene segmentation view

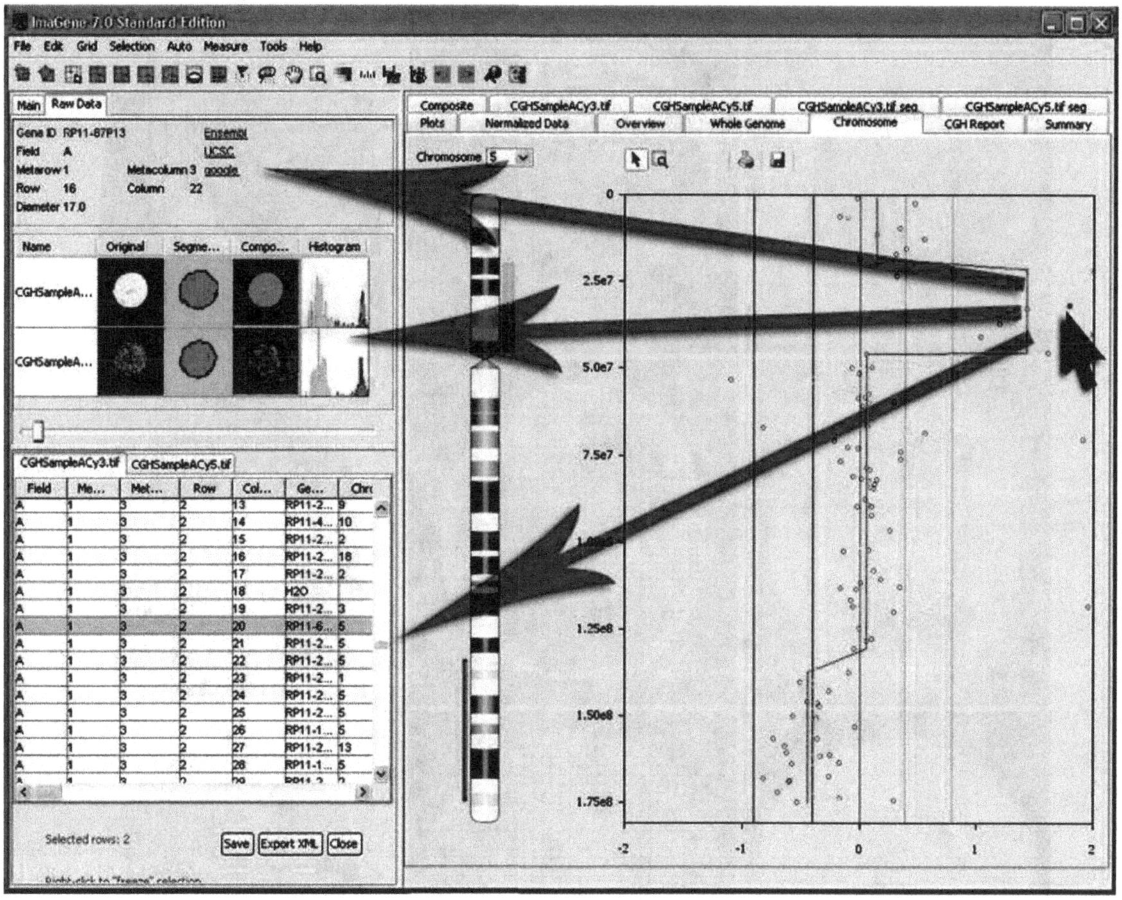

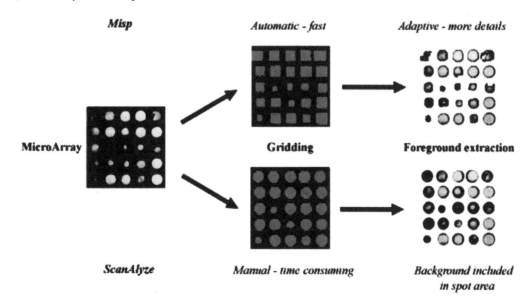

Figure 7. ScanAlyze technique

Figure 8. Segmentation by ScanArray Express

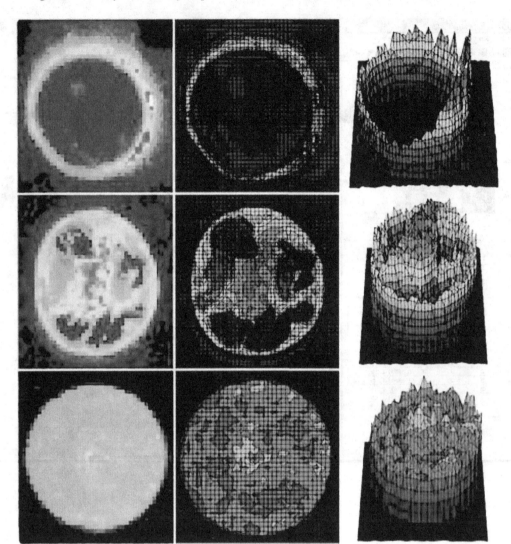

Image Analysis Methods

There are three steps for microarray image analysis as described in addressing, segmentation and information extraction. In our research, we will not focus on the addressing part, since we can get the grid information for the microarray data file from the Stanford website mentioned above. A spot is an area where printed cDNA is located. Segmentation is a process used to divide a spot area from a non-spot area. The spot area is called foreground and the non-spot area is called background (Qin, Rueda, Ali & Ngom, 2005). We will focus on four types of segmentation methods: fixed circle segmentation, adaptive circle segmentation, adaptive shape segmentation and histogram segmentation. Fixed circle segmentation is an ideal method; it assumes that each spot has the same size and a circular shape. The segmentation algorithm in this case is easy to implement, but the real spots may not have the ideal circular shape and the same size. Adaptive circle segmentation (Wang & Sun, 2011) permits for the diameter of each spot circle to be adjusted. It is better than the fixed circle, but still the spot shape is restricted to be a circle. Histogram segmentation uses the normal allocation of pixels intensity percentiles around and inside each spot to segment the spot from the background.

Obviously this method neglects the particular pixel locations. It will not give out the accurate spot intensity, but only return the trend. Adaptive shape segmentation is designed to improve the accuracy of the segmentation. This method is better than the fixed and adaptive circle segmentation methods. Watershed, seed region growing and globally optimal geodesic active contours (Appleton & Talbot, 2005) are the three algorithms usually used that fall into the adaptive shape segmentation method class. Watershed segmentation (PratimAcharjya & Ghoshal, 2012) defines an image as a topographic surface and assumes the water enters from the minima and floods the surface. The only visible surface after the flood is called the watershed lines. Watershed segmentation has the weakness of overlaying the original image. The segmentation area of watershed is always larger than that of the original image. Seeded region growing (SRG) segment is a method that starts with some seeds (starting points) and then includes the neighboring pixels to check if they have similar intensities. In the affirmative case, the pixels are "joined" together, if not, they will be in different classes. This process will continue until all the pixels have been included in a class containing one of the seeds. The weakness of the seed region growing is that if the seeds were chosen improperly the segmentation result will not be accurate. Globally Optimal Geodesic Active Contours (GOGAC) are the new segmentation method which was executed in Spot (Shan, He & Wang, 2014).The weakness of this method is that it prefers to produce circles, it cannot put off overlaps and it is slower than the SRG method.

Information Extraction and Segmentation

Information extraction and segmentation is the major foundation progression of image analysis. One microarray image can have thousands of spots and spots can vary in size, shape, intensity. The spots have to be quantified for further analysis . The Effortless closed curve of minimal energy represented through a metric, under the constraint to the geodesic must hold a particular internal point is produced by GOGAC. This limitation is a natural constraint to find a non-trivial global minimum and is also a natural alternative to different adhoc forces that put off contours from collapsing upon themselves.

Problem Statement

The problem involves finding the Correct Segmented Spots by GOGAC Method is solved by this Improved GOGAC Method. The thesis illustrates an approach to image segmentation based on deformable models to overcome incorrect spot segmentation of microarray images. In particular our method corrects segmentation errors of GOGAC.

Problem Description

Image segmentation has long been accepted as a complicated setback. A lot of programs, algorithms have been anticipated. In this progression a current prominent development is the Globally Optimal Geodesic Active Contour (GOGAC) (Ananth & Pannirselvam, 2012). Recently, Incorrect Segmentation results for microarray images have attracted much attention due to their inability of generating correctly segmented spots. Figure 9 presents the segmentation result image obtained by using the GOGAC.

Figure 9. Segmentation Results by GOGAC Method.

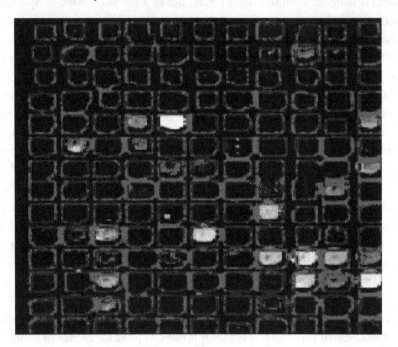

Consequently, using GOGAC for the segmentation of microarray image will affect next step of the cDNA microarray data analysis i.e. quantification and analysis (Figure 10)

Challenges

Globally Optimal GAC segmentation takes minimum time for segmentation of the image that is 2.5 seconds, it is faster than other deformable methods like Classic GAC and Multiscale GAC.While speed supports to do work quicker but it also poses challenges for the segmentation. These challenges include incorrect segmented spots, so we have to develop an approach to image segmentation based on deformable models to overcome incorrect spot segmentation of microarray images. This is achieved by first identifying 'under segmented' spots in the result of GOGAC.In order to quantify and analyze the patterns of spots, method must be able to recognize incorrect segmented spots as being distinct from other normal spots in the image.

Solution

We have developed an approach to image segmentation based on deformable models to overcome incorrect spot segmentation of microarray images.In particular our method corrects segmentation errors of GOGAC. Our goal is to find 'under segmented' spots in the result of GOGAC and improve it by border expansion method. We have used the Globally Optimal Geodesic Active Contours based segmentation algorithm proposed in which is implemented in MATLAB software. Globally Optimal Geodesic Active Contours method generates segmentation results quantifies shape of spots, area, perimeter, and circularity and the log ratios of the red and green channels based on median values mean of foreground for each

Figure 10. Steps of Microarray Image Analysis Process.

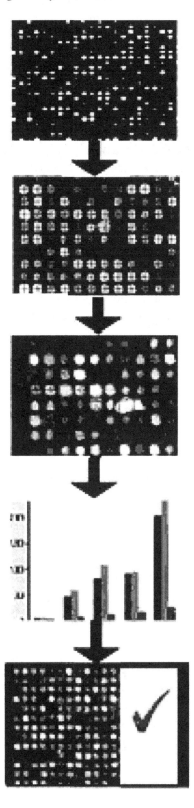

channel and background, inter quartile range of foreground for each channel and background are some important features that can be calculated. We have found that GOGAC generates an incorrect segmentation these types of incorrect spots are corrected by our proposed Improved GOGAC Segmentation method.

Experimental Results

In this section, we present the experimental results, indicating the different types of spots. The GOGAC experimental results using the deformable model implemented by Appleton are also presented for comparison. The sizes of all the test images are given in Table 1. Our Improved GOGAC segmentation results were tested on images from the microarray database of Stanford University. We have used the human peripheral blood mononuclear cellular images.

Gridding Result

The Spot software provides option for semi-automatic gridding. The user has to mark the center of the first spot of each and every block, which is a tedious task. Despite of this manual marking of start of block, gridding method is not very robust. Figure 12 below shows an example of incorrect gridding. In this figure a cross point of red lines, marks the center of a spot. A black arrow points to the entire column of spots skipped by gridding method.

Table 1. Details of Images Used in the Project

S. N.	Experiment ID	Image Dimensions	No of Blocks	Spots per Block
1	57536	1892x5500	48 blocks (12 rows with 4 blocks each)	30x30
2	57537	1948x5601	48 blocks (12 rows with 4 blocks each	30x30
3.	57540	1948x5601	48 blocks (12 rows with 4 blocks each	30x30
4.	57541	1948x5601	48 blocks (12 rows with 4 blocks each	30x30
5.	57538	1892x5500	48 blocks (12 rows with 4 blocks each	30x30
6.	57539	1892x5500	48 blocks (12 rows with 4 blocks each	30x30
7.	57542	1948x5601	48 blocks (12 rows with 4 blocks each	30x30
8.	57543	1948x5601	48 blocks (12 rows with 4 blocks each	30x30
9.	57546	1892x5500	48 blocks (12 rows with 4 blocks each	30x30
10.	57547	1948x5601	48 blocks (12 rows with 4 blocks each	30x30

Figure 11. Sample image from Stanford University.

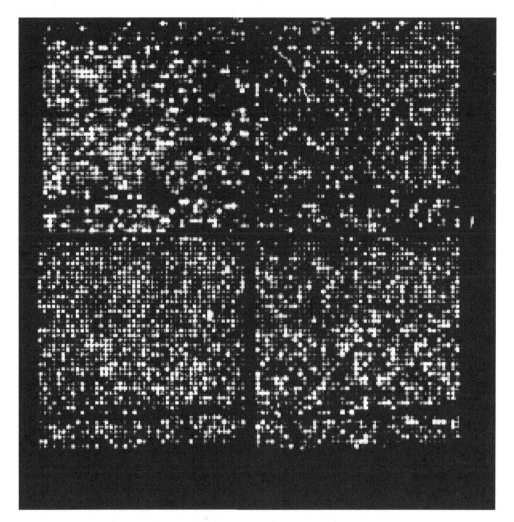

Segmentation Results

GOGAC from the Spot software has been applied to the considered images the segmentation results are visually analyzed. For manual segmentation of thousands of spots in a cDNA microarray image is extremely tedious task, therefore visual analysis has been widely used for checking the segmentation accuracy. The segmentation results are shown below. Notice in Figure 13 (a) the segmentation error due to incorrect gridding. When a spot is not processed by gridding and finding method it is also not processed by segmentation method.

The segmented results are robust in the case of correct segmentation particularly for those spot which pixels are outside the segmented region and, we found these results are very effective for accurate image analysis. Some of the incorrect segmentation is provided in Figures 14(a), 15(a), 16(a), 17(a), 18(a), 19(a) and 20(a).shows a case where the improvement in the spots is needed. In Figures 14(b), 15(b), 16(b), 17(b), 18(b), 19(b), and 20(b) the Improved GOGAC results for images are presented and we can easily observe that results are improved up to more than satisfaction level. The test examples include

Figure 12. Gridding results

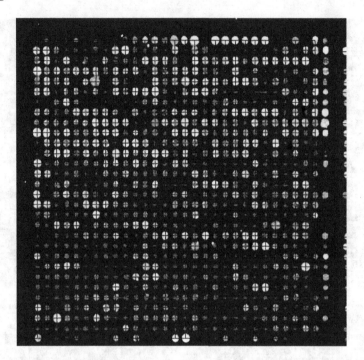

Figure 13. Segmentation results (a), (b), (c) and (d)

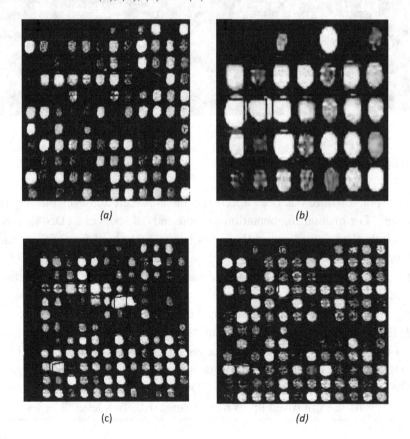

(a)

(b)

(c)

(d)

five image sets. The results of the first set of examples are shown in Figure 12(a), where we have taken 3×3 spots of GOGAC and compared with the improved GOGAC. The results of the Improved GOGAC method are shown in Figure 12 (b).

Which is better in spots whose pixels are outside the boundary than the other deformable model based segmentation:

Figure 14. The comparison of GOGAC with Improved GOGAC method. (a) GOGAC result for 3x3 spots (b) Improved GOGAC result for 3x3 spots.

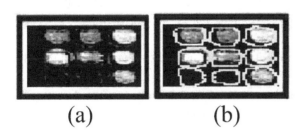

Figure 15. (a) GOGAC result for 2x2 spots (b) Improved GOGAC result for 2x2 spots

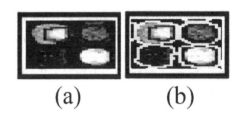

Figure 16. (a) GOGAC result for 2x2 spots from view1 (b) Improved GOGAC result for 2x2 spots

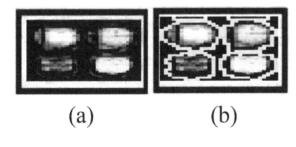

Figure 17. (a) GOGAC result for 2 spots (b) Improved GOGAC result for 2 spots

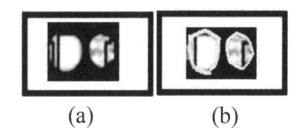

Figure 18. (a) GOGAC result for 2x2 spots from view2 (b) Improved GOGAC result for 2x2 spots

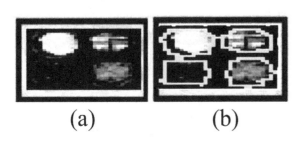

Figure 19. (a) GOGAC result for 2x2 spots from view3 (b) Improved GOGAC result for 2x2 spots

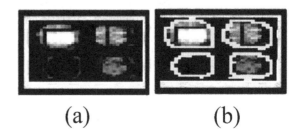

Figure 20. (a) GOGAC result for 2x2 spots from view4 (b) Improved GOGAC result for 2x2 spots.

Figure 21. (a) GOGAC result for 2x2 spots from view1 (b) Improved GOGAC result for 2x2 spots

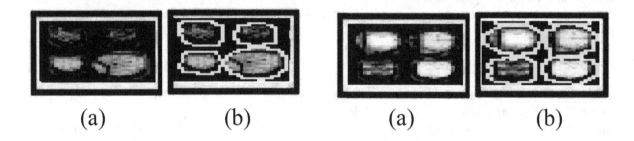

(a)   (b)   (a)   (b)

Here we compare the computational speed of the Caselles's classic GAC scheme, the proposed improved globally optimal GAC scheme. The test example is a 600×450 microarray image, the goal being to segment the image.

Figure 22 depicts the result of the classic GAC segmentation implemented by level set evolution. It converges in 21.5 seconds, the result of a multiscale GAC segmentation, converging in 3.1 seconds and the result of the globally optimal GAC segmentation presented here. The algorithm takes 2.5 seconds. But the result of an improved GOGAC segmentation proposed here takes 0.35 seconds for computation.

SUMMARY

In this chapter, we introduced a novel work to perform Image segmentation of under segmented spots of human peripheral blood cells from Stanford University. The method consists of GOGAC, Intensity thresholding, Identification of Unassigned Pixels, Image Subtraction operations and Assignment of Unassigned pixels to the spots by using Border Expansion Method. We have taken image of 1892x5500 and 1948x5601 dimensions and Experiments performed at 100 images of 48 blocks each contains 30×30 spots. After that we compared the results of GOGAC with Improved GOGAC.Here we also showed how our methods results are better than previous methods.

FUTURE RESEARCH DIRECTIONS

The future scope of the work is to make an automatic segmentation method for segmentation of medical images, including microarray,MRI and CT image. Afterwards the approach will be extended to get more robust segmentation results. The developed approach will be applied to segment cells in 2D and we can extend this for 3D images. Both static and dynamic image data can be investigated.The work can be extended to very fast image segmentation.

Figure 22. Comparison of computational speed

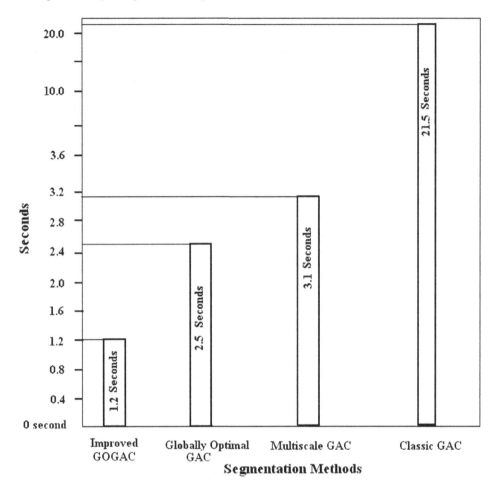

CONCLUSION

GOGAC method's performance is good in terms of time than Active Contours. So we will perform post processing operation on the results of GOGAC to correct the under segmented results and then we can make a better method than Active Contours. The GOGAC segmentation method based on deformable model can be applied to medical image analysis processes. But improper segmentation is a major problem. We have tested GOGAC method for segmentation of cDNA microarray images implemented in the Spot software for images from two different experiments. The results show that the GOGAC generates incorrect segmentation results for cDNA microarray images. The incorrect segmentation result will affect next step of the cDNA microarray data analysis .We implemented post processing process for automatic correction of spots In this work, an improved method with identification of unassigned pixels, assignment of unassigned pixels to the correct spot by border expansion approach is proposed to overcome the problem. The segmentation of microarray images is effective. Experiment results show that our method provides better results than other deformable models. The proposed method might be a better method for microarray image segmentation with better performance and less time consumes.

REFERENCES

Abdelsamea, M., Gnecco, G., & Medhat Gaber, M. (2015). A SOM-based Chanâ€"Vese model for unsupervised image segmentation. *Soft Computing*. doi:10.1007/s00500-015-1906-z

Ali, H., Badshah, N., Chen, K., & Khan, G. (2016). A variational model with hybrid images data fitting energies for segmentation of images with intensity inhomogeneity. *Pattern Recognition*, *51*, 27–42. doi:10.1016/j.patcog.2015.08.022

Ananth, K., & Pannirselvam, S. (2012). A Geodesic Active Contour Level Set Method for Image Segmentation. *International Journal of Image, Graphics, Signal Processing*, *4*(5), 31–37. doi:10.5815/ijigsp.2012.05.04

Appleton, B., & Talbot, H. (2005). Globally Optimal Geodesic Active Contours. *Journal of Mathematical Imaging and Vision*, *23*(1), 67–86. doi:10.1007/s10851-005-4968-1

Benninghoff, H., & Garcke, H. (2014). Efficient Image Segmentation and Restoration Using Parametric Curve Evolution with Junctions and Topology Changes. *SIAM Journal on Imaging Sciences*, *7*(3), 1451–1483. doi:10.1137/130932430

Bresson, X., & Esedog, Ì. (2007). Fast Global Minimization of the Active Contour/Snake Model. *Journal of Mathematical Imaging and Vision*, *28*(2), 151–167. doi:10.1007/s10851-007-0002-0

Can, A., Leclercq, L., Lelong, J., & Botteldooren, D. (2010). Traffic noise spectrum analysis: Dynamic modeling vs. experimental observations. *Applied Acoustics*, *71*(8), 764–770. doi:10.1016/j.apacoust.2010.04.002

Chen, A., Deeley, M., Niermann, K., Moretti, L., & Dawant, B. (2010). Combining registration and active shape models for the automatic segmentation of the lymph node regions in head and neck CT images. *Medical Physics*, *37*(12), 6338. doi:10.1118/1.3515459 PMID:21302791

Chen, D. (2013). A Novel Image Segmentation Algorithm: Region Merging Using Superpixel-based Local CRF Model. *J. Inf. Comput. Sci.*, *10*(16), 5145–5153. doi:10.12733/jics20103063

Chen, Y., & Chen, O. (2009). Image Segmentation Method Using Thresholds Automatically Determined from Picture Contents. *EURASIP Journal on Image and Video Processing*, *2009*, 1–15. doi:10.1155/2009/140492

Dawoud, A., & Netchaev, A. (2012). Fusion of visual cues of intensity and texture in Markov random fields image segmentation. *IET Computer Vision*, *6*(6), 603–609. doi:10.1049/iet-cvi.2011.0233

Diop, E., & Burdin, V. (2013). Bi-planar image segmentation based on variational geometrical active contours with shape priors. *Medical Image Analysis*, *17*(2), 165–181. doi:10.1016/j.media.2012.09.006 PMID:23168322

Drapikowski, P., & Domaga, Å. (2014). Semi-Automatic Segmentation of Ct/Mri Images Based on Active Contour Method for 3D Reconstruction of Abdominal Aortic Aneurysms. *Image Processing & Communications*, *19*(1). doi:10.1515/ipc-2015-0002

Fussenegger, M., Roth, P., Bischof, H., Deriche, R., & Pinz, A. (2009). A level set framework using a new incremental, robust Active Shape Model for object segmentation and tracking. *Image and Vision Computing*, *27*(8), 1157–1168. doi:10.1016/j.imavis.2008.10.014

Gao, Y., Kikinis, R., Bouix, S., Shenton, M., & Tannenbaum, A. (2012). A 3D interactive multi-object segmentation tool using local robust statistics driven active contours. *Medical Image Analysis*, *6*(6), 1216–1227. doi:10.1016/j.media.2012.06.002 PMID:22831773

Huang, G., & Pun, C. (2015). Robust Interactive Segmentation Using Color Histogram and Contourlet Transform. *IJCTE*, *7*(6), 489–494. doi:10.7763/IJCTE.2015.V7.1007

Jiang, G., & Lin, Y. (2010). Skin color segmentation algorithm combining adaptive model and fixed model. *Journal Of Computer Applications*, *30*(10), 2698–2701. doi:10.3724/SP.J.1087.2010.02698

Jung, Y., Kang, M., & Heo, J. (2014). Clustering performance comparison using K -means and expectation maximization algorithms. *Biotechnology & Biotechnological Equipment*, *28*(sup1), S44-S48.10.1080/13102818.2014.949045

Karasulu, B. (2013). An approach based on simulated annealing to optimize the performance of extraction of the flower region using mean-shift segmentation. *Applied Soft Computing*, *13*(12), 4763–4785. doi:10.1016/j.asoc.2013.07.019

Kass, M., Witkin, A., & Terzopoulos, D. (1988). Snakes: Active contour models. *International Journal of Computer Vision*, *1*(4), 321–331. doi:10.1007/BF00133570

Kim, D., & Park, J. (2005). Connectivity-based local adaptive thresholding for carotid artery segmentation using MRA images. *Image and Vision Computing*, *23*(14), 1277–1287. doi:10.1016/j.imavis.2005.09.005

Kocher, M., & Leonardi, R. (1986). Adaptive region growing technique using polynomial functions for image approximation. *Signal Processing*, *11*(1), 47–60. doi:10.1016/0165-1684(86)90094-0

Lankton, S., & Tannenbaum, A. (2008). Localizing Region-Based Active Contours. *IEEE Transactions on Image Processing*, *17*(11), 2029–2039. doi:10.1109/TIP.2008.2004611 PMID:18854247

Li, Y., Luo, S., & Zou, Q. (2010). Active Contour Model Based on Salient Boundary Point Image for Object Contour Detection in Natural Image. *IEICE Transactions on Information and Systems*, *E93-D*(11), 3136–3139. doi:10.1587/transinf.E93.D.3136

Li, Y., Luo, S., & Zou, Q. (2010). Active Contour Model Based on Salient Boundary Point Image for Object Contour Detection in Natural Image. *IEICE Transactions on Information and Systems*, *E93-D*(11), 3136–3139. doi:10.1587/transinf.E93.D.3136

Li, Z., & Weng, G. (2011). Segmentation of cDNA Microarray Image Using Fuzzy c-Mean Algorithm and Mathematical Morphology. *KEM*, *464*, 159–162. doi:10.4028/www.scientific.net/KEM.464.159

Liu, S., & Peng, Y. (2012). A local region-based Chanâ€"Vese model for image segmentation. *Pattern Recognition*, *45*(7), 2769–2779. doi:10.1016/j.patcog.2011.11.019

Maciejewski, M., Surtel, W., Maciejewska, B., & Małecka-Massalska, T. (2015). Level-set image processing methods in medical image segmentation. *Bio-Algorithms And Med-Systems, 11*(1). doi:10.1515/bams-2014-0017

Majewski, J., & Rosenblatt, D. (2012). Exome and whole-genome sequencing for gene discovery: The future is now! *Human Mutation, 33*(4), 591–592. doi:10.1002/humu.22055 PMID:22411407

Ortiz, A., Gorriz, J., Ramirez, J., & Salas-Gonzalez, D. (2012). Unsupervised Neural Techniques Applied to MR Brain Image Segmentation. *Advances in Artificial Neural Systems, 2012*, 1–7. doi:10.1155/2012/457590

Petitjean, C., & Dacher, J. (2011). A review of segmentation methods in short axis cardiac MR images. *Medical Image Analysis, 15*(2), 169–184. doi:10.1016/j.media.2010.12.004 PMID:21216179

PratimAcharjya, P., & Ghoshal, D. (2012). A Modified Watershed Segmentation Algorithm using Distances Transform for Image Segmentation. *International Journal of Computers and Applications, 52*(12), 46–50. doi:10.5120/8258-1791

Pratondo, A., Chui, C., & Ong, S. (2016). Robust Edge-Stop Functions for Edge-Based Active Contour Models in Medical Image Segmentation. *IEEE Signal Processing Letters, 23*(2), 222–226. doi:10.1109/LSP.2015.2508039

Qin, L., Rueda, L., Ali, A., & Ngom, A. (2005). Spot Detection and Image Segmentation in DNA??Microarray Data. *Applied Bioinformatics, 4*(1), 1–11. doi:10.2165/00822942-200504010-00001 PMID:16000008

Rahman, M. (2012). Unsupervised Natural Image Segmentation Using Mean Histogram Features. *Journal Of Multimedia, 7*(5). doi:10.4304/jmm.7.5.332-340

Reddy, G., Ramudu, K., Srinivas, A., & Rao, R. (2011). Fast Level Set Evolution of Region Based Segmentation of Satellite and Medical Imagery on Noisy Images. *International Journal Of Applied Physics And Mathematics*, 78-81. doi:10.7763/ijapm.2011.v1.15

Renka, R. (2009). Image segmentation with a Sobolev gradient method. *Nonlinear Analysis: Theory. Methods & Applications, 71*(12), e774–e780. doi:10.1016/j.na.2008.11.070

Shan, H., He, C., & Wang, N. (2014). MCA aided geodesic active contours for image segmentation with textures. *Pattern Recognition Letters, 45*, 235–243. doi:10.1016/j.patrec.2014.04.018

Shang, S. (2010). *DNA microarray analysis of the gene expression profile of kidney tissue in a type 2 diabetic rat model*. Mol Med Rep. doi:10.3892/mmr.2010.367

Shao, G., Li, T., Zuo, W., Wu, S., & Liu, T. (2015). A Combinational Clustering Based Method for cDNA Microarray Image Segmentation. *PLoS ONE, 10*(8), e0133025. doi:10.1371/journal.pone.0133025 PMID:26241767

Shi, C. (2006). A Parametric Active Contour Model for Medical Image Segmentation Using Priori Shape Force Field. *Journal Of Computer Research And Development, 43*(), 2131. doi:10.1360/crad20061215

Soria, D., Garibaldi, J., Ambrogi, F., Biganzoli, E., & Ellis, I. (2011). A 'non-parametric' version of the naive Bayes classifier. *Knowledge-Based Systems, 24*(6), 775–784. doi:10.1016/j.knosys.2011.02.014

Sun, S. (2013). High Precision Infrared Image Data Rendering Algorithm Based on Probability Sequence. *J. Inf. Comput. Sci.*, *10*(16), 5293–5299. doi:10.12733/jics20102304

Tao, W., & Tai, X. (2011). Multiple piecewise constant with geodesic active contours (MPC-GAC) framework for interactive image segmentation using graph cut optimization. *Image and Vision Computing*, *29*(8), 499–508. doi:10.1016/j.imavis.2011.03.002

Vard, A., Jamshidi, K., & Movahhedinia, N. (2012). An automated approach for segmentation of intravascular ultrasound images based on parametric active contour models. *Australasian Physical & Engineering Sciences in Medicine*, *35*(2), 135–150. doi:10.1007/s13246-012-0131-7 PMID:22415899

Vard, A., Monadjemi, A., Jamshidi, K., & Movahhedinia, N. (2011). Fast texture energy based image segmentation using Directional Walshâ€"Hadamard Transform and parametric active contour models. *Expert Systems with Applications*, *38*(9), 11722–11729. doi:10.1016/j.eswa.2011.03.058

Vlachos, M., & Dermatas, E. (2013). Finger vein segmentation in infrared images using supervised and unsupervised clustering algorithms. *Pattern Recognition and Image Analysis*, *23*(2), 328–334. doi:10.1134/S1054661813020168

Wang, H., & Liu, M. (2012). Medical Images Segmentation Using Active Contours Driven By Global And Local Image Fitting Energy. *International Journal of Image and Graphics*, *12*(02), 1250015. doi:10.1142/S0219467812500155

Wang, H., Zhang, H., & Ray, N. (2013). Adaptive shape prior in graph cut image segmentation. *Pattern Recognition*, *46*(5), 1409–1414. doi:10.1016/j.patcog.2012.11.002

Wang, L., Li, C., Sun, Q., Xia, D., & Kao, C. (2009). Active contours driven by local and global intensity fitting energy with application to brain MR image segmentation. *Computerized Medical Imaging and Graphics*, *33*(7), 520–531. doi:10.1016/j.compmedimag.2009.04.010 PMID:19482457

Wang, Y., & Sun, Y. (2011). Adaptive Mean Shift Based Image Smoothing and Segmentation. *Acta Automatica Sinica*, *36*(12), 1637–1644. doi:10.3724/SP.J.1004.2010.01637

Wee-Chung Liew, A., Yan, H., & Yang, M. (2003). Robust adaptive spot segmentation of DNA microarray images. *Pattern Recognition*, *36*(5), 1251–1254. doi:10.1016/S0031-3203(02)00170-X

Xu, C., & Zhang, Y. (2014). Cell Contour Irregularity Feature Extraction Methods based on Linear Geometric Heat Flow Curve Evolution. *International Journal Of Signal Processing, Image Processing. Pattern Recognition*, *7*(3), 181–192. doi:10.14257/ijsip.2014.7.3.15

Xu, X., & He, C. (2013). Implicit Active Contour Model with Local and Global Intensity Fitting Energies. *Mathematical Problems in Engineering*, *2013*, 1–13. doi:10.1155/2013/367086

Yang, H., Zhao, L., & Tang, S. (2014). Brain Tumor Segmentation Using Geodesic Region-based Level Set without Re-initialization. *International Journal Of Signal Processing, Image Processing. Pattern Recognition*, *7*(1), 213–224. doi:10.14257/ijsip.2014.7.1.20

Ye, K., & Zhan, Y. (2009). Image segmentation algorithm based on mathematical morphology and active edgeless contour model without edges. *Journal Of Computer Applications*, *29*(9), 2398–2401. doi:10.3724/SP.J.1087.2009.02398

Yuan, J. (2012). Active contour driven by region-scalable fitting and local Bhattacharyya distance energies for ultrasound image segmentation. *IET Image Processing, 6*(8), 1075–1083. doi:10.1049/iet-ipr.2012.0120

Yuasa, M., Watanabe, M., Nishiura, M., Yamaguchi, K., Kondo, T., Anno, H., & Muto, K. (2003). Automatic heart wall contour extraction from MR images using active contour models: Initial contour setting based on principal component analysis. *Systems and Computers in Japan, 34*(4), 72–82. doi:10.1002/scj.1202

Zheng, Q. (2012). New local segmentation model for images with intensity inhomogeneity. *Optical Engineering (Redondo Beach, Calif.), 51*(3), 037006. doi:10.1117/1.OE.51.3.037006

Zou, X. (2013). Improved Dcut and its application in image segmentation. *Journal Of Computer Applications, 32*(8), 2291–2295. doi:10.3724/SP.J.1087.2012.02291

KEY TERMS AND DEFINITIONS

Active Contour Model (ACM): Active contour model, also called snakes, is a framework in computer vision for delineating an object's outline from a possibly noisy 2D image.

Globally Optimal Geodesic Active Contour (GOGAC): An approach to optimal object segmentation in the geodesic active contour framework.

Gridding: Gridding is a mathmatical process to make an image bigger, smaller or the same size (copy it).

Histogram: A histogram is a graphical representation of the distribution of numerical data.

Level Set Methods (LSM): Level set methods (LSM) are a conceptual framework for using level sets as a tool for numerical analysis of surfaces and shapes.

Local Binary Fitting (LBF): Its robust and efficient level set method Image Segmentation method.

Seeded Region Growing (SRG): Region growing is a simple region-based image segmentation method. It is also classified as a pixel-based image segmentation method.

Segmentation: In computer vision, image segmentation is the process of partitioning a digital image into multiple segments (sets of pixels, also known as superpixels).

Chapter 4
Towards Parameterized Shared Key for AVK Approach

Shaligram Prajapat
Maulana Azad National Institute of Technology, India & Devi Ahilya University, India

Ramjeevan Singh Thakur
Maulana Azad National Institute of Technology, India

ABSTRACT

"Key" plays a vital role in every symmetric key cryptosystem. The obvious way of enhancing security of any cryptosystem is to keep the key as large as possible. But it may not be suitable for low power devices since higher computation will be done for longer keys and that will increase the power requirement which decreases the device's performance. In order to resolve the former specified problem an alternative approach can be used in which the length of key is fixed and its value varies in every session. This is Time Variant Key approach or Automatic Variable Key (AVK) approach. The Security of AVK based cryptosystem is enhanced by exchanging some parameters instead of keys between the communicating parties, then these parameters will be used to generate required keys at the receiver end. This chapter presents implementation of the above specified Mechanism. A model has been demonstrated with parameterized scheme and issues in AVK approach. Further, it has been analyzed from different users' perspectives. This chapter also highlights the benefits of AVK model to ensure two levels of security with characterization of methods for AVK and Estimation of key computation based on parameters only. The characteristic components of recent styles of key design with consideration of key size, life time of key and breaking threshold has also been pointed out. These characteristics are essential in the design of efficient symmetric key cryptosystem. The novel approach of AVK based cryptosystem is suitable for low power devices and useful for exchanging very large objects or files. This scheme has been demonstrated with Fibonacci-Q matrix and sparse matrix based diffused key information exchange procedures. These models have been further tested from perspective of hackers and cryptanalyst, to exploit any weakness with fixed size dynamic keys.

DOI: 10.4018/978-1-5225-0536-5.ch004

INTRODUCTION

"Sending and receiving information securely" is the sole objective of every communication system. The medium on which information is propagated has been transformed drastically due to growth in communication technology. As the transmission over public network takes places between unknown entities, ensuring security of information is a challenging task due to vulnerability of the public systems (Diffe & Hellman, 1977). Hence, ensuring security of information between participating entities is essential. Similarly, protection of data of interconnected machines within networked system from malicious damage is also desirable aspect of a successful cryptosystem. Since, the cryptosystem is exposed publicly in networked system. All of its components like plaintext, cipher text, key, enciphering algorithm and deciphering algorithms are available on the network either in hidden formats or exposed in some other way(depending upon mechanism) (Chakrabarti, et. al., 2008). Except the original text i.e. the plain text before leaving sender's machine, all other information is available in encrypted or hidden format. Among these components of symmetric key based cryptosystem, secrecy of key is important because if key is compromised, then rest other components are of no use. Using brute force attacks mechanism, weakness of these cryptosystems can be exploited, where cryptanalyst or attacker tries each possible key until the right key is found to decrypt the message (Prajapat & Thakur, *2015*). According to Moore's law, the power of personal computers has historically doubled approximately every 18 months. In addition, well equipped attackers often develop new techniques and algorithms to improve the efficacy of key search attacks. Therefore, estimate of the time required for successful key search attacks must be revised downward as the computing power and resources which are available to attacker's increases. Most of the time they are successful due to: availability and accessibility of fast computing resources, capability to use power of AI enabled algorithms, availability of sender/receiver's personal information to prune the search space making task of cryptanalyst and hacker's job easier (A. Nadeem et. al., 2005). With the growth of multi course processing, availability of CPU-GPU pairs parallel and grid based computing algorithms, the search time can be reduced to polynomial time from exponential (infeasible) in near future. Presently, to enhance the success rate of brute force attack best alternatives are:

- Reduce the life time of key.
- Increase the key length. In former approach by choosing the shorter key lifetime, one can reduce the possible potential damage even if one of the keys is known.

In later approach, choosing longer key length one can decrease the probability of successful attacks by increasing the number of combinations that are possible (Prajapat & Thakur, *2015*). The state of art symmetric key based cryptosystem trends towards increasing length of key for enhancing security, but it has certain side effects. It increases processing, resource utilization, and time consumption. In the next section of this chapter, we will learn the model of AVK, as a solution to the above problem. And subsequently we will learn to add extra security provision for this model of key exchange using exchange parameters only mechanism. The chapter also highlights novel methods for generating keys using parameterized key based cryptosystem.

BACKGROUND OF KEY SIZE SELECTION PROBLEM

The traditional approach of choosing key is actually deciding the string of characters consisting of digits, numbers, special symbols etc. (depending upon the type of implementation and system need) which is checked by source or destination. If the supplied key matches with the one which is associated with the actual user's resource (files, databases, etc), access is granted to all the resources of the authorized user (Shaligram Prajapat, R.S. Thakur, 2015).

- **Worst Case***:* It is obvious, simple, straightforward and inexpensive style of choosing key length. In this scheme, user will be frequently choosing a relatively short string of characters. The user may be allowed to choose these keys, but, in such situations, the chosen key would be easy to remember. It implies that key can be easily cracked with a predictable set of permutations and combinations. Thus, it becomes easier for an intruder to guess the key and breach into system.
- **Best Case***:* In this scheme, when difficult key or less obvious key is chosen, it breaks the comfort zone of user. The key is difficult to remember. So, the users save the key in the form of writing or recording the key somewhere noted on paper or may be in the system also, thus making it equally vulnerable.

One alternative to above mentioned problems is that, we can increase the length of key making the system relatively more secure against exhaustive search performed by cryptanalyst. But, before dealing with increment aspects of key length, it would be worth mentioning the notion of Safe Period and Breaking Period. The concept of probable expected *Safe period* and *Breaking period* or *Threshold* to prevent a key from systematic attacks can be computed from equation(1) and(2), This can be used as an indicator of the effectiveness of a selected length of key used in a given cryptosystem.

- **Safe Period:** It is the maximum time required to guess actual key using brute force method. It can be computed from following expression.

$$\text{Safe Time} = \frac{\text{Total number of keys} \quad \times \quad \text{Time to enter one key}}{2} \tag{1}$$

- **Breaking Period:** For any given key, it is the *optimistic time* to break the key, selected from characters set domain of size N, *Breaking period* for a given key can be computed from following expression:

$$\text{Breaking Threshold} = \frac{N^x \quad * \quad L}{R} \tag{2}$$

where:

x = length of key (in number of characters)
R = Character transmission rate. *R* characters per minute. (Computed from time required to enter data)

N = Size of character-set (domain-set) (i.e. number of letters and numeric from which the key is selected in number of characters involved for entry and replying in a log- in attempt is N characters)

Situation: 1

Consider a hypothetical cryptic communication system where sender or receiver uses keys of length 6 characters with the key entry rate 60 characters per minute. The key is constructed from a character set, a domain of size 20 characters (this means that only a limited set of infrequent characters are being used), the key-length x is 6 characters(Bytes), and the number of characters L in the session log-in is 15 characters(Bytes). For an operator working on a keyboard for the exhaustive key search, the expected Safe period would be:

$$\text{Safe Time} = \frac{\text{All number of keys} \quad * \quad \text{Time to enter a key}}{2}$$

$$\text{Safe Time} = \frac{20^6 \quad * \quad 15}{2 * 60} \text{ Minutes}$$

$$\text{Safe Time} = 8 \quad * \quad 10^6 \text{ Minutes}$$

$$\text{Safe Time} \approx 15 \text{ Years}$$

Situation: 2 (Usage of Parallel Node)

Further, extending the idea of previous case, with the assumption of using more systems (for simplicity, n=2). If two systems are used in parallel to solve the problem of situation-1, what would be effect over the performance of Safe period? Obviously, this may result in reduction in computation of expected Safe period because exhaustive search is empowered by the use of additional computing node connected to the first computing node.

We further assume that the two computers are connected by a high-speed line on which the data transmission rate (R) *is* 1200 characters per second (CPS) the expected Safe period would be:

$$\text{Safe Time} = \frac{20^6 \quad * \quad 15}{2 * 36000} \text{ Minutes}$$

Safe time= 13334.34 minutes

Safe time $\approx$ 9.523 days.

This reduces the effort from infeasible (result of situation 1) to feasible region (result of situation 2).

Situation: 3 (Using Delay to Prevent Guessing)

Allowing 'delay' between successive failure attempts also has an impact on breaking threshold. In other words, by adding automatic delay after each unsuccessful attempt can enhance the security, this can be elucidated as follows:

If a delay of 5 seconds is added between 2 unsuccessful attempts, then the time for each entry increases from 0.0125 second to 5.0125 second and the expected Safe period becomes greater than 5 years. In this way, the delay between each unsuccessful guessing makes it harder or infeasible to guess.

Formulation of Basis for Deciding the Length of a Key

The discussion of situation-1, situation-2 and situation-3 can be extended to form the baseline for deciding optimum key size. To compute the key length of suitable performance, let us assume that p is the probability that a correct key will be found by a cryptanalyst, *and* the time period in months over which systematic attempts are to be made over each 24 hours per day of operation is *M,* so *p* will have an upper bounded of p_0 where:

$$P_0 = \frac{\text{Number of possible attempts to break the key in M months}}{\text{Number of Possible Keys}} \tag{3}$$

$$\text{The number of possible attempts in M months} = \frac{T * M * 30 * 24 * 60}{L}$$

The number of possible key is N^x, Therefore

$$p = \frac{4.32 * 10^4 * T * M}{L * N^x}$$

The probability that a proper key will be found is *p,* where $p \geq p_0$, which gives

$$N^x \geq \frac{4.32 * 10^4 * T * M}{L * p_0} \tag{4}$$

This is Anderson's formula and can be used to decide the length of key i.e. x, so that an intruder has a limited possibility of guessing the valid key, that is not greater than p. This can be explained with following illustrations:

Example: 1

Consider a set of alphabets with 26 characters to create a key, it is desirable that it will have the probability of not greater than 0.001 of being discovered or interpolated after systematic attack of one month. If data entry rate is 300 characters per minute (CPS) and maximum key entry requires 15 characters, then estimate the length of a key. Using the equation (4),

$$20^x \geq \frac{4.32 * 10^4 * 300 * 1}{15 * 0.001}$$

$$20^x \geq 8.64 * 10^8$$

For $x = 2$, $26^2 \leq 8.64 * 10^8$

For $x = 3$, $26^3 \leq 8.64 * 10^8$

For $x = 4$, $26^4 \leq 8.64 * 10^8$

For $x = 5$, $26^5 \leq 8.64 * 10^8$

For $x = 6$, $26^6 \leq 8.64 * 10^8$

For $x = 7$, $26^7 \geq 8.64 * 10^8$

Thus optimum key size is 7.Thus above situations infer following facts can be inferred.

1. The critical factor for preventing an intruder from discovering a key by an exhaustive search is the length of the key.
2. For optimum key size, only five or six characters in length are relatively safe from systematic attack,
3. Key will generally not fail because of systematic attack, but, as a result of the carelessness of person who is using it.

MAIN FOCUS OF THE CHAPTER

Enhancement of Symmetric Key Based Cryptosystem by Increasing Key Size

Consider the following table, showing some symmetric key based cryptosystems and key size for encryption and decryption of plaintext information. DES was used widely in the financial industries. DES is a block cipher with 64-bit block size and 56-bit keys (Nadeem et. al., 2005; Prajapat & Thakur, 2014). This algorithm is still strong but, new versions with increased key length; 3DES have been developed to make it more secure. International Data Encryption Algorithm –IDEA uses 128 bit key and is considered very secure. RC2, RC4 are also fast cipher but, requires large keys. It accepts keys of variable length (Elminaam at. al., 2008).

Table 1. Some Symmetric algorithms and their key lengths

S.no.	Algorithm	Key Length
1	DES	64-bit block size and 56-bit keys
2	3DES	64 bit block size with 192 bits key size
3	RC2	64-bits block size with a variable key size, ranges from 8 to128 bits
4	Blowfish	64-bit block –size with variable length key, ranging from 32 bits to 448 bits; default 128
5	AES	128-bit block size with variable key length of 128, 192, or 256 bits; default 256.
6	RC6	128 bit block size of with key sizes of 128, 192 and 256 bits.

(Shaligram Prajapat at. al.,2013)

AVK Based Model for Symmetric Key Based Cryptosystem

In literature, various studies have been conducted to analyze the performance of algorithms for fixing the key and varying its length like 128 bit, 192 bit and 256 bit key. The significant observation was that increasing key size requires more battery and time consumption (D. S. A. Elminaam at. al., 2008). Simulation based results also shows that effect of changing the key size of AES on power consumption reduces performance .The performance comparison for AES and RC6 algorithm (with128 bit, 192 bits and 256 bit keys) over processing time and energy also highlights similar impact on increasing key sizes. It can be seen that going from 128 bits key to 192 bits causes increase in power and time consumption about 8% and going from 192 bits to 256 bits, key causes an increase of 16% .Results were similar in case of RC6. Alternative approach for improving security instead of using long keys of variable length to minimize time complexity and high power consumption AVK concept can be introduced, where the secret key will vary from session to session. Subsequent section will discuss this alternative AVK based strategy, where efficient transmission of data from source to destination will be achieved by using dynamic key.

Table 2. AVK approach for Symmetric key based cryptosystem (P.Chakrabarti. 2007)

Session ID	Alice Sends	Bob Receives	Bob Sends	Alice Receives	Remarks
1	Secret key (say 2)	2	Secret key (say 6)	6	For next slot, Alice will use 6 as key and Bob 2 as key for transmitting data.
2	Alice sends Bob first data as: 3 xor 6	Bob gets back original data as: (3 xor 6)xor 6 = 3	Bob sends first data as: 7 xor 2	Alice gets back original data as: (7 xor 2) xor 2 = 7	Alice will create new key 6 xor 7 for next slot. Bob will create new key (2xor 3).
3	Alice sends next data as: 4 xor (6 xor7)	Bob gets back original data as: ((4 xor(6xor 7)) (6 xor 7)) = 4	Bob sends next data as: 8xor (2xor 3)	Alice recovers data as: ((8 xor(2xor 3)) (2 xor 3)) = 8	Thus, Alice and Bob respectively exchange data 34 and 78.

Fibonacci-Q Matrix Based Information Exchange

The working of encryption based on Fibonacci-Q matrix based cryptosystem (Shaligram at. al. 2012) is described below.

Encryption Process

Step 1: $M = \begin{bmatrix} m_1 & m_2 \\ m_3 & m_4 \end{bmatrix}$ where $m_i > 0$ and $i = 1,2,3,4,..$

Step 2: With parameters $n = 4$ we construct Keys as $Q^4 = \begin{bmatrix} 00005 & 00003 \\ 00003 & 00002 \end{bmatrix}$

or key $= \begin{bmatrix} 00000101 & 00000011 \\ 00000011 & 00000010 \end{bmatrix}$

Step3: Generate Cipher text matrix $C = M*K = \begin{bmatrix} m_1 & m_2 \\ m_3 & m_4 \end{bmatrix} * \begin{bmatrix} 00000101 & 00000011 \\ 00000011 & 00000010 \end{bmatrix}$

$e_1 = 00000101 * m_1 + 00000011 * m_2$

$e_2 = 00000011 * m_1 + 00000010 * m_2$

$e_3 = 00000101 * m_3 + 00000011 * m_4$

$e_4 = 00000011 * m_3 + 00000010 * m_4$

Decryption Process

Stakhov (2006), have explained the decryption process as follows:

Step 1: $E = \begin{bmatrix} e_1 & e_2 \\ e_3 & e_4 \end{bmatrix}$ where $m_i > 0$ and $i = 1,2,3,4,..$

Step 2: Compute the reversible deciphering function with shared parameters $n = 4$ we construct Keys as

$Q^{-4} = \begin{bmatrix} 00002 & -00003 \\ -00003 & 00005 \end{bmatrix}$

$$\text{or key} = \begin{bmatrix} 00000010 & -00000011 \\ -00000011 & 00000101 \end{bmatrix}$$

Step3: Recover plain text matrix $M = C*K = \begin{bmatrix} e_1 & e_2 \\ e_3 & e_4 \end{bmatrix} * \begin{bmatrix} 00000010 & -00000011 \\ -00000011 & 00000101 \end{bmatrix}$

$m_1 = 00000101 * e_1 - 00000011 * e_2$

$m_2 = 00000011 * e_1 + 00000010 * e_2$

$m_3 = 00000101 * e_3 - 00000011 * e_4$

$m_4 = 00000011 * e_3 + 00000010 * e_4$

Above process has been analyzed, implemented and tested. (See details Shaligram et.al. 2012, 2013, 2014 and 2015).The algorithm has been analyzed, implemented and tested in the form of a symmetric key from both user and hackers or cryptanalyst's perspective. To support AVK model, it is recommended that parameter n and p must be changed from session to session to compute key of a particular session. In the next section, another approach for AVK based symmetric cryptosystem is discussed.

Sparse Matrix Based Information Exchange

Consider secure transmission of information of moving objects over noisy channel. Assume that desirable data of our interest are the non-zero entries of sparse matrix, using row major form (assuming standard representation scheme) at transmission end. The location coordinate (i, j) of nonzero element would serve as a key for encryption/ decryption using a linear curve, where a and b are row and column indexes of non-zero data respectively (Shaligram Prajapat, at. al., 2014). The assumption of proposed algorithms is that row and column indexes starts from 1.so reconsidering the original compact sparse matrix representation:

Linear AVK (LAVK) Based Encryption Scheme

Algorithm LSAVK-Encrypt (Matrix CSM[ ])

{ // Receive plain text from sender with location information, generate cipher and transmit

    for each i from 1 to CSM[0][3] in steps of 1 do

      { a ← CSM[i][0], b ← CSM[i][1], plaintext ← CSM[i][2];

      Generate Cipher Text CSM'[i][2] ← a+b*plaintext;

      Transmit Cipher Text(CSM'[ ])

      }

}

Algorithm LSAVK-Decrypt (Matrix CSM'[ ])

{ // Receive compact sparse matrix(cipher text) and recover plaintext information

    for each i from 1 to CSM[0][2] in steps of 1 do

      { a ← CSM'[i][0], b ← CSM'[i][1], plaintext ← CSM'[i][2];

      Generate Plain Text CSM'[i][3] ← $(CSM'[i][3] - CSM'[i][0]) / CSM'[i][1]$;

      return Plain-Text(CSM'[ ])

      }

}

The LAVK-Encrypt() is a linear method that accepts compact form of sparse matrix entries (containing information to be transmitted)and uses location (index position) as parameter for Cipher generation i.e. it exploits information of nonzero element(information content) and converts the information into cipher text in linear time. Similarly, LAVK-Decrypt () receives cipher text of data item and based on its key (using position co-ordinate of element as parameter).It recovers plaintext information. Since, key is diffused into the block of data (Compact Sparse Matrix) which is being transferred and no key exchange takes place separately, so it becomes highly difficult to interpolate any information regarding plaintext or key.

    Each element or datum (data) is having a different location, such as the key. The location index or coordinate will act as parameter to construct key for encryption or decryption of data. Following table demonstrates the working of proposed scheme:

    The sparse matrix recovered by intruder or hacker would by as follows:

[1,3,19; 2,1,15; 2,4,11; 2,6,18; 3,2,12; 3,5,14; 4,2,11; 4,3,29; 5,1,11; 5,2,15; 5,5,16; 6,3,9]

Table 3. LAVK approach for secure information transmission

Index	I	Generated Cipher by (Man in middle)	M(i,j)	Data from Node-1 (Binary Plaintext)	Message bits on Noisy Channel	Decimal Equivalent	Data Received by Node-2 (Received Plaintext)
00	06	06	12	00001100	01001110	078	00001100
01	01	03	19	00010011	00111010	058	00010011
02	02	01	15	00001111	00010001	017	00001111
03	02	04	11	00001011	00101110	046	00001011
04	02	06	18	00010010	01101110	110	00010010
05	03	02	12	00001100	00011011	027	00001100
06	03	05	14	00001110	01001010	073	00001110
07	04	02	11	00001011	00011010	026	00001011
08	04	03	29	00011101	01011011	091	00011101
09	05	01	11	00001011	00010000	016	00001011
10	05	02	15	00001111	00100011	035	00001111
11	05	05	16	00010000	01010101	085	00010000
12	06	03	09	00001001	00100001	033	00001001

The advantage of LAVK based algorithms can be studied from the above table. It is noticed that for similar data, (Row-id. 3, 7 and 9) encrypted information would be different-bit strings, so patterns of original plain text cannot be generated; this adds an addition level of security. The data is encrypted by position of the device; hence, the key would be different for different locations. So, same information would have different ciphers making position based variability in data items. The algorithm is memory efficient $O(p+1) = O(p)$ and takes $O(n)$ time for processing, where p is number of nonzero items.

PARAMETERS ONLY SCHEME FOR AUTOMATIC VARIABLE KEY

So far during the discussions, in the previous sections, we have pointed out about state-of-art cryptographic algorithms that rely on increasing the key size. Thus, it would require more time, computation and battery power. Automatic Variable Key (AVK) has been devised to explore alternative approach. Two methods have been discussed to demonstrate how AVK based cryptosystem can be developed. Both methods use some parameters to construct key. Fibonacci method (for a particular session, with given n and p values computations can be done for f_{n-1}, f_n and f_{n+1}) (Shaligram Prajapat, R.S.Thakur., 2015) and Sparse Matrix (Location co-ordinate (i, j) will act as parameter for encryption /Decryption) based approach can be modeled for automatic variability of key for secure information exchange. For these AVK based cryptosystem, parameters (n, p) or location (i, j) can vary from session to session. So, even if the intruder gets unwanted access to the key of session at time slot t, it would not be valid for original message extraction in session slot at time (t+1) onwards. In this model, since key is not transmitted in the data transfer. So, it becomes highly difficult to interpolate any information regarding plaintext or key. This entire process can be modeled in the form of parameterized-AVK model as Figure 1:

In this model, (shown below) node-1 and node-2 (Can be extended to node-n) are communicating with each other by sharing parameters instead of key exchange. The model also demonstrates that for same parameters different approaches may generate same key. Thus, additional level of security may be achieved by parameterized model. The two approaches for computation of key from parameters have been demonstrated by approach-1 and approach-2.

Figure 1. Parameterized-AVK model

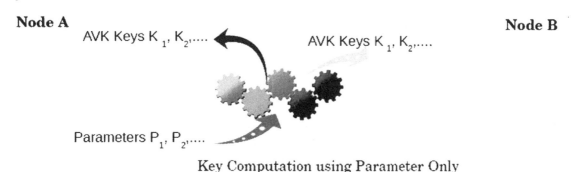

Computing Keys from Geometric Mean

Following algorithm demonstrates working of information exchange based on 'parameters only' scheme:

Algorithm parameters4Key − node − 1$\left(parameters\ p_1,\ p_2 \right)$

{

1.   Sense parameters p_1, p_2;
2.   Compute the key for information exchange by: $key_i = \left(p_1 * p_2 \right)^{1/2}$;
3.   Sense the information to exchange $= D_i$;

4.   If $\left(mode == transmit \right)$ Generate Cipher text $C_i = Encrypt\left(D_i,\ key_i \right)$;
Transmit Ci;

      Receive Plain text $P_i = Decrypt\left(D_i,\ key_i \right)$;

5. else Use P_i;

    }

Computing Keys from Arithmetic and Harmonic Mean

Algorithm Parameters4Key − node − 2 $\left(parameters\ p_1,\ p_2 \right)$

{

1.   *Sense parameters p_1, p_2;*
2.   *Compute the Arithmetic Mean A.M. = $\left(p_{1+}p_2 \right) / 2$;*
3.   *Compute the Harmonic Mean H.M. = $2 * p_1 * p_2 / \left(p_1 + p_2 \right)$*

4.   *Compute the $Key_i = \left(A.M. * H.M \right)^{1/2}$*
5.   *If $\left(mode == transmit \right)$ Generate Cipher text $C_i = Encrypt\left(D_i,\ key_i \right)$; Transmit C_i;*

      Receive Plain text $P_i = Decrypt\left(D_i,\ key_i \right)$;

6.   *else Use P_i;*

    }

The major advantage of approach-1 and approach-2 can be noted here, without exchanging entire key, node-1 and node-2 will securely communicate with each other. Both the nodes are computing the same key using different function, which in turn enhances the level of security.

    Hence, even if the parameters or method at any one node for key computation is known, it will not work for next node or parameter set (Shaligram Prajapat, R.S.Thakur, 2014).

EVALUATION OF CRYPTOSYSTEM: HACKERS / CRYPTANALYST PERSPECTIVE

The strength and weakness of cryptosystem can be evaluated by exploiting them and identifying degree of damage or loss of information. Harder the exploitation of system, weakness will make the cryptosystem more secure. By collecting or recording parameter information in log, noticing availability of captured cipher text, some guessed plaintext may be used by cryptanalyst or hacker for pattern discovery, and guessing the vulnerability of system, will measure the degree of success.

Analyzing Parameter Passing through Queries

Consider log of session information in the form of a database consisting of information about key with corresponding set of parameters, $P = \{ p_1, p_2, p_3, p_4 \}$ and it is possible to submit queries about the composition of key for any key, then a series of request and replies in the following format can be achieved:

$$Request_1 \left(p_1 + p_2 + p_3 \right) \ Reply \ key \ k_1$$
$$Request_2 \left(p_1 + p_2 + + p_4 \right) \ Reply \ key \ k_2$$
$$Request_3 \left(p_1 \quad + p_3 + p_4 \right) \ Reply \ key \ k_3$$
$$Request_4 \left(p_2 + p_3 + p_4 \right) \ Reply \ key \ k_4$$

The augmented matrix of request response set would be:
$$\begin{bmatrix} 1 & 1 & 1 & 0 & key_1 \\ 1 & 1 & 0 & 1 & key_2 \\ 1 & 0 & 1 & 1 & key_3 \\ 0 & 1 & 1 & 1 & key_3 \end{bmatrix}$$

Table 4. Types of patterns needed by cryptanalysis

Input for Cryptic Mining	Information assumed to be available for pattern mining		
	Encryption Algorithm	Cipher text (for decoding)	Addition Requirements
Cipher text only	Yes	Yes	Only patterns from cipher text have to be explored or scanned, due to randomization of ciphers, it is relatively harder, but some information like key size can be interpolated.
Known plaintext	Yes	Yes	Identification of patterns from log of (P, C) pairs, where: P = plain text, C= Cipher text
Chosen plaintext	Yes	Yes	Patterns for CP can be explored i.e. Cipher text chosen by cryptanalyst and corresponding decrypted plain text i.e. (C, p = (C)) and learning from these patterns for future prediction can be attempted.
Chosen text	Yes	Yes	Patterns for training and cross validation are decided by cryptanalyst. Plain text chosen by cryptanalyst corresponding cipher text(PC), Cipher text chosen by cryptanalyst & corresponding decrypted plain text(CP)

Simplification of these four equations values of all the unknowns can be solved, for example:

$$p_1 = \left(key_1 + key_2 + key_3 - 3 * key_4\right)/3$$
$$p_2 = \left(key_1 + key_2 - 2 * key_3 + 2 * key_4\right)/3$$
$$p_3 = \left(key_1 + key_3 + key_4 - 2 * key_{2)}\right)/3$$
$$p_4 = \left(key_2 + key_3 + key_4 - 2 * key_1\right)/3$$

Thus, it is clear that parameters p_1, p_2, p_3, p_4 are known, that are being propagated over the network. Known parameters, known cipher text pairs log can be used to predict future parameters. Hence, several attempts will be made to predict the probable key or plain text.

- **Improvement:** For protecting the system, request must be set small and with zero or minimum overlapping. If requests have no overlapping the database cannot be compromised through the use of simultaneous equations. Following algorithm may be used for solving n equations or n parameters,

$Algorithm\, GEMSAE\left(\; A[\;]\;,\; n,\; X\;\right)$

Begin

for $i = 1$ *to* n *in steps of* 1 *do*

        for $j = 1$ *to* $\left(n + 1\right)$ *in steps of* 1 *do*

                Read A_{ij}

        end for

end for

//Forward elimination with partial pivoting

for $k = 1$ *to* $n - 1$ *in steps of* 1 *do*

$max \leftarrow \left| A_{kk} \right|$

$p \leftarrow k$

for $m = \left(k + 1\right)$ *to* n *in steps of* 1 *do*

        if $\left(\; \left| A_{mk} \right| > \; max \;\right)$ *then*

        $\{ max \leftarrow \left| A_{mk} \right|; \; p \leftarrow m; \}$

end for

$$if \ \Big(\ max \ \leq \ e \Big)$$

$$\Big\{ \ Print \ ``Ill - Conditioned \ matrix" \ ;exit\Big\}$$

$$else \ if \ \Big(p = k\Big)then \ go \ to \ ****$$

$$for \ q = k \ to \ \Big(n+1\Big) \ in \ steps of \ 1 \ do$$

$$\{ \ tmp \leftarrow A_{kq}; \ A_{kq} \leftarrow A_{pq}; \ A_{pq} \leftarrow tmp \ ;\}$$

end for

$$for \ m \ = \ \Big(k+1\Big) \ to \ n$$

$$*** \quad for \ i = \Big(k+1\Big) \ to \ n \ in \ steps of \ 1 \ do$$

$$u \leftarrow A_{ik} \ / \ A_{kk}$$

$$for \ j = \ k \ to \ \Big(n+1\Big) \ in \ steps of \ 1 \ do$$

$$A_{ij} \leftarrow A_{ij} \ - u * A_{kj}$$

end for

endfor

endfor

// Back Substitution

$$X_n \leftarrow A_{n(n+1)} \ / \ A_{ii};$$

$$for \ i = \Big(n-1\Big) \ to \ 1 \ in \ steps \ of \ -1 \ do$$

$$sum \leftarrow 0;$$

$$for \ j = \Big(\ i+1\Big) \ to \ n \ in \ steps \ of \ 1 \ do$$

$$sum \leftarrow sum \ + \ A_{ij} * X_j$$

end for

$$X_i \leftarrow \Big(\ A_{i(n+1)} - sum \ \Big) / A_{ii}$$

end for

End

GEMSAE receives linear equations $A \, x \ = \ b$ and converts it into upper triangular system $U \ x \ = \ b'$. The matrix 'U' occupies upper triangular element positions of A. The algorithm ensures that $A_{kk} = 0$.

- **Complexity Analysis:** For k from 0 to n-1, GEMSAE systematically eliminates variable $X[k]$ from equations (k+1) to n-1, so that coefficient matrix becomes upper triangular. In k^{th} iteration, an appropriate multiple is subtracted from each of equation k+1 to n-1.The multiple of kth equation is selected in such a manner that the kth coefficient becomes zero from k+1 to n, eliminating X_k from these equations.

- **Computations:** Assume that each scalar arithmetic takes a unit time. The kth iteration of the outer loop does not involve any computation on rows 1 to k-1; or columns 1 to k-1.So, only lower right F_{n-1}, F_n and F_{n+1} $((n-k)*(n-k)$ sub matrix of A will be computationally active. GEMSAE involves approx. $n^2/2$ divisions and approx. $\left[(n^3/3) - (n^2/2)\right]$ subtractions and multiplications. For large n, sequential run time of the GEMSAE is approx. $2n^3/3$..So, sequential complexity $T(n) = O(n^3)$.

CONCLUSION

This chapter highlights the significance of key, key size, life time of key and breaking threshold with suitable examples. These characteristics are essential in the design of every symmetric key cryptosystem. Both key length, key life time play a crucial role in security of cryptosystems. The obvious way of enhancing security of any cryptosystem is to keep the key as large as possible which may be suitable for low power devices. AVK scheme is in development phase, and various models are being evolved and suggested with fixed size dynamic keys empowered by 'parameters only' approach. Various parameterized security models without key exchange among communicating entities has been discussed with their merits and demerits. These schemes have been discussed in the light of exploiting patterns of ciphers, parameters and log of session wise captured information. This chapter also paves way for application of mining algorithms in cryptographic domain.

FUTURE RESEARCH DIRECTIONS

The choice of key length must be from 4 to 6 characters for optimum size with respect to time and power issue. Larger size of AVK would not be significant, and shorter key length would compromise the strength of cryptosystem. Performance analysis of AVK approach with state of art methods needs to be analyzed carefully. Choosing key as Fibonacci Q matrix may have several issues, such as, over what range of n and p cryptosystem will give optimum performance, beyond which it may have slow performance and easy guessing issues. From security point of view, it would be better to have matrix elements of 4 to 6 digits that is minimum 32 bit to maximum key size of 48 bits. The Sparse approach for AVK can be extended for three and higher dimensions. For cipher generation of any input size, encryption of plaintext or decryption of cipher text can be explored with various nonlinear curves and can be compared for efficiency with LAVKencrypt() and LAVKdecrypt(). Any cryptosystem which is working properly for encryption and decryption task always needs to be passed through proper screen-test from hackers or intruder's perspective to rectify against weaknesses. So, for how long it fights against brute force attack and AI based tests? It needs to be investigated. It is assumed that output of encryption process is always random, free from patterns. But, in reality this is not the case. Patterns may be discovered, attempts can be made based on: cipher classification and similarity. Ciphers may be arranged into clusters based upon key size, plaintext-cipher text correlations, association rule base can be formulated for predictions based on frequent patterns. So, metric to describe efficiency of cryptosystem w.r.t. systematic attack has to be tested also from these AI based tests.

REFERENCES

Nadeem, A., & Javed, M. Y. (2005, Aug). A Performance comparison of data encryption algorithms. *IEEE-International Conference of Information and Communication Technologies*. doi:10.1109/ICICT.2005.1598556

Schneier. (1996). *Applied cryptography: Protocols, Algorithms, and Source Code in C*. Wiley.

Elminaam, Kader, & Hadhoud. (2008). Performance Evaluation of Symmetric Encryption Algorithms. *International Journal of Computer Science and Network Security, 8*(12), 280–286.

Sutherland et al. (2010). *Cracking Codes and Cryptograms for Dummies*. Wiley.

Hellman. (2002). An Overview of Public Key Cryptography. IEEE Communication Magazine, 16(6), 24-32.

Chakrabarti, P., Bhuyan, B., Chowdhuri, A., & Bhunia, C. (2008). A novel approach towards realizing optimum data transfer and Automatic Variable Key (AVK) in cryptography. IJCSNS, 8(5), 241-250.

Prajapat, S., & Thakur. (2015a). Optimal Key Size of the AVK for Symmetric Key Encryption. *Covenant Journal of Information & Communication Technology, 71*.

Prajapat, S., & Thakur. (2015b). Various Approaches towards Crypt-analysis. *International Journal of Computer Applications, 127*(14), 15-24.

Prajapat, S., & Thakur, R. S. (2016a). Cryptic Mining for Automatic Variable Key Based Cryptosystem. *Elsevier Procedia Computer Science*, 78(78C), 199–209. doi:10.1016/j.procs.2016.02.034

Prajapat, S., & Thakur. (2016b). Realization of information exchange with Fibo-Q based Symmetric Cryptosystem. *International Journal of Computer Science and Information Security*.

Prajapat, S., & Thakur. (2016c). Cryptic Mining: Apriori Analysis of Parameterized Automatic Variable Key based Symmetric Cryptosystem. *International Journal of Computer Science and Information Security*.

Chakrabarti. (2007). Application of Automatic Variable Key (AVK) in RSA. *International Journal HIT Transactions on ECCN, 2*(5), 301-305.

Chakraborty, Mondal, Chaudhuri, & Bhunia. (2006). Various new and modified approaches for selective encryption (DES, RSA and AES) with AVK and their comparative study. International Journal HIT Transaction on ECCN, 1(4), 236-244.

Prajapat, Parmar, & Thakur. (2015). Investigation of Efficient Cryptosystem Using SGcrypter. *IJAER*, 853-858.

Prajapat et al. (2012). A Novel Approach For Information Security With Automatic Variable Key Using Fibonacci Q-Matrix. *International Journal of Computer & Communication Technology, 3*(3).

Prajapat, Rajput, & Thakur. (2013, Oct). Time variant approach towards Symmetric Key. *IEEE- Science and Information Conference 2013.*

Prajapat, & Thakur. (2014a, Mar). Time variant key using exact differential equation model. *National Conference in Emerging Trends in cloud Computing and Digital Communication* (ETCDC-2014).

Prajapat, & Thakur. (2014b, Jun). *Sparse approach for realizing AVK for Symmetric Key Encryption.* Presented on second days, International Research Conference on Engineering, Science and Management (IRCESM 2014), Dubai, UAE.

Prajapat, & Thakur. (2014c, Oct). *Time variant key using Fuzzy differential equation model.* Oriental Bhopal, India.

Prajapat, & Thakur. (2015a). Towards Optimum size of key for AVK based cryptosystem. Covenant Journal of Informatics and Communication Technology, 3(2).

Prajapat, & Thakur. (2013, Sep). *Recurrence relation approach for key prediction.* 18th International Conference of Gwalior Academy of Mathematical Science (GAMS), MANIT, Bhopal, India.

Prajapat, Swami, Singroli, Thakur, Sharma, & Rajput. (2014). Sparse approach for realizing AVK for Symmetric Key Encryption. *International Journal of Recent Development in Engineering and Technology, 2*(4), 13-18.

Prajapat, & Thakur. (2015b, Jun). Markov Analysis of AVK Approach of Symmetric Key Based Cryptosystem. *LNCS, 9159,* 164-176.

Prajapat, & Thakur. (2014d, Oct). Association Rule Extraction in AVK based cryptosystem. *International Conferences on Intelligent Computing and Information System* (ICICIS-2014).

Ross. (2010). Introduction to Probability models (10th ed.). Academic Press.

Stakhov, A. P. (2006). Fibonacci matrices, a generalization of the 'Cassini formula', and a new coding theory. Chaos, Solutions & Fractals, 30(1), 56–66.

Chapter 5
Innovative Approach for Improving Intrusion Detection Using Genetic Algorithm with Layered Approach

Aditi Nema
BIRT, India

ABSTRACT

The detection portion of Intrusion Detection System is the most complicated. The IDS goal is to make the network more secure, and the prevention portion of the IDS must accomplish that effort. After malicious or unwanted traffic is identified, using prevention techniques can stop it. When an IDS is placed in an inline configuration, all traffic must travel through an IDS sensor. In this paper the reduced the features and perform layered architecture for identify various attack (DoS, R2L, U2R, Probe) and show accuracy using SVM with genetic approach.

INTRODUCTION

Intrusion detection systems are the 'burglar alarms' (or rather 'intrusion alarms') of the computer security field. The aim is to defend a system by using a combination of an alarm that sounds whenever the site's security has been compromised, and an entity—most often a site security officer (SSO)—that can respond to the alarm and take the appropriate action, for instance by ousting the intruder, calling on the proper external authorities, and so on. This method should be contrasted with those that aim to strengthen the perimeter surrounding the computer system. We believe that both of these methods should be used, along with others, to increase the chances of mounting a successful defence, relying on the age-old principle of defence in depth.

It should be noted that the intrusion can be one of a number of different types. For example, a user might steal a password and hence the means by which to prove his identity to the computer. We call such a user a masquerader, and the detection of such intruders is an important problem for the field.

DOI: 10.4018/978-1-5225-0536-5.ch005

Other important classes of intruders are people who are legitimate users of the system but who abuse their privileges, and people who use pre-packed exploit scripts, often found on the Internet, to attack the system through a network. This is by no means an exhaustive list, and the classification of threats to computer installations is an active area of research.

Early in the research into such systems two major principles known as anomaly detection and signature detection were arrived at, the former relying on flagging all behavior that is abnormal for an entity, the latter flagging behavior that is close to some previously defined pattern signature of a known intrusion. The problems with the first approach rest in the fact that it does not necessarily detect undesirable behavior, and that the false alarm rates can be high. The problems with the latter approach include its reliance on a well defined security policy, which may be absent, and its inability to detect intrusions that have not yet been made known to the intrusion detection system. It should be noted that to try to bring more stringency to these terms, we use them in a slightly different fashion than previous researchers in the field.

An intrusion detection system consists of an audit data collection agent that collects information about the system being observed. This data is then either stored or processed directly by the detector proper, the output of which is presented to the SSO, who then can take further action, normally beginning with further investigation into the causes of the alarm.

Intrusion detection systems (IDSs) are software or hardware systems that automate the process of monitoring the events occurring in a computer system or network, analyzing them for signs of security problems. As network attacks have increased in number and severity over the past few years, intrusion detection systems have become a necessary addition to the security infrastructure of most organizations. Although firewalls have traditionally been seen, as the "first line of defense" against would be attackers, intrusion detection software is rapidly gaining ground as a novel but effective approach to making your networks more secure. Intrusion detection operates on the principle that any attempt to penetrate your systems can be detected and the operator alerted - rather than actually stopping them. This is based on the assumption that it is virtually impossible to close every potential security; intrusion detection takes a very "real world" viewpoint, emphasizing instead the need to identify attempts at breaking in and to assess the damage they have caused.

Intrusion detection involves determining that some entity, an intruder, has attempted to gain, or worse, has gained unauthorized access to the system.

Intruders are classified into two groups:

- External intruders do not have any authorized access to the system they attack.
- Internal intruders have at least some authorized access to the system. Internal intruders are further subdivided into the following three categories.

Masqueraders are external intruders who have succeeded in gaining access to the system and are acting as an authorized entity.

Legitimate intruders have access to both the system and the data but misuse this access (misfeasors).

Clandestine intruders have or have obtained supervisory (root) control of the system and as such can either operate below the level of auditing or can use the privileges to avoid being audited by stopping, modifying, or erasing the audit records [Anderson80]

Evolution of Intrusion Detection

Intrusion detection has been an active field of research for about two decades, starting in 1980 with the publication of John Anderson's(Anderson,1980) and then improved by D. Denning (Denning 1987). Computer Security Threat Monitoring and Surveillance, which was one of the earliest papers in the field. Dorothy Denning's seminal paper, "An Intrusion Detection Model," published in 1987, provided a methodological Framework that inspired many researchers. The intruder identify through the intrusion detection system (IDS), the description of IDS is given below-

INTRUSION DETECTION SYSTEMS (IDS)

An IDS is a computer security system which detects misuse, attacks against, or compromise of computers connected to a network. They operate by passively examining network packets as they travel over the wire and alerting administrators when they see something unusual or malicious. IDS monitors packets on the network wire and attempts to discover if a hacker/cracker is attempting to break into a system (or cause a denial of service attack). A typical example is a system that watches for large number of TCP connection requests (SYN) to many different ports on a target machine, thus discovering if someone is attempting a TCP port scan. Before getting started with describing trends in the IDS design, it should be noted that IDS has a classifier kernel. The kernel of the IDS is responsible for classifying the acquired features into two groups namely normal and anomaly, where the anomaly pattern is likely to be an attack. Nevertheless, there are occasions where a legitimate use of the network resources may lead to a positive classification result for the anomaly or signature based intrusion detection. As a result of this wrong classification, IDS will wrongly raise the alarm and will signal an attack. This is a common problem with the IDS and is called False Positive (FP). One of the parameters to measure the quality of IDS is the number of its FP alarms. The smaller is the number of false positives, the better is the IDS.

IDS TECHNOLOGIES

IDS Technology is defined in various ways, on the basis of network type and their behavior, that are as follows:

- **Network-Based:** A Network Intrusion Detection System (NIDS) is one common type of IDS that analyzes network traffic at all layers of the Open Systems Interconnection (OSI) model and makes decisions about the purpose of the traffic, analyzing for suspicious activity. Most NIDSs are easy to deploy on a network and can often view traffic from many systems at once. A term becoming more widely used by vendors is "Wireless Intrusion Prevention System" (WIPS) to describe a network device that monitors and analyzes the wireless radio spectrum in a network for intrusions and performs countermeasures.
- **Wireless:** A wireless local area network (WLAN) IDS is similar to NIDS in that it can analyze network traffic. However, it will also analyze wireless-specific traffic, including scanning for external users trying to connect to access points (AP), rogue APs, users outside the physical area of the company, and WLAN IDSs built into APs. As networks increasingly support wireless technol-

ogies at various points of a topology, WLAN IDS will play larger roles in security. Many previous NIDS tools will include enhancements to support wireless traffic analysis.

- **Network Behavior Anomaly Detection:** Network behavior anomaly detection (NBAD) views traffic on network segments to determine if anomalies exist in the amount or type of traffic. Segments that usually see very little traffic or segments that see only a particular type of traffic may transform the amount or type of traffic if an unwanted event occurs. NBAD requires several sensors to create a good snapshot of a network and requires benchmarking and base lining to determine the nominal amount of a segment's traffic.
- **Host-Based**: Host-based intrusion detection systems (HIDS) analyze network traffic and system-specific settings such as software calls, local security policy, local log audits, and more. A HIDS must be installed on each machine and requires configuration specific to that operating system and software.

IDS MODELS

Classification of IDS essentially falls under two models:

1. Misuse or signature-based model
2. Anomaly based model

Misuse or Signature-Based Model

The misuse or signature-based is the most-used IDS model. Signatures are patterns that identify attacks by checking various options in the packet, like source address, destination address, source and destination ports, flags, payload and other options. The collection of these signatures composes a knowledge base that is used by the IDS to compare all packet options that pass by and check if they match a known pattern. Misuse detectors analyze system activity, looking for events or sets of events that match a predefined pattern of events that describe a known attack. As the patterns corresponding to known attacks are called signatures, misuse detection is sometimes called "signature-based detection." The most common form of misuse detection used in commercial products specifies each pattern of events corresponding to an attack as a separate signature. However, there are more sophisticated approaches to doing misuse detection (called "state-based" analysis techniques) that can leverage a single signature to detect groups of attacks.

Figure 1. Misuse detection system

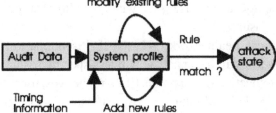

A typical misuse detection system

Advantages

Misuse detectors are very effective at detecting attacks without generating an overwhelming number of false alarms.

Misuse detectors can quickly and reliably diagnose the use of a specific attack tool or technique. This can help security managers prioritize corrective measures.

Misuse detectors can allow system managers, regardless of their level of security expertise, to track security problems on their systems, initiating incident handling procedures.

Disadvantages

Misuse detectors can only detect those attacks they know about –therefore they must be constantly updated with signatures of new attacks.

Many misuse detectors are designed to use tightly defined signatures that prevent them from detecting variants of common attacks. State-based misuse detectors can overcome this limitation, but are not commonly used in commercial IDS.

Anomaly Based Model

The anomaly based model tries to identify new attacks by analyzing strange behaviors in the network. It learn how the traffic in the network works and later try to identify different patterns to then send some kind of alert to the sensor or console. IDS made using this model have higher tendency for raising false alarm, as they often suspicious about all network behavior irrespective of malicious or legitimate. Anomaly detectors identify abnormal unusual behavior (anomalies) on a host or network. They function on the assumption that attacks are different from "normal" (legitimate) activity and can therefore be detected by systems that identify these differences. Anomaly detectors construct profiles representing normal behavior of users, hosts, or network connections. These profiles are constructed from historical data collected over a period of normal operation. The detectors then collect event data and use a variety of measures to determine when monitored activity deviates from the normal.

The measures and techniques used in anomaly detection include:

Threshold detection, Statistical measures, Rule-based measures

Figure 2. Anomaly detection system

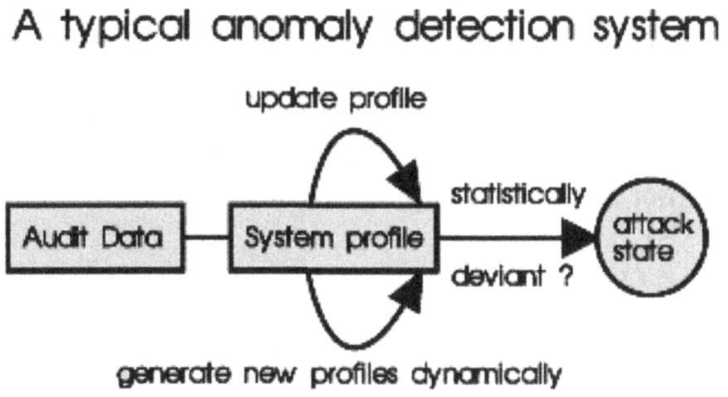

Advantages

IDSs based on anomaly detection detect unusual behavior and thus have the ability to detect symptoms of attacks without specific knowledge of details.

Anomaly detectors can produce information that can in turn be used to define signatures for misuse detectors.

Disadvantages

Anomaly detection approaches usually produce a large number of false alarms due to the unpredictable behaviors of users and networks.

Anomaly detection approaches often require extensive "training sets" of system event records in order to characterize normal behavior patterns.

Audit Records

A fundamental tool for intrusion detection is the audit record. Some record of ongoing activity by users must be maintained as input to an intrusion detection system. Basically, two plans are used:

1. **Native Audit Records:** Virtually all multiuser operating systems include accounting software that collects information on user activity. The advantage of using this information is that no additional collection software is needed. The disadvantage is that the native audit records may not contain the needed information or may not contain it in a convenient form.
2. **Detection-Specific Audit Records:** A collection facility can be implemented that generates audit records containing only that information required by the intrusion detection system. One advantage of such an approach is that it could be made vendor independent and ported to a variety of systems. The disadvantage is the extra overhead involved in having, in effect, two accounting packages running on a machine.

Comparison with Firewalls

Though they both relate to network security, an intrusion detection system (IDS) differs from a firewall in that a firewall looks outwardly for intrusions in order to stop them from happening. Firewalls limit access between networks to prevent intrusion and do not signal an attack from inside the network. An IDS evaluates a suspected intrusion once it has taken place and signals an alarm. An IDS also watches for attacks that originate from within a system. This is traditionally achieved by examining network communications, identifying heuristics and patterns (often known as signatures) of common computer attacks, and taking action to alert operators. A system that terminates connections is called an intrusion prevention system, and is another form of an application layer firewall.

KDD DATASET

The KDD 99[5] Intrusion detection datasets are based on the 1998 DARPA initiative to provide designers of intrusion detection systems (IDS) with a benchmark on which to evaluate different methodologies. That is used to spoof different IP addresses, thus generating traffic between different IP addresses. Finally, there is a sniffer that records all network traffic using the TCP dump format. This was processed into about five million connection records. The data set contains a total of 24 attack types (connections) that fall into 4 major categories: Denial of service (DoS), Probe, User to Root (U2R), Remote to User (R2L). Each record is labeled either as normal, or as an attack, with exactly one specific attack type [2].

1. **Denial of Service (DoS):** Attacker tries to prevent legitimate users from using a service. These attacks are probably the nastiest, most difficult to address and most horrible, because they are very easy to launch, difficult (sometimes impossible) to track, and it is not easy to refuse the requests of the attacker.
2. **Remote to Local (R2L):** Attacker does not have an account on the victim machine, hence tries to gain access. The goal of these attacks is to access some resources that machine should not provide the attacker. Host should provide command shell access without being sure that the person making such a request is someone who should get it, such as a local administrator.
3. **User to Root (U2R):** It is obviously undesirable for an unknown person to be able to execute commands on your server machines. Attacker has local access to the victim machine and tries to gain superuser privileges.
4. **Probe:** Attacker tries to gain information about the target host. An attacker might wish to make configuration changes to host perhaps changing its IP address, putting a start-up script in place to cause the machine. In this case, the attacker will need to gain administrator's privileges on the host.
5. **Knowledge Discovery in Databases (KDD):** The process of identifying these valid, novel, potentially useful, and ultimately understandable patterns in data We consider a pattern as the relationship between two variables that could be linear or not-linear. In our case these variables are called features because they are characteristics for a given concept. A possible definition of knowledge concerns the information from multiple domains that has been synthesized, through inference or deduction, into meaning or understanding that was not previously known. Knowledge is derived from information but is richer and more meaningful than information. In fact, it includes familiarity, awareness and understanding gained through experience or study, and results from making comparisons, identifying consequences, and making connections.

NSL KDD Dataset

NSL KDD is a data set suggested to solve some of the inherent problems of the KDD'99 data set. The number of records in the NSL-KDD train and test sets are reasonable. This advantage makes it affordable to run the experiments on the complete set without the need to randomly select a small portion. Consequently, evaluation results of different research work will be consistent and comparable.

The NSL KDD data set has the following advantages over the original KDD data set:-

It does not include redundant records in the train set, so the classifiers will not be biased towards more frequent records.

There are no duplicate records in the proposed test sets; therefore, the performance of the learners is not biased by the methods which have better detection rates on the frequent records.

The number of selected records from each difficulty level group is inversely proportional to the percentage of records in the original KDD data set. As a result, the classification rates of distinct machine learning methods vary in a wider range, which makes it more efficient to have an accurate evaluation of different learning techniques.

The numbers of records in the train and test sets are reasonable, which makes it affordable to run the experiments on the complete set without the need to randomly select a small portion. Consequently, evaluation results of different research works will be consistent and comparable.

In this context, the term Data Mining (Lee & Stolfo, 2000) is somewhat overloaded. It sometimes refers to the whole process of knowledge discovery, sometimes to the specific Machine Learning phase. We adopt the first perspective for which a possible definition of Data Mining relies to the extraction of implicit, previously unknown, and potentially useful knowledge from data. Knowledge, if found, must be meaningful in that it leads to some advantage, usually an economic one. In fact, it could be generalized to make accurate predictions on future data. Moreover, problems increase when the dimensionality of the considered data is relevant. The search of patterns in databases, which are collections of data with dozens of features, is in fact a complex activity because the presence of redundant, noisy or not correlated information's that can badly affect the extraction of the correct knowledge from the data.

The number of feature is thus a critical aspect in discovering knowledge and tries to reapply it on unseen examples, because not all the dataset's features are really informative. This parameter influences therefore both the accuracy and the speed of the classification algorithms. Thus, to adopt techniques to reduce the number of features involved in the mining algorithm we can use Feature Selection (FS), also known as subset selection or variable selection, which is a common preprocessing step(Blum & Langley,1997)(Liu &Motoda,2001) used in Machine Learning. In some cases, accuracy on future classification can be improved; in others, the result is a more compact, easily interpretable representation of the target concept.

False Positives and Negatives

The impossible for IDS to be perfect, primarily because network traffic is so complicated. The erroneous results in IDS are divided into two types: false positives and false negatives.

False positives occur when the IDS erroneously detects a problem with traffic. False negatives occur when unwanted traffic is undetected by the IDS. Both create problems for security administrators and may require that the system be calibrated. A greater number of false positives are generally more acceptable but can burden a security administrator with some amounts of data. However, because it is undetected, false negatives do not afford a security administrator an opportunity to review the data.

A NIDS can detect many types of events, from benign to malicious. Reconnaissance events alone are not dangerous, but can lead to dangerous attacks. Reconnaissance events can originate at the TCP layer, such as a port scan. Running services have open ports to allow legitimate connections. During a port scan, an attacker tries to open connections on every port of a server to determine which services are running. Reconnaissance attacks also include opening connections of known applications, such as Web servers, to gather information about the server's OS and version. NIDS can also detect attacks at the network, transport, or application layers. These attacks include malicious code that could be used for denial of service (DoS) attacks and for theft of information. Lastly, NIDS can be used to detect less dangerous but nonetheless unwanted traffic, such as unexpected services (i.e., backdoors) and policy violations and calculating these following parameters-

Accuracy

The accuracy of a measurement system is the degree of closeness of measurements of a quantity to that quantity's actual (true) value.

$$\text{Accuracy} = \frac{\text{Number of true positives} + \text{Number of true negatives}}{\text{true positives} + \text{false positives} + \text{false negatives} + \text{true negatives}} \quad (1)$$

Precision

The precision of a measurement system, also called reproducibility or repeatability, is the degree to which repeated measurements under unchanged conditions show the same results

$$\text{Precision} = \frac{\text{Number of true positives}}{\text{Number of true positives} + \text{false positives}} \quad (2)$$

Recall

Recall is the probability that a (randomly selected) relevant document is retrieved in a search. Note that the random selection refers to a uniform distribution over the appropriate pool of documents; i.e. by randomly selected retrieved document, we mean selecting a document from the set of retrieved documents in a random fashion.

The random selection should be such that all documents in the set are equally likely to be selected.

$$\text{Recall} = \frac{\text{True positives}}{\text{true positives} + \text{false negatives}} \quad (3)$$

F-Measure

The F-measure was derived by van Rijsbergen (1979) so that "measures the effectiveness of retrieval with respect to a user who attaches β times as much importance to recall as precision

$$F^2 = \frac{\left(1 + \beta^2\right)\left(\text{precision.recall}\right)}{\beta^2.\text{precision} + \text{recall}} \quad (4)$$

Confusion Matrix

Confusion matrix is a specific table that allows visualization of the performance of an algorithm, typically a supervised learning one (in unsupervised learning it is usually called a matching matrix). Each column of the matrix represents the instances in a predicted class, while each row represents the instances in an actual class. In predictive analytics, a table of confusion (sometimes also called a confusion matrix), is a table with two rows and two columns that reports the number of false positives, false negatives, true positives, and true negatives. This allows more detailed analysis than mere proportion of correct guesses (accuracy). Accuracy is not a reliable metric for the real performance of a classifier, because it will yield misleading results if the data set is unbalanced (that is, when the number of samples in different classes vary greatly.

Support Vector Machine

Support vector machines (SVM) (Hui,Hong &Xin,2003) were first suggested by Vapnik (1995) and have recently been used in a range of problems including pattern recognition (Pontil and Verri, 1998), bioinformatics (Yu, Ostrouchov, Geist, & Samatova, 1999), and text categorization (Joachims, 1998). SVM classifies data with different class labels by determining a set of support vectors that are members of the set of training inputs that outline a hyper-plane in the feature space. SVM provides a generic mechanism that fits the hyper-plane surface to the training data using a kernel function. The user may select a kernel function (e.g. linear, polynomial, or sigmoid) for the SVM during the training process that selects support vectors along the surface of this function.

Extensions of the SVM concept have been made by several authors, for example Mangasarian's generalized SVMs. Particularly interesting is the development of a system, called the Bayes Point Machine that enforces another inductive principle given by Bayesian generalization theory. More recently, a number of practical applications of SVMs have been reported, in fields as diverse as bioinformatics, computational linguistics and computer vision. Intrusion detection is essentially a pattern recognition and classification problem. It is used to distinguish the normal data from the abnormal through detection. SVM is a new method for designing classifier based on small sample learning applied over small sample data.

Layered Approach

In layered model three layers used for detecting DOS, probe, R2L and U2R attacks. Each layer is separately trained with a small set of relevant features and then deployed sequentially. However some researchers have proposed four layer models to detect each type of attack separately (Gupta &Nath, 2010). The layered model is reducing computation and time required to detect anomalous events. The time required to detect an intruder is significant and can be reduced burden for communication over the different layer. This can be achieved by making the layers autonomous and self-sufficient to block an attack without the need of a central decision-maker. This approach includes Probe layer, DOS layer, R2L layer, and U2R layer. Each layer has separately set of feature for filter of intruder and selects a small set of features for rather than using all the 41 features. The performance layered CRFs (Gupta & Nath, 2007), is comparable to that of the decision trees and the naive Bayes and layer system has higher attack detection accuracy. Layered model is used for reduce computation and the overall time required to detect anomalous events.

Genetic Algorithm

Genetic Algorithm (GA) is one of meta-heuristic optimization techniques, which include simulated annealing, tabu search, and evolutionary strategies. These are applied to function optimization problems. Genetic algorithm will be able to create a high quality solution and use the principles of selection and evolution to produce several solutions to a given problem. It is used recently to support intrusion detection systems, by creating new rule from available rules. The functioning of a GA can be described by using specific data structure and by defining the set of genetic operators and the reproduction procedure Genetic algorithm used by Researchers for explore the use of GAs in intrusion detection, and reported very high success rates, but on data sets other than the KDD 99 Cup, such as the DARPA data set. In this research designed a GA that generates a set of rules, wherein each rule is generated to classify every attack type in the training and testing data set.

GA has been demonstrated to converge to the optimal solution for many diverse and difficult problems as a powerful and stochastic tool based on principles of natural evolution (Eiben & Smith, 2001). The details of our implementation of GA are described as Follows: The first step in GAs is to define the encoding allowing describing any potential solution as a numerical vector, and then we can generate a population randomly.

The briefly describe some concept and operation in GA:

- **Selection Operator:** The selection process selects individuals from population directly based on fitness values (Eiben & Smith, 2001).
- **Recombination:** The role of the crossover operation is to create new individuals from old ones. Crossover often is a probabilistic process that exchanges information between some (usually two) parent individuals in order to generating some new child individual.
- **Mutation Operator:** Mutation is applied to one individual and produces a modified mutant child.
- **Fitness Function:** The role of the Fitness function is to measure the quality of solutions.

Fitness Function

GAs mimics the survival-of-the-fittest principle of nature to make a search process. Therefore, GAs is naturally suitable for solving maximization problems. Maximization problems are usually transformed into minimization problem by suitable transformation. In general, a fitness function F(i) is first derived from the objective function and used in successive genetic operations. Fitness in biological sense is a quality value which is a measure of the reproductive efficiency of chromosomes. In genetic algorithm, fitness is used to allocate reproductive traits to the individuals in the population and thus act as some measure of goodness to be maximized. This means that individuals with higher fitness value will have higher probability of being selected as candidates for further examination. Certain genetic operators require that the fitness function be non-negative, although certain operators need not have this requirement. For maximization problems, the fitness function can be considered to be the same as the objective function or F(i)=o(i). For minimization problems, to generate non-negative values in all the cases and to reflect the relative fitness of individual string, it is necessary to map the underlying natural objective function to fitness function form.

GA Operators

The operation of GAs begins with a population of random strings representing design or decision variables. The population is then operated by three main operators; reproduction, crossover and mutation to create a new population of points. GAs can be viewed as trying to maximize the fitness function, by evaluating several solution vectors. The purpose of these operators is to create new solution vectors by selection, combination or alteration of the current solution vectors that have shown to be good temporary solutions. The new population is further evaluated and tested till termination. If the termination criterion is not met, the population is iteratively operated by the above three operators and evaluated. This procedure is continued until the termination criterion is met.

Reproduction

Reproduction (or selection) is an operator that makes more copies of better strings in a new population. Reproduction is usually the first operator applied on a population. Reproduction selects good strings in a population and forms a mating pool. This is one of the reasons for the reproduction operation to be sometimes known as the selection operator. Thus, in reproduction operation the process of natural selection causes those individuals that encode successful structures to produce copies more frequently. To sustain the generation of a new population, the reproduction of the individuals in the current population is necessary. For better individuals, these should be from the fittest individuals of the previous population. There exist a number of reproduction operators in GA literature, but the essential idea in all of them is that the above average strings are picked from the current population and their multiple copies are inserted in the mating pool in a probabilistic manner.

Crossover

A crossover operator is used to recombine two strings to get a better string. In crossover operation, recombination process creates different individuals in the successive generations by combining material from two individuals of the previous generation. In reproduction, good strings in a population are probabilistic-ally assigned a larger number of copies and a mating pool is formed. It is important to note that no new strings are formed in the reproduction phase. In the crossover operator, new strings are created by exchanging information among strings of the mating pool. A crossover operator is mainly responsible for the search of new strings.

Many crossover operators exist in the GA literature. One site crossover and two site crossover are the most common ones adopted. In most crossover operators, two strings are picked from the mating pool at random and some portions of the strings are exchanged between the strings. Crossover operation is done at string level by randomly selecting two strings for crossover operations. A one site crossover operator is performed by randomly choosing a crossing site along the string and by exchanging all bits on the right side of the crossing site as shown in Figure 3.

In one site crossover, a crossover site is selected randomly (shown as vertical lines). The portion right of the selected site of these two strings is exchanged to form a new pair of strings. The new strings are thus a combination of the old strings. Two site crossovers is a variation of the one site crossover, except that two crossover sites are chosen and the bits between the sites are exchanged as shown in Figure 4.

Figure 3. One site crossover operation

String 1 | 011|01100
String 2 | 110|11001

011|11001
011|01100

Before crossover   After crossover

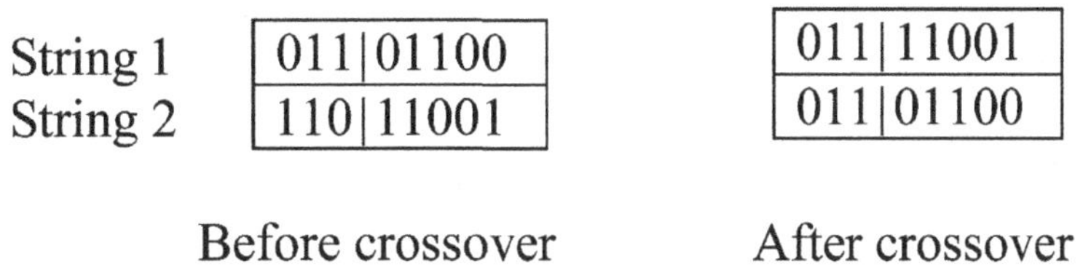

Figure 4. Two site crossover operation

String 1 | 011 |011| 00
String 2 | 110 |110| 01

011 |110| 00
011 |011| 01

Before crossover   After crossover

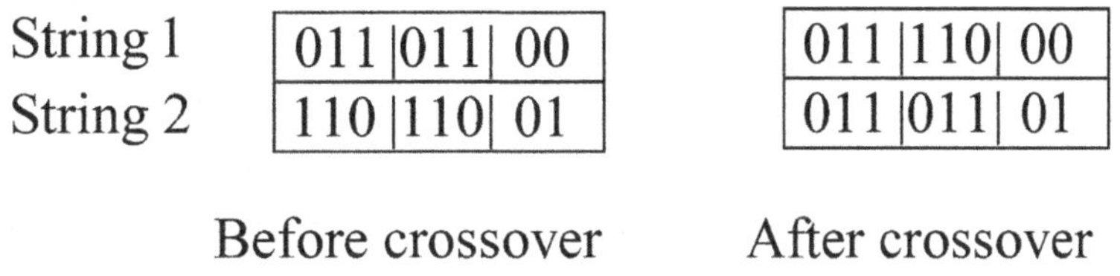

One site crossover is more suitable when string length is small while two site crossovers are suitable for large strings. Hence the present work adopts a two site crossover. The underlying objective of crossover is to exchange information between strings to get a string that is possibly better than the parents.

Mutation

Mutation adds new information in a random way to the genetic search process and ultimately helps to avoid getting trapped at local optima. It is an operator that introduces diversity in the population whenever the population tends to become homogeneous due to repeated use of reproduction and crossover operators. Mutation may cause the chromosomes of individuals to be different from those of their parent individuals.

Classification Rules

Classification rules are an alternative to decision trees used for representing knowledge. This rule are discovered from the training examples and then reapplied in case of unseen example classification to assign the class value at the new instances. Thus, they are "learned" from the knowledge inside the known data.

Classification rules present a certain structure composite of an antecedent and a consequent: The antecedent, or precondition, of a rule is a series of tests just like the tests at nodes in decision trees, and the consequent (or conclusion) gives the class or classes that apply to instances covered by that rule, or perhaps gives a probability distribution over the classes. An example of classification rules is providing just below:-

If Humidity== 40% and Temperature == 20C then Play = yes

If Humidity== 90% and Temperature == 40C then Play = no

Generally, the preconditions are logically and all the tests must succeed if the rule is to fire. However, in some rule formulations the preconditions are general logical expressions rather than simple conjunctions. We often think of the individual rules as being effectively logically or-end together: if anyone applies, the class (or probability distribution) given in its conclusion is applied to the instance.

It is easy to read a set of rules directly off a decision tree. The produced rules are unambiguous in that the order in which they are executed is irrelevant. However, rules that are read directly off a decision tree are far more complex than necessary, and rules derived from trees are usually pruned to remove redundant tests.

One reason why rules are popular is that each rule seems to represent an independent "nugget" of knowledge. New rules can be added to an existing rule set without problems, whereas to add to a tree structure may require reshaping the whole tree. However, this independence is something of an illusion, because it ignores the question of how the rule set is executed. In fact, if rules are meant to be interpreted in order, some of them, taken individually and out of context, may be incorrect. On the other hand, if the order of interpretation is supposed to be casual, then it is not clear what to do when different rules lead to different conclusions for the same instance. This situation cannot arise for rules that are read directly of a decision tree because the redundancy included in the structure of the rules prevents any ambiguity in interpretation.

A different problem occurs when an instance is encountered that the rules fail to classify at all. Again, this cannot occur with decision trees, or with rules read directly off them, but it can easily happen with general rule sets. Individual rules are simple, and sets of rules seem deceptively simple, but given just a set of rules with no additional information, it is not clear how it should be x interpreted (P. Langley, 1994).

Machine learning algorithms that generate rules invariably produce ordered rule sets in multi-class situations, and this sacrifices any possibility of modularity because the order of execution is critical. Thus, we have chosen not to apply this approach for the testing of our algorithm.

BACKGROUND

GA achieves a high prediction accuracy rate and minimal false positive rate on the KDD Cup 99 data set (Gupta & Nath, 2010)(Tavalaee,Ebrahim,Lu &Ghorbani,2009). The Stanford Research Institute's next-generation real-time intrusion detection expert system statistical component (NIDES/STAT) observes behaviors of subjects on a monitored computer system and adaptively learns what is normal for individual subjects, such as users and groups (Axelsson, 1999). The 1999 KDDCup data set contains a set of records that represent connections to a military computer network where there have been multiple intrusions and attacks. KDD dataset contains symbolic as well as continuous features. Attacks fall into four main categories DoS (Denial of Service), R2L (Remote to Local), U2R (User to Root) and Probe. This data set was obtained from the UCI KDD archive. (Tavalaee, Ebrahim, Lu &Ghorbani, 2009)(Blake &Merz, 1998)

Feature selection is an important issue in many research areas, such as bio-informatics, chemistry, and text categorization. There are some reasons for selecting important features:

- Reducing the number of features decreases the learning time and storage requirements.
- Removing irrelevant features and keeping informative ones usually improve the accuracy and performance.
- The subset of selected features may help to discover more knowledge about the data.

List of Features with Their Descriptions and Data Types

Following is the data set that was obtained from the UCI KDD archive (Tavalaee, Ebrahim, Lu & Ghorbani, 2009; Blake &Merz, 1998):

The prediction accuracy rate sets the benchmark for test the performance of the GA. Genetic Algorithm comes from biology but it is very influential on computational sciences in optimization. This method is very effective to get optimal or sub optimal solutions of problems as it have only few constraints (Sawah, 2007). It uses generate and test mechanism over a set of probable solutions (called as population in GA) and bring optimal acceptable solution. It executes its three basic operations (Reproduction, Crossover and Mutation) iteratively on population. At present, fitness criterion to select fit individuals is based on the eight fields that match exactly with the attack connection.

PCA (Principal component analysis) transform used for dimensionality reduction which is used for dealing with high dimensional space of features. Recently research on machine learning for intrusion detection has standard much attention in the computation intelligence community. In intrusion detection algorithm, immense strength of audit data must be analyzed in order to conception new detection rule

Table 1. Field of NSL KDD dataset

Feature Number	Feature Name	Description	Type
1	Duration	Duration of the connection (in seconds)	Continuous
2	Protocol type	Type of the connection Protocol	Discrete
3	Service	Destination service	Discrete
4	Flag	Status flag of the connection	Discrete
5	Source bytes	Number of bytes sent from source to destination	Continuous
6	Destination bytes	Number of bytes sent from destination to source	Continuous
7	Land	1 if connection is from/to the same host/port; 0 otherwise	Discrete
8	Wrong fragment	Number of wrong fragments	Continuous
9	Urgent	Number of urgent packets	Continuous
10	Hot	Number of "hot" indicators	Continuous
11	Failed logins	Number of failed logins	Continuous
12	Logged in	1 if successfully logged in; 0 Otherwise	Discrete
13	Num Compromised	Number of "compromised" conditions	Continuous
14	Root shell	1 if root shell is obtained; 0 Otherwise	Continuous
15	Su attempted	1 if root shell is obtained; 0 Otherwise	Continuous
16	Num Root	Number of "root" accesses	Continuous
17	Num File creations	Number of file creation operations	Continuous
18	Num Shells	Number of shell prompts	Continuous
19	Num Access files	Number of operation on access control files	Continuous
20	Num Outbound commands	Number of outbound commands in an ftp session	Continuous

continued on following page

Table 1. Continued

Feature Number	Feature Name	Description	Type
21	Is hot login	1 if the login belongs to the "hot" list; 0 otherwise	Discrete
22	Is guest login	1 if the login is a guest login 0 Otherwise	Discrete
23	Count	Number of connections to the same host as the current connection in the past two seconds	Continuous
24	Srv count	Number of connection to the same service as the current connection in past two seconds	Continuous
25	Serror rate	Percentage of connection that have "SYN" error	Continuous
26	Srv serror rate	Percentage of connection that have "SYN" error	Continuous
27	Rerror rate	Percentage of connection that have "REJ" error	Continuous
28	Srv rerror rate	Percentage of connection that have "REJ" error	Continuous
29	Same srv rate	Percentage of connection to the same service	Continuous
30	Diff srv rate	Percentage of connection to different service	Continuous
31	Srv diff host rate	Percentage of connection to host	Continuous
32	Dst host count	Count of connection having same destination host	Continuous
33	Dst host srv count	Count of connection having the same destination host and using same service	Continuous
34	Dst host same srv rate	Percentage of connection having the same destination host and using same service	Continuous
35	Dst host diff srv	Percentage of different service on the current host	Continuous
36	Dst host same src port rate	Percentage of connection to the current hot having same src port	Continuous
37	Dst host srv diff	Percentage of connection to the same service coming from different host	Continuous
38	Dst host serror rate	Percentage of connection to the current host that have an S0 error	Continuous
39	Dst host srv serror rate	Percentage of connection to the current host and specified service that have an S0 error	Continuous
40	Dst host rerror rate	Percentage of connection to the current host that have an RST error	Continuous
41	Dst host srv rerror rate	Percentage of connection to the current host and specified service that have an RST error	Continuous

for increasing number of novel attack in high speed network. An anomaly model for SQL must take into account specific characteristics of the database query language. The decision tree initially constructed from a set of pre-defined data. The size of decision tree is depending upon the data set, if data set is large the number of branches of tree is large (Kumar,2012). A node of a decision tree specifies an attribute by which the data is to be partitioned. Each node has a number of edges, which are labeled according to a possible value of the attribute in the parent node. There are various decision algorithms, such as: ID3, SLIQ, CART, CHAID and so on. But J48 algorithm is the most representative and widely used. It is proposed by Quinlan in 1993. The ID3 algorithm is a first algorithm for build decision trees. It was designed to handle problems with discrete attributes and has an iterative and very simple structure applicable in training set without error classification and without no-value attributes. J48 classification has increased performance using feature reduction method and classification accuracy increase better after feature selection [18]. The problem in this technique is that it is difficult to find rule and accuracy should be reduced when dataset or category is large. The researcher said that the output from the decision tress, naive Bayes, and a number of other classification methods classifiers can be combined to generate a better classifier rather than selecting the best one.

The Layered Approach with the CRFs to gain the benefits of computational efficiency and high accuracy of detection in a single system (Gupta &Nath, 2010).The other researcher works on layered approach (Dzeroski & 2002)(Ji & Ma, 1997)(Tombini,Debar,Me,Ducasse, 2004).Compare the Layered Approach with the works in (Langley,1994), (Mukkamala,Janoski,2002), and (Lee & Stolfo,1998). The authors in (Hui,Xiao-hong &Xin 2003) describe the combination of "strong" classifiers using stacking, where the decision tress, naive Bayes and a number of other classification methods are used as base classifiers. The authors show that the output from these classifiers can be combined to generate a better classifier rather than selecting the best one. In (Mukkamala,Janoski,2002),, the authors use a combination of "weak" classifiers. The individual classification power of weak classifiers is slightly better than random guessing. The authors show that a number of such classifiers when combined using simple majority voting mechanism, provide good classification. In(Lee & Stolfo,1998) the authors apply a combination of anomaly and misuse detectors for better qualification of analyzed events.

FITNESS FUNCTION FOR ACCURACY

The value of Fitness function to decide whether a chromosome is good or not in a population. In this research accuracy of result decide which chromosome is good or not.

Anomaly network intrusion detection based on data mining techniques such as decision tree (DT), naïve Bayesian classifier (NB), neural network (NN), support vector machine (SVM), k-nearest neighbors (KNN), fuzzy logic model, and genetic algorithm have been widely used by researchers to improve the process of intrusion detection(Shon,Seo & Moon,2005). However, there exist various problems that induce the complexity of detection systems such as low accuracy; unbalanced detection rates different attack types, and high false positives.

MAIN FOCUS OF THE CHAPTER

Layers for Select Features

Normal and DoS
Normal and U2R
Normal and R2L
Normal and Probe

DoS Layer

The DoS attacks are meant to target to stop the service(s) that is (are) provided by flooding it with illegitimate requests. Hence, for the DoS layer, traffic features such as the "percentage of connections having same destination host and same service" and packet level features such as the "source bytes" and "percentage of packets with errors" is significant.

U2R Layer

The U2R attacks involve the semantic details that are very difficult to capture at an early stage. Such attacks are often content based and target an application. Hence, for U2R attacks, selected features such as "number of file creations" and "number of shell prompts invoked.

R2L Layer

The R2L attacks are one of the most difficult to detect as they involve the network level and the host level features, such as the "duration of connection" and "service requested" and the host level features such as the "number of failed login attempts" among others for detecting R2L attacks.

Probe Layer

The probe attacks are aimed at acquiring information about the target network from a source that is often external to the network. Hence, basic connection level features such as the "duration of connection" and "source bytes" are significant while features like "number of files creations" and "number of files accessed" are not expected to provide information for detecting probes.

The implementation of the layered approach by selecting small set of features for every layer rather than using all the 41 features. This is because all the 41 features are not required for detecting attacks belonging to a particular attack group. All above layers are also applied in (Gupta & Nath, 2010) but in proposed work, we are using above layers with genetic algorithm (GA) and with SVM that improve the confusion matrix. Our work follows following steps:

1. **Data Preprocessing:** The main advantage of preprocessing is to avoid attributes in greater numeric ranges dominating those in smaller numeric ranges. Numerical difficulties avoid during the calculation. Feature value preprocessing can help to increase SVM accuracy that is shown in our experimental results.
2. **Converting Genotype to Phenotype:** This step will convert each Parameter and feature chromosome from its genotype into a phenotype.
3. **Feature Subset:** After the applying genetic operations that convert each feature subset chromosome from the genotype into the phenotype and then feature subset can be determined.
4. **Fitness Evaluation:** training dataset is used to train the svm classifier, while the testing dataset is used to calculate classification accuracy. When the classification accuracy is obtained, each chromosome is evaluated by fitness function.
5. **Termination Criteria:** When the termination criteria are satisfied, the process ends; otherwise, we proceed with the next generation.
6. **Genetic Operation:** In this step, the system searches for better solutions by genetic operations, including selection, crossover, mutation, and replacement.

Problem Identify in Previous Algorithm

Training

Step 1: Select the number of layers, n, for the complete system.

Step 2: Separately perform features selection for each layer.

Step 3: Train a separate model with CRFs for each layer using the features selected from Step 2.

Step 4: Plug in the trained models sequentially such that only the connections labeled as normal are passed to the next layer.

Testing

Step 5: For each (next) test instance perform Steps 6 through 9.

Step 6: Test the instance and label it either as attack or normal.

Step 7: If the instance is labeled as attack, block it and identify it as an attack represented by the layer name at which it is detected and go to Step 5. Else pass the sequence to the next layer.

Step 8: If the current layer is not the last layer in the system Test the instance and go to **Step 7**: Else go to Step 9.

Step 9: Test the instance and label it either as normal or as an attack. If the instance is labeled as an attack, block it and identify it as an attack corresponding to the layer name.

In previous algorithm (Gupta & Nath, 2010), the researcher used layered approach with feature selection. In our work, combined layered approach is used with SVM and GA using feature reduction.

Proposed Algorithm

Training

Step 1: Select number of record or feature from dataset.

Step 2: Differentiate the training and testing dataset.

Step 3: Preprocessing perform over training and testing dataset.

Step 4: Select the number of layers, n, for the system.

Step 5: Convert genotype to phenotype.

Step 6: Separately perform features selection for each layer.

Step 7: Train a separate model with GA for each layer using the features selected from Step 5.

Step 8: Selecting feature subset

Step 9: Training dataset with feature selection is given in SVM classifier.

Step 10: Accuracy is obtained or Evaluate fitness.

Step 11: If fitness is better than terminate the process else go to next step.

Step 12: Perform Genetic operation

Step 13: go to step 5

Step 14: Trained models sequentially such that only the connections labeled as normal are passed to the next layer.

Testing

Step 1: Test the instance and label it either as attack or normal.

Step 2: If the instance is labeled as attack, block it and identify it as an attack represented by the layer name at which it is detected and go to Step 1. Else pass the sequence to the next layer.

Step 3: If the current layer is not the last layer in the system, test the instance and go to Step 2. Else go to Step 4.

Step 4: Test the instance and label it either as normal or as an attack. If the instance is labeled as an attack, block it and identify it as an attack corresponding to the layer name.

Step 5: Gcnotype to phenotype.

Step 6: Selecting feature subset for each layer.

Step 7: Test a separate model with GA for each layer using the features selected from Step 5.

Step 8: Testing dataset with feature selection is given in SVM classifier for classification accuracy.

Step 9: Accuracy is obtained or Evaluate fitness.

Step 10: If fitness is better than terminate the process else go to next step.

Step 11: Perform Genetic operation

Step 12: go to step 5

It makes intrusion detection with high resource consumption, as well as results in poor performance of real-time processing and intrusion detection rate. Without loss of generality feature selection can effectively improve the classification model performance, study on the feature selection-based intrusion detection method is therefore very necessary. This work proposes a simple and quick inconsistency-based feature selection method. Data inconsistency is firstly employed to find the optimal features, and the sequential forward search is then utilized to facilitate the selection of subset feature.

Benefits of Proposed GA

- **Assures Compliance**: Facilitates regular review and reporting on enterprise security information, monitors security controls to validate their effectiveness and provides real-time enforcement of policies and best practices.

- **Boosts Operational Performance:** Improve consolidating security information from across the organization into a central location, filtering out noise and false positives, and presenting real incidents. This enables a focused monitoring and response capability.

- **Reduces Exposure Time:** Optimizes reaction times with real time monitoring for security incidents, extensive notification and information capabilities and automated responses.

- **Improves Security Knowledge:** Delivers a comprehensive Knowledge Base that automatically builds security knowledge and internalizes new and updated information. This helps ensure that the knowledge needed to understand and respond to incidents is available when needed.

- **Increases Protection Levels:** Integrates and correlates real time and archived data from all security systems and processes. By tracking incidents to ensure they are handled correctly and on time, customers achieve true incident life cycle management for optimal protection.

Figure 5. Architecture for genetic operation used in feature selection and parameteroptimization for support vector machine

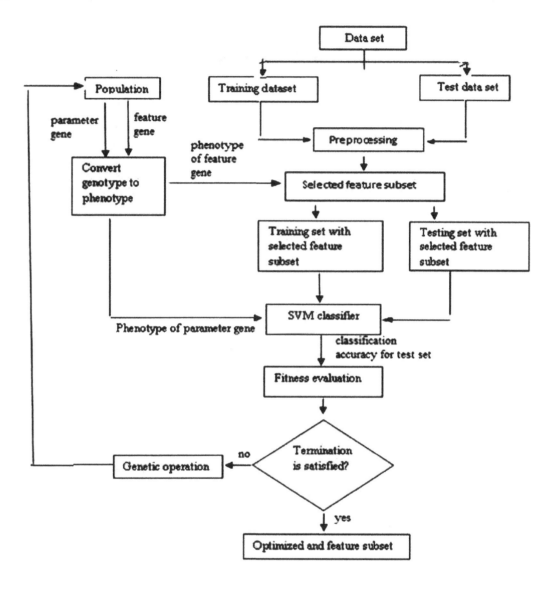

RESULTS

Apply Support Vector Machine with All Fields

Confusion matrix is a specific table that allows visualization the performance of an algorithm. Each column of the matrix represents the instances in a predicted class, while each row represents the instances in an actual class. In figure 6 the confusion matrix shows the 384 sample belong to normal and 27 sample are actual normal but predicted as R2L similar as the other rows and columns.

Figure 6. Resultant of confusion matrix between various types of attacks

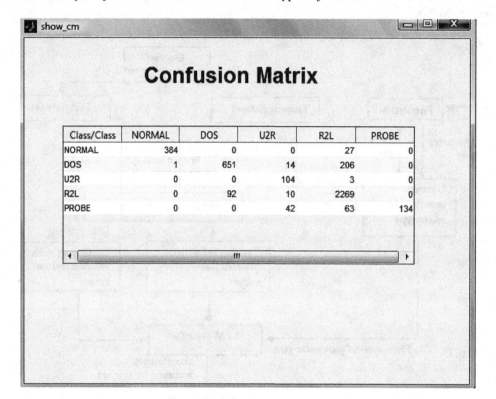

Apply Support Vector Machine with Reduced Fields

Confusion matrix is a specific table that allows visualization the performance of an algorithm. Each column of the matrix represents the instances in a predicted class, while each row represents the instances in an actual class.

In Figure 7 the confusion matrix shows the 387 sample belong to normal and 24 sample are actual normal but predicted as R2L similar as the other rows and columns.

CONCLUSION

This work proposed a GA-based strategy to select the feature subset and set the parameters for SVM classification. As far as we know, previous researches did not perform simultaneous feature selection and parameters optimization for support vector machines. We conducted experiments to evaluate the classification accuracy of the proposed GA-based approach with SVM and the SVM on datasets from UCI database. Generally, compared with the SVM, the proposed GA-based approach has good accuracy performance with fewer features.

Figure 7. Resultant of confusion matrix between various classes of attacks

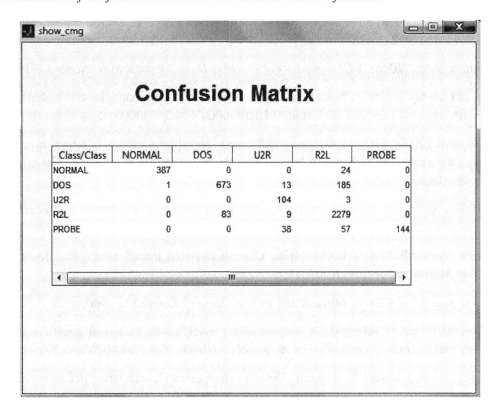

FUTURE RESEARCH DIRECTIONS

In future work various methods should be develop for feature reduction and identify intruder accurately and quickly because work with all 41 feature is time consuming so various improvement perform in feature reduction. Classification is one of the most researched tasks in computer science; some new issues still arise, like the problem of learning from imbalanced data. Data is said to be imbalanced when some classes differ significantly from others with respect to the number of instances available. The problem appears because learning algorithms tend to overlook less frequent classes, leading to poor classification rates in the less frequent classes.

REFERENCES

Anderson. (1980). *Computer Security Threat Monitoring and Surveillance*. Technical Report. James P. Anderson Co.

Barbara, D., Couto, J., Jajodia, S., & Wu, N. (2001). *Special section on data mining for intrusion detection and threat analysis*, Adam: A testbed for exploring the use of data mining in intrusion detection. *SIGMOD Record*, *30*, 15–24. doi:10.1145/604264.604266

Barbara, D., Wu, N., & Jajodia, S. (2001). Detecting novel network intrusions using bayes estimators. In *Proceedings of the First SIAM International Conference on Data Mining* (SDM 2001). doi:10.1137/1.9781611972719.28

Blake, Keogh, & Merz. (2008). *UCI repository of machine learning databases*. Academic Press.

Blum, A. L., & Langley, P. (1997). Selection of Relevant Features and Examples in Machine Learning. *Artificial Intelligence, 97*(1-2), 245–271. doi:10.1016/S0004-3702(97)00063-5

Bridges & Rayford. (2000). Fuzzy data mining and genetic algorithms applied to intrusion detection. In *Proceedings of the Twenty-third National Information Systems Security Conference*. National Institute of Standards and Technology.

Denning. (1987). An Intrusion Detection Model. *IEEE Transactions on Software Engineering, 13*(2), 222–232.

Dzeroski, S., & Zenko, B. (2002). Is Combining Classifiers Better than Selecting the Best One. *Proc. 19th Int'l Conf. Machine Learning (ICML '02)*.

Eiben, A.E., & Smith, J.E. (2001). *Introduction to Evolutionary Computing*. Springer.

Frohlich, H. (2003). Feature selection for support vector machines by means of genetic algorithm. In *15th IEEE International Conf. on Tools with Artificial Intelligence*. doi:10.1109/TAI.2003.1250182

Fugate, M., & Gattiker, J. R. (2002). Anomaly Detection Enhanced Classification in Computer Intrusion Detection. In *Pattern Recognition with Support Vector Machines, First International Workshop* (LNCS), (vol. 2388, pp. 186-197). Springer. doi:10.1007/3-540-45665-1_15

Gupta, K. K., Nath, B., & Kotagiri, R. (2007). Conditional Random Fields for Intrusion Detection. *Proc. 21st Int'l Conf. Advanced Information Networking and Applications Workshops (AINAW '07)*. doi:10.1109/AINAW.2007.126

Gupta, & Nath. (2010). Layered Approach Using Conditional Random Fields for Intrusion Detection. *IEEE Transactions on Dependable and Secure Computing, 7*(1).

Hu, C., Yu, Q., Li, Y., & Ma, S. (2000). *Extraction of Parametric Human model for posture recognition using Genetic Algorithm*. 4th IEEE international conference on automatic face and gesture recognition, Grenoble, France.

Hu, W., Liao, Y., & Rao Vemuri, V. (2003). Robust Support Vector Machines for Anomaly Detection in Computer Security. In *Proceedings of 2003 International Conference on Machine Learning and Applications*.

Ji, C., & Ma, S. (1997). Combinations of Weak Classifiers. *IEEE Transactions on Neural Networks, 8*(1), 32–42. doi:10.1109/72.554189 PMID:18255608

Kim, D. S., & Park, J. S. (2003). Network-based Intrusion Detectio with Support Vector Machines. In *Information Networking, Networking Technologies for Enhanced Internet Services International Conference* (ICOIN 2003), (LNCS), (vol. 2662, pp. 747-756). Springer.

Lakhina, Joseph, & Verma. (2010). Feature Reduction using Principal Component Analysis for Effective Anomaly-Based Intrusion Detection on NSL-KDD. *International Journal of Engineering Science and Technology, 2*(6), 1790-1799.

Langley. (1994). Selection of Relevant Features in Machine Learning. *Proc. AAAI Fall Symp. Relevance.*

Lee, W., Stolfo, & Mok. (1998). Mining audit data to build intrusion detection models. In *Proceedings of the Fourth International Conference on Knowledge Discovery and Data Mining* (KDD '98).

Lee, W., Stolfo, S., & Mok, K. W. (2000). Adaptive Intrusion Detection: A Data Mining Approach. *Artificial Intelligence Review, Kluwer Academic Publishers, 14*(6), 533–567. doi:10.1023/A:1006624031083

Lee, W., & Stolfo, S. J. (1998). Data Mining Approaches for Intrusion Detection. In *Proc. of the 7th USENIX Security Symp.*

Lee, W., & Stolfo, S. J. (1998). Data Mining Approaches for Intrusion Detection. In *Proc. of the 7th USENIX Security Symp.*

Li, Guan, & Zan. (2003). Network intrusion detection based on support vector machine. *Journal of Computer Research and Development, 6*, 800-807.

Liu, H., & Motoda, H. (Eds.). (2001). *Feature Extraction, Construction and Selection a Data Mining Perspective*. Kluwer Academic.

Mukkamala, S., Janoski, G., & Sung, A. H. (2002). Intrusion Detection Using Neural Networks and Support Vector Machines. In *Proceedings of IEEE International Joint Conference on Neural Networks*. IEEE Computer Society Press. doi:10.1109/IJCNN.2002.1007774

Mukkamala, S., Janoski, G., & Sung, A. H. (2002). Intrusion Detection Using Neural Networks and Support Vector Machines. In *Proceedings of IEEE International Joint Conference on Neural Networks*. IEEE Computer Society Press. doi:10.1109/IJCNN.2002.1007774

Nguyen, H., Franke, K., & Petrovic, S. (2010). Improving Effectiveness of Intrusion Detection by Correlation Feature Selection. *2010 International Conference on Availability, Reliability and Security*. IEEE. doi:10.1109/ARES.2010.70

NSL KDD Dataset. (n.d.). Available at http://nsl.cs.unb.ca/NSL-KDD/

Overview of Attack Trends. (2002). Retrieved from http://www.cert.org/archive/pdf/attack_trends.pdf

Park, J. S., Lee, J., Kim, D. S., & Chi, S.-D. (2002). Using Support Vector Ma-chine to Detect the Host based Intrusion. In *IRC International Conference on Internet Information Retrieval*.

Sawah, A. E. (2007). A framework for 3D hand tracking and gesture recognition using elements of genetic programming. *4th Canadian conference on Computer and robot vision*, Montreal, Canada. doi:10.1109/CRV.2007.3

Shon, T., Seo, J., & Moon, J. (2005). SVM approach with a genetic algorithm for network intrusion detection. In *Proc. of 20th International Symposium on Computer and Information Sciences (ISCIS 2005)*. Berlin: Springer-Verlag. doi:10.1007/11569596_25

Sivanandam, S. N., & Deepa, S. N. (2007). *Principles of soft computing*. New Delhi: Wiley India.

Srinivasulu, Satya Prasad, & Ramesh Babu. (2010). Intelligent Network Intrusion Detection Using DT and BN Classification Techniques. *Int. J. Advance. Soft Compute. Appl., 2*(1).

Sung, A. H., & Mukkamala, S. (2004). The Feature Selection and Intrusion Detection Problems. In *Proceedings of the 9th Asian Computing Science Conference*, (LNCS) (vol. 3029). Springer. doi:10.1007/978-3-540-30502-6_34

Tavallaee, M., Bagheri, E., Lu, W., & Ghorbani, A. A. (2009). A Detailed Analysis of the KDDCUP 99 Data Set. *Proceedings of the 2009 IEEE Symposium on Computational Intelligence in Security and Defense Application (CISDA 2009)*. IEEE. doi:10.1109/CISDA.2009.5356528

Tombini, E., Debar, H., Me, L., & Ducasse, M. (2004). A Serial Combination of Anomaly and Misuse IDSes Applied to HTTP Traffic. *Proc. 20th Ann. Computer Security Applications Conf. (ACSAC '04)*. doi:10.1109/CSAC.2004.4

Upendra & Kumar. (2012). An Efficient Intrusion detection based on Decision Tree Classifier Using Feature Reduction. *International Journal of Scientific and Research, 2*(1).

Zaman, S., & Karray, F. (2009). Features selection for intrusion detection systems based on support vector machines. In *Proceedings of the 6th IEEE Conference on Consumer Communications and Networking Conference*.

KEY TERMS AND DEFINITIONS

Genetic Algorithm (GA): Genetic Algorithm (GA) is one of meta-heuristic optimization techniques, which include evolutionary strategies.

Intrusion Detection System (IDS): Intrusion detection systems (IDSs) are software or hardware systems that automate the process of monitoring the events occurring in a computer system or network.

KDD Dataset: The KDD 99 Intrusion detection datasets are based on the 1998 DARPA initiative to provide designers of intrusion detection systems (IDS).

Layered Approach: Each layer is separately trained with a small set of relevant features and then deployed sequentially.

Support Vector Machine (SVM): SVM classifies data with different class labels.

Section 2
Knowledge Visualization and Big Data

Chapter 6
Knowledge Extraction from Domain-Specific Documents

Ram Kumar
Barkatullah University, India

Shailesh Jaloree
SATI, India

R. S. Thakur
MANIT, India

ABSTRACT

Knowledge-based systems have become widespread in modern years. Knowledge-base developers need to be able to share and reuse knowledge bases that they build. As a result, interoperability among different knowledge-representation systems is essential. Domain ontology seeks to reduce conceptual and terminological confusion among users who need to share various kind of information. This paper shows how these structures make it possible to bridge the gap between standard objects and Knowledge-based Systems.

INTRODUCTION

In this paper, we proposed a technique for Knowledge extraction from domain specific documents using ontology and K-Means. Clustering for automatic extraction of Knowledge from the various sources (web, databases etc...) on (from) specific documents and for organize them. The documents collected according to (the) user specifications and are organized in form of ontology. The system offers support to the user during the extraction process by extracting keywords and groups them into classes & concepts by using K-Means Clustering. Web characteristics, such as dimension and dynamics (Levene, 2004) place many difficulties to users willing to explore it as an information source. Moreover, information retrieved from the Web is typically a large collection of documents. A query in Google for "Artificial Intelligence" gives, today, a list of 95.000.000 results. Organizing this information conveniently improves the efficiency of its exploitation. To take advantage of the value contained in this huge information system there is a need

DOI: 10.4018/978-1-5225-0536-5.ch006

for tools that help people to explore it and to retrieve, organize and analyze relevant information. It is also important to give the user the possibility of specifying how he or she requires the retrieved documents to be organized. When working with large corpora of documents it is hard to comprehend and process all the information contained in them. Standard text mining and information retrieval techniques usually rely on word matching and do not take into account the similarity of words and the structure of the documents within the corpus. We try to overcome that by automatically extracting the keywords covered within the documents in the corpus and helping the user to organize them into ontology.

BACKGROUND

Ontology, in its original meaning, is a branch of philosophy (specifically, metaphysics) concerned with the nature of existence. It includes the identification and study of the categories of things that exist in the universe. One scenario of ontology is in Artificial Intelligence, where it is defined as "An ontology is a formal, explicit specification of shared conceptualization. This definition is given by Gruber (Gruber, 1993) which is most commonly used by knowledge engineering community. Here Conceptualization is a "world view" that often present as a set of concepts and their relations. It is the abstract representation of a real world entity (view) with the help of domain relevant concepts (Bhowmick, 2010). Since the ontologist has huge amount of knowledge which is unstructured and it should be organized. Conceptualization helps to organize and structures the acquired knowledge using external representations that are independent of the implementation languages and environments (Arabshian, 2012). Ontology refers to the shared understanding of a domain of interest and is represented by a set of domain relevant concepts, the relationships among the concepts, functions and instances (Bhowmick, 2010).Ontology is used for representing the knowledge of a domain in a formal and machine understandable form in areas like intelligent information processing. Thus it provides the platform for effective extraction of information and many other applications (Choudhary, 2012). It is very useful for expressing and sharing the knowledge of semantic web.

Ontology is a set of concepts connected with different types of relations. Each topic includes a set of related documents. Construction of such ontology from a given corpus can be a very time consuming task for the user. In order to get a feeling on what the topics in the corpus is, what the relations between topics are and, at the end, to assign each document to some certain topics, the User has to go through all the documents. This system aims at assisting the user in a fast extraction of keywords and semi-automatic construction of the ontology from a large document collection. Domain Ontology refers to a specific vocabulary used to describe a certain reality. It presupposes the identification of the key concepts and relationships in the domain of interest. Domain ontology seeks to reduce or eliminate conceptual and terminological confusion among the members of a user community who need to share various kinds of electronic documents and information. It does so by identifying and properly defining a set of relevant concepts that characterize a given application domain, say, for travel agents or medical practitioners. An ontology specifies a shared understanding of a domain. It contains a set of generic concepts (such as "object," "process," "accommodation," and "single room"), together with their definitions and inter-relationships. The construction of its unifying conceptual framework fosters communication and cooperation among people, better enterprise organization, and system interoperability. It also provides such system- engineering benefits as reusability, reliability, and Specification. Ontologies can have different degrees of formality, but they must include metadata such as concepts, relations, axioms, instances, or terms that lexicalize concepts. From the terminological viewpoint, ontology can even be seen as a vocabulary containing a set of formal descriptions (made up of axioms) that approximate term meanings and enable a consistent interpretation of the terms and their relationships.

What Principles should be Followed to Build Ontologies?

Here we summarize some design criteria and a set of principles that have been proved useful in the development of ontologies:

- **Clarity and Objectivity** (Gruber, 1995): The ontology should provide the meaning of defined terms by providing objective definitions and also natural language documentation.
- **Completeness** (Gruber, 1995): A definition expressed in terms of necessary and sufficient conditions is preferred over a partial definition (defined only through necessary or sufficient condition).
- **Coherence** (Gruber, 1995): To permit inferences that are(those are) consistent with the definitions.
- **Maximum Monotonic Extendibility** (Gruber, 1995): It means that new general or specialized terms should be included in the ontology in a (such a) way that is does not require the revision of existing definitions.
- **Minimal Ontological Commitments** (Gruber, 1995): To make as few claims as possible about the world being modeled, giving the parties committed to the ontology freedom to specialize and instantiate the ontology as required.
- **Ontological Distinction Principle** (Borgo, 1996): Classes in ontology should be disjoint.
- **Diversification of Hierarchies**: Increase the power provided by multiple inheritance mechanisms (Arpirez, 1998).
- **Modularity** (Bernaras,1996): Minimize coupling between modules.
- **Minimization of the Semantic Distance Between Sibling Concepts** (Arpirez, 1998): Similar concepts are grouped and represented using the same primitives.
- **Standardization** of names whenever is possible (Arpirez, 1998)

What are the Components of Ontologies?

Knowledge in ontologies is formalized using five kinds of components: classes, relations, functions, axioms and instances (Gruber, 1993). Classes in the ontology are usually organized in taxonomies. Sometimes, the notion of ontology is diluted, in the sense that taxonomies are considered to be full ontologies (Studer, 1998). Concepts are used in a broad sense. A concept can be anything about which something is said and, therefore, could also be the description of a task, function, action, strategy, reasoning process, etc. Relations represent a type of interaction between concepts of the domain. They are formally defined as any subset of a product of n sets, that is: R: C1 x C2 x ... x Cn. Examples of binary relations include: subclass-of and connected-to.

Functions are a special case of relations in which the n-th element of the relationship is unique for the n-1preceding elements. Formally, functions are defined as: F: C1 x C2 x ... x Cn-1 Cn. Examples of functions are Mother-of and Price-of-a-used-car that calculates the price of a second-hand car depending on the car-model, manufacturing date and number of kilometers.

Axioms are used to model sentences that are always true. Instances are used to represent elements.

To construct ontology, specialists from several fields must thoroughly analyze the domain by:-

Examining the vocabulary that describes the entities that populate it Developing formal descriptions of the terms (formalized into concepts, relationships, or instances of concepts) in that vocabulary characterizing the conceptual relations that hold among or within those terms.

RELATED WORK

Ontology is to build a domain ontology based on different heterogeneous sources. It has the following steps. First, generic core ontology is used as a top level structure for the domain-specific ontology. Second, a dictionary is used to acquire domain concepts. Third, domain-specific and general corpora of texts are used to remove concepts that were not domain specific. This method can quickly construct aim ontology for a specific domain, but for the lack of domain generic core ontology and the efficient method of pruning still now, the effect of exist application is not so good (Kietz,2000). Conceptual clustering, concepts are grouped according to the semantic distance between each other to make up hierarchies. But because of lack the domain context to instruct in the process of distance computation, the conceptual clustering process can't be efficiently controlled. Furthermore, by this method, only taxonomic relations of the concepts in the ontology can be generated (Faure,2000). Concept learning, a given taxonomy is incrementally updated as new concepts are acquired from real-world texts. Concept learning is a part of the process of ontology learning (Hahn, 2000). Text2Onto (Maedche, 2000)creates an ontology from annotated texts. This system incorporates probabilistic ontology models (POMs). It shows a user different model ranked according to the certainty ranking and does linguistic preprocessing of the data. It also finds properties that distinguish a class from another.Text2Onto uses an annotated corpus for term generation It is also based on shallow NLP tools, was able to extract key concepts and semantic relations from texts. Selection of concepts was based on the tf/idf measure used in the field of information retrieval. Semantic relations were extracted using an association rule mining algorithm and predefined regular expression rules. However, as tf/idf was designed primarily for IR, the system extracted both domain-specific and common concepts. Also, the identification of semantic relations is based on POS tags, limiting the accuracy of the relations extracted.

Association rules, the association rules have been used to discover non-taxonomic relations between concepts, using a concept hierarchy as background knowledge. Association rules are most used on the data mining process to discover information stored on database. Ontology learning mostly uses unstructured texts but not the structure data in database. So, association rule is just an assistant method to help the ontology generation (Maedche, 2001). OntoLearn (Navigli,2003) uses an unstructured corpus and external knowledge of natural language definitions and synonyms to generate terms. However, the ontology that external knowledge of natural language definitions and synonyms to generate them. However the ontology that is generated is a hierarchical classification and does not involve property assertions. Wen Zhou (Zhou,2006) have proposed a semi-automatic technique that starts form small core ontology constructed by domain experts and learns the concepts and relations by use of the general ontology WordNet and event based natural language processing technologies automatically to construct the domain ontology. Relations learning for ontology are based on event extraction that finds out the verb relations between concepts. This method is fully based on WordNet to discover relationship between concepts. H. Kong (Kong,2006) gave the methodology for building the ontology automatically based on the frame ontology from the WordNet concepts and existing knowledge data. The ontology building method is divided into two parts. One part is to make the possibility for building the ontology automatically based on the frame ontology from the WordNet concepts that are the standard structured knowledge data. Other part is to make the more complete ontology using the specific input data made by the do-main experts. This method is not totally automatic, here first core concepts are taken from Wordnet and relation-ship between concepts are limited to Wordnet only. Iqbal (Iqbal,2001) proposed a semi automated algorithm to transform data to the ontology language, OWL, while taking advantage of the actual data stored in a database schema. Transforming database schemas into an ontology language opens the door wide to the many advantages offered by the Semantic Web. They described Ontology, as the vocabulary and core component of the Semantic Web, provides a re-usable logical representation of real-world things in a particular domain or application area. The biggest research challenge is to enable intelligent systems without having to make any changes in their existing relational database schemas. To solution to problem is dealing with the underlying difference between a database schema and an ontology – namely, the 'closed-world assumption' of a database schema vs the 'open-world assumption' of an ontology. Hence they proposed a semi-automated approach to transform a database schema into the ontology language, OWL-DL.

In Sowa's Top Level Ontology (Sowa,1995), the categories and distinctions are derived from the sources like logic, linguistics, artificial intelligence and philosophy. The ontology has a lattice structure where the top level concept is of universal type and the bottom level concepts are absurd type. The primitive concepts are taken from the set: independent, continuant, occurrent, concrete and abstract.

Wordnet (Goerge,1995) is the largest lexical database for English. It is categorized into synsets each representing one lexical concept. The synsets are related to each other by a set of linguistic relationships like hypernymy and hyponymy, meronymy and holonymy, hynonymy and antonymy.Wordnet represents lexical entries into five categories: nouns, verbs, adjectives, adverbs and functional words. It is used in natural language processing based applications. Maedche and Staab (Maedche, 2000) distinguished different ontology learning approaches focus on the type of input used for learning, such as semi-structured text, structured text, unstructured text. In this sense, they proposed the following classification: ontology learning from text, from dictionary, from knowledgebase, from semi-structured schemata and from relational schemata. Now, most of the domains haven't so much existed semi-structured text, structured text, but there are many unstructured text, such as domain literature, web page. OntoEdit (Sure,2002) provides an environment for the development and modification of ontologies with the help of a graphical user interface. The concept hierarchy can be edited or created in which the concepts may be abstract or concrete. The decision of making direct instances of a concept depends upon the type of the concept. The support for handling synonymous concepts is evident. It has support for several plugins for including domain lexicons, inference engine and import-export facilities.

OntoLT (Buitelaar,2004) allows a user to define mapping rules which provides a precondition language that annotates the corpus. Preconditions are implemented using XPATH expressions and consist of terms and functions. According to the preconditions that are satisfied, candidate classes and properties are generated. Again, OntoLT uses pre-defined rules to find these relationships. CRCTOL (Jiang, 2005) Concept Tuple based Ontology Learning (CRCTOL) for mining rich semantic knowledge in the form of ontology from domain-specific documents, in this paper novel system, known as Concept Relation. By using a full text parsing technique and incorporating statistical and lexico-syntactic methods, the knowledge extracted by our system is more concise and contains a richer semantics compared with alternative systems. By using a full text parsing technique and incorporating both statistical and lexico-syntactic methods, the knowledge extracted by our system is more concise and contains a richer semantics compared with alternative systems. The CRCTOL system consists of three core components, namely Natural

Language Processing, Algorithm Library, and Domain Lexicon. J. Wang (Wang,2006) used rule-based information extraction as a method to learn ontology instances. It automatically extracts the wanted factors of the instances, with the help of the definition in domain ontology. A key technique for the use of IE is rule generation. they put forward a rule generation algorithm RGA-CIE which applies supervised learning with bottom-up strategy and uses a heuristic method to decide rule generalization path and laplacian* formula to evaluate the performance of rules. Wu yuhuang (Yuhuang,2009) proposes a web based ontology learning model. This approach concerns realizing the ontology's automatic extraction from the Web page and discovering the pattern and the relations of the ontology semantics concept from the Web page data. It semi-automatically extracts the Web ontology through the analysis of Web page collection in the identical application domain. Q. Yang (Yang, 2010) present an Ontology Learning method which combines personalized recommendation with concept extraction and stable domain concept extraction method. This method uses machine learning for extraction of field concept. Recommendation study is used to domain concept extraction. It largely improves the accuracy of the concept extraction and the stability. There are still many issues to be resolved in the field of ontology learning like relationship learning. The main lacks for all the methods and tools presented in this overview are that there are not integrated methods and tools that combine different techniques and heterogeneous knowledge sources with existing ontologies to accelerate the learning process.

MAIN FOCUS OF THE CHAPTER

Text Mining is fairly broad in its research, addressing a large range of problems and developing different approaches. Here we present only a very small subset of the available methods, namely only those that we found the most suitable for the problem addressed in this paper. Text mining is an interdisciplinary field which draws on information retrieval, data mining, machine learning, statistics, and computational linguistics. Preprocessing of document collection (text categorization, information extraction, term extraction), storing the intermediate representations, analyzing the intermediate representation using a selected technique such as distribution analysis, clustering, trend analysis, and association rules, and visualizing the results are considered necessary processes in designing and implementing a text mining tool. Among the features of text mining systems/tools are:

- A user centric process which leverages analysis technologies and computing power to access valuable information within unstructured text data sources.
- Text mining processes are driven by natural language processing and linguistic based algorithm.
- Eliminate the need to manually read unstructured data sources.

Natural Language Processing (NLP)

NLP is a technology that concerns with natural language generation (NLG) and natural language understanding (NLU). NLG uses some level of underlying linguistic representation of text, to make sure that the generated text is grammatically correct and fluent. Most NLG systems include a syntactic releaser to ensure that grammatical rules such as subject-verb agreement are obeyed, and text planner to decide how to arrange sentences, paragraph, and other parts coherently. The most well known NLG application is machine translation system. The system analyzes texts from a source language into grammatical or conceptual representations and then generates corresponding texts in the target language. NLU is a system that computes the meaning representation, essentially restricting the discussion to the domain of computational linguistic. NLU consists of at least of one the following components; tokenization, morphological or lexical analysis, syntactic analysis and semantic analysis. In tokenization, a sentence is segmented into a list of tokens. The token represents a word or a special symbol such an exclamation mark. Morphological or lexical analysis is a process where each word is tagged with its part of speech. The complexity arises in this process when it is possible to tag a word with more than one part of speech. Syntactic analysis is a process of assigning a syntactic structure or a parse tree, to a given natural language sentence. It determines, for instance, how a sentence is broken down into phrases, how the phrases are broken down into sub-phrases, and all the way down to the actual structure of the words used.

Semantic analysis is a process of translating a syntactic structure of a sentence into a semantic representation that is precise and unambiguous representation of the meaning expressed by the sentence. A semantic representation allows a system to perform an appropriate task in its application domain. The semantic representation is in a formally specified language. The language has expressions for real world objects, events, concepts, their properties and relationships, and so on. Semantic interpretation can be conducted in two steps: context independent interpretation and context interpretation. Context independent interpretation concerns what words mean and how these meanings combine in sentences to form sentence meanings. Context interpretation concerns how the context affects the interpretation of the sentence. The context of the sentence includes the situation in which the sentence is used, the immediately preceding sentences, and so on.

Information Extraction (IE)

IE involves directly with text mining process by extracting useful information from the texts. IE deals with the extraction of specified entities, events and relationships from unrestricted text sources. IE can be described as the creation of a structured representation of selected information drawn from texts. In IE natural language texts are mapped to be predefine, structured representation, or templates, which, when it is filled, represent an extract of key information from the original text (Rao,2003; Karanikas,2000). The goal is to find specific data or information in natural language texts. Therefore the IE task is defined by its input and its extraction target. The input can be unstructured documents like free texts that are written in natural language or the semi-structured documents that are pervasive on the Web, such as tables or itemized and enumerated lists. Using IE approach, events, facts and entities are extracted and stored into a structured database. Then data mining techniques can be applied to the data for discovering new knowledge. Unlike information retrieval (IR), which concerns how to identify relevant documents from a document collection, IE produces structured data ready for post-processing, which is crucial to many text mining applications. IE allows for mining the actual information present within the text, rather than the limited set of tags associated to the documents. The work of (Karanikas,2000; Nahm,2002), have presented how information extraction is used for text mining. According to Hobbs (1997) and Cowie (2000) typical IE are developed using the following three steps:

- **Text Pre-Processing:** Level ranges from text segmentation into sentences and sentences into tokens, and from tokens into full syntactic analysis;
- **Rule Selection:** The extraction rules are associated with triggers (e.g. keywords), the text is scanned to identify the triggering items and the corresponding rules are selected;

- **Rule Application:** Checks the conditions of the selected rules and fill in the form according to the conclusions of the matching rules. Furthermore Singh (2004) and Hale (2005) emphasized that information extraction is based on understanding of the structure and meaning of the natural language in which documents are written, and the goal of information extraction is to accumulate semantic information from text. Technically, extracting information from texts requires two pieces of knowledge: lexical knowledge and linguistic grammars. Using the knowledge we are able to describe the syntax and semantic of the text (Nedellec, 2005).A common approach to information extraction is to use patterns which match against text and identify items of interest. Patterns are applied to texts which have undergone various levels of linguistic analysis, such as phrase chunking (Soderland,1999) and full syntactic parsing (Gaizauskas,1996).The approaches may use different definition of what constitutes a valid pattern. For example, (Yangarber,2000) use subject-verb-object tuples derived from a dependency parse, followed by (Jones,2003) uses patterns which match certain grammatical categories, mainly nouns and verbs, in phrase chunked text. Reference (Charniak,2001) reported in identifying the parts of a person name through analysis of name structure. For example, the name Doctor Paul R. Smith is composed of a person title, a first name, a middle name, and a surname. It is presented as a preprocessing step for entity recognition and for the resolution of co references to help determine, for instance, that John F. Kennedy and President Kennedy are the same person, while John F. Kennedy and Caroline Kennedy are two distinct persons. Research work in (Smith,2002) applied IE for detecting events in text. Event detection consists of detecting temporal entities in conjunction with other entities. For example, conferences are usually made up of four parts: one conference name, one location, and two dates (e.g., name:"AAAI," location: "Boston," start date: "July 16th 2006,"end date: "July 20th 2006"). A person birth or death is a person name and date pair (e.g., name: "John Lennon," date: "December 8th, 1980"). Smith used event detection to draw maps where war locations and dates are identified.

Clustering

Clustering (Liritano, 2001) is a technique used to group similar documents, but it differs from categorization in that documents are clustered on the fly instead of through the use of predefined topics. Another benefit of clustering is that documents can appear in multiple subtopics, thus ensuring that a useful document will not be omitted from search results. A basic clustering algorithm creates a vector of topics for each document and measures the weights of how well the document fits into each cluster. Clustering technology can be useful in the organization of management information systems, which may contain thousands of documents. Clustering is a technique for partitioning data so that each partition (or cluster) contains only points which are similar according to some predefined metric. In the case of text this can be seen as finding groups of similar documents that is documents which share similar words.

K-Means Clustering

In K-means clustering algorithm (Zhao, 2008) , while calculating Similarity between text documents, not only consider eigenvector based on algorithm of term frequency statistics, but also combine the degree of association between words, then the relationship between keywords has been taken into consideration, thereby it lessens sensitivity of input sequence and frequency, to a certain extent, it considered semantic understanding, effectively raises similarity accuracy of small text and simple sentence as well as preciseness and recall rate of text cluster result.

The first step in text clustering is to transform documents, which typically are strings of characters into a suitable representation for the clustering task:

1. **Remove Stop-Words**: The stop-words are high frequent words that carry no information (i.e. pronouns, prepositions, conjunctions etc.). Remove stop-words can improve clustering results.
2. **Stemming**: By word stemming it means the process of suffix removal to generate word stems. This is done to group words that have the same conceptual meaning, such as work, worker, worked and working.
3. **Filtering**: Domain vocabulary V in ontology is used for filtering. By filtering, document is considered with related domain words (term). It can reduce the documents dimensions. A central problem in statistical text clustering is the high dimensionality of the feature space. Standard clustering techniques cannot deal with such a large feature set, since processing is extremely costly in computational terms. We can represent documents with some domain vocabulary in order to solving the high dimensionality problem. In the beginning of word clustering, one word randomly is chosen to form initial cluster. The other words are added to this cluster or new cluster, until all words are belong to m clusters. This method allow one word belong to many clusters and according with the fact. This method implements word clustering by calculating word relativity and then implements text classification.

K-Means (Jain, 1999). is an iterative algorithm which partitions the data into k clusters. It has already been successfully used on text documents (Steinbach, 2000) to cluster a large document corpus based on the document topic and incorporated in an approach for visualizing a large document collection (Grobelnik, 2002). You can see the algorithm roughly in Algorithm 1.

Algorithm 1: K-Means.
Input: A set of data points, a distance metric, the desired number of clusters k
Output: Clustering of the data points into k clusters
    1. Set k cluster centers by randomly picking k data points as
    2. cluster centers
    3. Repeat
    4. Assign each point to the nearest cluster center
    5. Recompute the new cluster centers
    6. Until the assignment of data points has not changed

In this paper, we present methodology that aims to extract knowledge from Domain specific documents and to derive ontology. This methodology assists users in the processing different resources and extracts keywords from domain specific documents, with the following characteristics:

- Allow for the broad specification of any class, including its ontological structure
- Enable the effective exploration of large document collections by the end-user;

SOLUTIONS AND RECOMMENDATIONS

Two Layer Architectural Approach

To meet the above mentioned requirements we have proposed a two Layer Architectural Approach to represent the domain specific ontology (Figure 1). Ontology usually helps to define basic kinds and structures of concepts considered to be domain independent. These include Meta properties and topmost categories of entities and relationships. Identifying these few basic principles creates a foundational ontology and supports a model's generality to ensure reusability across different domains. Then domain ontology helps to identify key domain conceptualizations and describe them according to the organizational structure established by the top ontology. The result, the core ontology, usually includes a few hundred application-domain concepts.

- **Common Upper Ontology**: This layer capture general concepts. Concepts in this layer are not domain specific.
- **Domain Specific Ontology**: It's a collection of low level ontologies which apply to different domains. E.g. "The doctor removes a pluster."What is the relation between 'doctor, 'removing' and 'driving'? How can I think, abstractly, about removing? What are relevant questions? What are fixed elements, such as: There is movement (What kind of movement?); Something/ someone moves (Who or what?); Something/ someone provokes movement (Who or what?); The movement has a goal (Which goal?)

DOMAIN KNOWLEDGE ACQUISITION FOR BUILDING ONTOLOGY

Its aims to find and retrieve (from the Web and other sources) as many relevant documents as possible while retrieving as few non-relevant documents as possible. Human experts provide the system with

Figure 1. Two Layer Architectural Approach

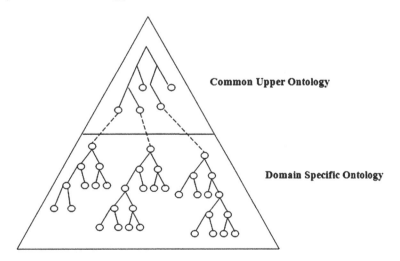

a small number of domain-specific concepts that represent high-level concepts and are used as seed concepts to discover new concepts and relations. Those concepts and their relations are viewed as the core ontology of the system. Ordinarily, the domain's name can be the top concept of the core ontology. Core ontology which is used as a base in the learning process includes the domain concepts and their taxonomic relations mostly organized as concept hierarchy. So the process of ontology enrichment starts with this generic (top-level) ontology. This system suggests knowledge for specific Domain based on extracting keywords from a set of documents inside the concept.The overall architecture of ontology building using domain Knowledge Acquisition is shown in Figure 2.

Terminological Extraction

Terminology extraction refers to discovery of terms that are good candidates for the concepts in ontology. It can be facilitated by the exploitation of learning objects as the primary source of knowledge: learning objects are purely didactic documents, providing definitions and explanations about concepts to be learned. These concepts share the properties of low ambiguity and high specificity, due to their natural engagement in learning. This system needs to determine the content of each document. It works on plain text documents and partitions them into a set of paragraphs, containing a set of sentences.

Figure 2. Ontology building using domain knowledge acquisition

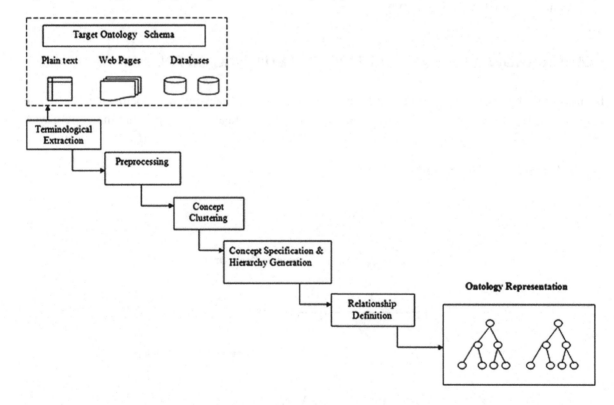

Preprocessing

First, the documents in domain corpus need to be preprocessed and converted into plain text format that natural language process tools can conduct. Preprocessing comprises any transformation process that is applied to the retrieved documents to generate appropriate document models. The expert should provide a domain corpus as sources which should be used in the following steps to refine and extend the ontology we obtain in last step? The corpus is important knowledge resource of ontology learning has to cover the entire domain specified by the application. Sources are heterogeneous in their formats and contents. Sources can be free text documents, semi-structured text, domain text, and generic text.

Concept Clustering

Conceptual clustering, concepts are grouped according to the semantic distance between each other to make up hierarchies. But because of lack the domain context to instruct in the process of distance computation, the conceptual clustering process can't be efficiently controlled. Furthermore, by this method, only taxonomic relations of the concepts in the ontology can be generated .Here K means Algorithm can be used for Concept Clustering.

Concept Specification and Hierarchy Generation

Concept will be specified by the domain expert (Figure 3). The most relevant features of the Concept specification include: − a set of representative keywords, which will be used to generate the queries to submit at the meta-search process − for instance "IT",

- A taxonomy, representing the ontological structure of the topic − for instance ("media", "hardware", "software") and
- A partially classified set of documents that should include labeled documents on every taxonomy categories.

Figure 3. Domain oriented concept specification

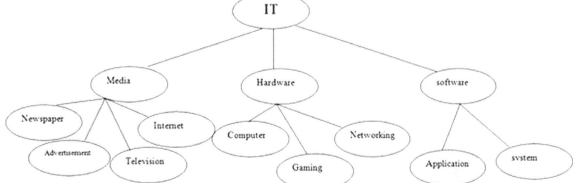

The Concept taxonomy is a hierarchy of concepts specifying the ontological structure of the resource. The root is the keyword itself. The taxonomy is merely a way of structuring the resource according to user specific needs. Web documents are multi-faceted and it is not possible to know which particular facet the user is interested in unless specified. Each document in the resource is associated to just one category – the most specific category in the taxonomy adequately representing the document. We assume that there is no uncertainty as to which particular facet is the user interested in and that the topic categories are not ambiguous. Under these assumptions a singular category might be associated to each document without ambiguity.

There are several possible approaches in developing a class hierarchy (Uschold & Gruninger 1996):

1. A top-down development process starts with the definition of the most general concepts in the domain and subsequent specialization of the concepts. For example, we can start with creating classes for the general concepts of IT. Then we specialize the IT class by creating some of its subclasses: Media, Hardware and software. We can further categorize the Hardware class, for example, into Computer, Gaming Networking and so on. A bottom-up development process starts with the definition of the most specific classes, the leaves of the hierarchy, with subsequent grouping of these classes into more general concepts. For example, we start by defining classes newspaper, Television and advertisement. We then create a common superclass for these two classes—Media—which in turn is a subclass of IT.
2. A combination development process is a combination of the top-down and bottom up approaches: We define the more salient concepts first and then generalize and specialize them appropriately. We might start with a few top-level concepts such as IT, and a few specific concepts, such as Advertment. We can then relate them to a middle-level concept, such as Media. Then we may want to generate all of the IT classes from different perspective, thereby generating a number of middle-level concepts.

Relationship Definition

Defining Relationship is a very difficult and challenging part of ontology building process. Most of the ontology keeps a very few relationships among concepts such as' is-a' and 'Part-of'. However, the relationship list should be broad enough to cover most important forms so that the ontology can be utilized widely by different applications. Moreover, the list of relationships is different in different domains. The types of relationships are decided according to the requirement of the applications. These Relationships allows defining rules about semantic relationship categories hence constituting progressively a linguistic knowledge base. For the moment, we define the following generic categories as shown in Figure 4.

- Taxonomical relationships (is-a, is-a-kind–of, appositions)
- Composition relationships (compose, contain, etc.)
- Description relationships (describes, is-described-by)
- Definition relationships (defines, is-defined-as …)
- Explanation relationships (explains, is-explained-by)
- Causal relationships (causes, leads-to, is-caused-by, etc.)
- Reference relationships (refers-to, is-referenced-by, is-associated-with), etc.

Figure 4. Ontology representation using taxonomical relationships

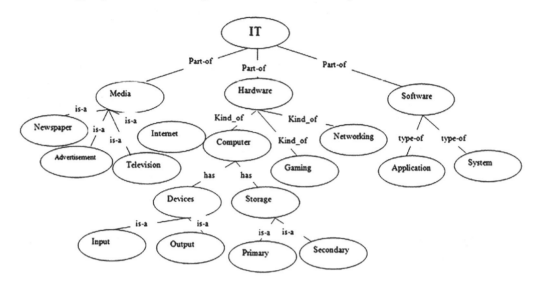

The human expert is free to create new categories in the editor and to provide lexicon-semantic patterns denoting them or to enrich the available categories with new patterns. The same domain knowledge can then be "adapted" to fit particular needs. For example, in an IT context, some kinds of links are usually represented such as composition links and aggregation links. A concept would insist on the available objects and their relationship to each other's whereas other domains may focus on attributes and characteristics.

FURTHER RESEARCH DIRECTIONS

We will focus the future research on extracting event using Link mining which can mine the correlation between semantic units.So the semantic units can be combined to form stronger semantic attribute which will highly improve the quality of ontology and efficiency of ontology creation.

CONCLUSION

In this paper, we presented a solution to domain ontology that seeks to reduce conceptual and terminological confusion among users who need to share various kind of information. This paper shows how these structures make it possible to bridge the gap between standard objects and ontology.

REFERENCES

Anick, P. G., & Tipirneni, S. (1999). The paraphrase search assistant: terminological feedback for iterative information seeking. In *SIGIR '99: Proceedings of the 22nd annual international ACM SIGIR conference on Research and development in information retrieval*. New York, NY:ACM Press. doi:10.1145/312624.312670

Arabshian, K., Danielsen, P., & Afroz, S. (2012, March). Lexont: Semiautomatic ontology creation tool for programmable web. In *AAAI 2012 Spring Symposium on Intelligent Web Services Meet Social Computing*.

Arpirez, J., G'omez-P'erez, A., Lozano, A., & Pinto, S. (1998). (onto)2agent: An ontology-based www broker to select ontologies. In A. Gomez-Perez, & V. R. Benjamins (Eds.), *Proceedings of the Workshop on Applications of Ontologies and Problem-Solving Methods, held in conjunction with ECAI-98*. Brighton, UK: ECAI.

Bernaras, A., Laresgoiti, I., & Corera, J. (1996). Building and reusing ontologies for electrical network applications. In *Proceedings of the 12th ECAI*.

Bhowmick, Roy, Sarkar, & Basu. (2010). *A Framework For Manual Ontology Engineering For Management Of Learning Material Repository*. Academic Press.

Borgo, Guarino, & Masolo. (1996). Stratified ontologies: the case of physical objects. In *Proceedings of the Workshop on Ontological Engineering, held in conjunction with ECAI-96*. Budapest: ECAI.

Buitelaar, S., & Olejnik, D. (2004). *A protege plug-in for ontology extraction from text based on linguistic analysis*. Academic Press.

Charniak, U. (2001). Unsupervised learning of name structure from conference data. In *Proceedings of the 2nd Meeting of the North American Chapter of the Association for Computational Linguistics*.

Choudhary, J., & Roy, D. (2012, May). An Approach to Build Ontology in Semi-Automated way. *Journal of Information and Communication Technologies*, *2*(5).

Cowie, J., & Wilks, Y. (2000). *Information extraction*. New York: Academic Press.

Faure, D., & Poibeau, T. (2000). First experiments of using semantic knowledge learned by ASIUM for information extraction task using INTEX. In S. Staab, A.Maedche, C. Nedellec, & P. Wiemer-Hastings (Eds.), *Proceedings of the Workshop on Ontology Learning,14th European Conference on Artificial Intelligence ECAI'00*.

Gaizauskas, R., Wakao, T., Humphreys, K., Cunningham, H., & Wilks, Y. (1996).Description of the lasie system as used for muc-6. In *Proceedings of the Sixth Message Understanding Conference* (MUC-6).

Goerge, M. A. (1995). Wordnet: A Lexical Database for English. *Communications of the ACM*, *38*(11), 39–41. doi:10.1145/219717.219748

Grobelnik, M., & Mladenic, D. (2002). Efficient visualization of large text corpora. In *Proceedings of the 17th TELRI seminar*.

Gruber, T. R. (1993). A Translation Approach to Portable Ontology Specifications. *Knowledge Acquisition*, *5*, 199–220.

Gruber, T. R. (1995). Towards principles for the design of ontologies used for knowledge sharing. *International Journal of Human-Computer Studies*, *43*(5-6), 907–928. doi:10.1006/ijhc.1995.1081

Hahn, U., & Schulz, S. (2000). Towards Very Large Terminological Knowledge Bases: A Case Study from Medicine. In *Canadian Conference on AI 2000*. doi:10.1007/3-540-45486-1_15

Hale, R. (2005). Text mining: Getting more value from literature resources. *Drug Discovery Today, 10*(6), 377–379. doi:10.1016/S1359-6446(05)03409-4 PMID:15808812

Hearst, M. A. (1998, May). Automated discovery of wordnet relations. In WordNet: An Electronic Lexical Database. MIT Press.

Hobbs, R., Appelt, D., Bear, J., Israel, D., Kameyama, M., Stickel, M., & Tyson, M. (1997). *FASTUS: A cascaded finite-state transducer for extraction information from natural language text.*In E. Roche & Y. Schabes (Eds.), *Finite States Devices for Natural Language Processing* (pp. 383–406).

Irbil, A. M., Moh'd, A., & Khan, Z. (2011). *A Semi-Automated Approach To Transforming Database Schemas Into Ontology Language.* IEEE.

Jain, A. K., Murty, M. N., & Flynn, P. J. (1999). Data Clustering: A Review. *ACM Computing Surveys, 31*(3), 264–323. doi:10.1145/331499.331504

Jiang, X., & Tan, A. H. (2005). Mining Ontological Knowledge from Domain-Specific Text Documents. *Proceedings of the Fifth IEEE International Conference on Data Mining.* IEEE. doi:10.1109/ICDM.2005.97

Jones, R., Ghani, R., Mitchell, T., & Riloff, E. (2003).Active learning for information extraction with multiple view feature sets. *Conference on Machine Learning (ICML 2003).*

Karanikas, H., Tjortjis, C., & Theodoulidis, B. (2000). An approach to text mining using information extraction. In *Proceedings of Workshop of Knowledge Management: Theory and Applications in Principles of Data Mining and Knowledge Discovery 4th European Conference.*

Kietz, J. U., Maedche, A., & Volz, R. (2000). A Method for Semi-Automatic Ontology Acquisition from a Corporate Intranet. In N. Aussenac-Gilles, B. Biebow, & S. Szulman (Eds.), *EKAW'00 Workshop on Ontologies and Texts.* Juan-Les-Pins, France: CEUR. Available: http://CEURWS.org/Vol-51

Kong, H., Hwang, M., & Kim, P. (2006). Design of the automatic ontology building system about the specific domain knowledge. *8th International Conference on Advanced Com-munication Technology (ICACT).*

Levene, M., & Poulovassilis, A. (2004). *Adapting to Change in Content,Size, Topology and Use* (W. Dynamics, Ed.). Springer.

Liritano, S., & Ruffolo, M. (2001). Managing the Knowledge Contained in Electronic Documents: a Clustering Method for Text Mining. IEEE.

Maedche, A., & Staab, S. (2001). *Ontology Learning for the Semantic Web.* IEEE.

Maedche, A., & Staab, S. S. (2000). Semi-automatic engineering of ontologies from text. In *12th International Conference on Software Engineering and Knowledge Engineering.*

Nahm, U., & Mooney, R. (2002). Text mining with information extraction. In *Proceedings of the AAAI 2002 Spring Symposium on Mining Answers from Texts and Knowledge Bases.*

Navigli, R., Gangemi, A. & Velardi, P. (2003). *Ontology learning and its application.* Academic Press.

Nedellec, C., & Nazarenko, A. (2005). *Ontologies and information extraction: A necessary symbiosis. In Ontology Learning from Text: Methods, Evaluation and Applications.* IOS Press Publication.

Rao, R. (2003). From unstructured data to actionable intelligence. In *Proceedings of the IEEE Computer Society.*

Singh, N. (2004). *The use of syntactic structure in relationship extraction.* (Master's thesis). MIT.

Smith, D. (2002). Detecting and browsing events in unstructured text. In *Proceedings of ACM SIGIR Conference on Research and Development in Information Retrieval.* doi:10.1145/564376.564391

Soderland, S. (1999). Learning information extraction rules for semi-structured and free text. *Machine Learning, 34*(1/3), 233–272. doi:10.1023/A:1007562322031

Sowa, J. F. (1995). Top-level Ontological Categories. *International Journal of Human-Computer Studies, 43*(5-6), 669–685. doi:10.1006/ijhc.1995.1068

Steinbach, M., Karypis, G., & Kumar, V. (2000). A comparison of document clustering techniques. In *Proceedings of KDD Workshop on Text Mining,6th ACM SIGKDD International Conference on Knowledge Discovery and Data Mining* (KDD).

Studer, R., Benjamins, V. R., & Fensel, D. (1998). Knowledge engineering, principles and methods. *Data & Knowledge Engineering, 25*(1-2), 161–197. doi:10.1016/S0169-023X(97)00056-6

Sure, Y., Angele, J., & Staab, S. (2002). OntoEdit: Guiding Ontology Development by Methodology and Inferencing. *Proceedings of the 1st International Conference on Ontologies, Databases and Applications of Semantics for Large Scale Information Systems.* doi:10.1007/3-540-36124-3_76

Wang, J., Wang, C., Liu, J., & Wu, C. (2006). Information Extraction forlearning of Ontology Instances. *IEEE International Conference on Industrial Informatics.*

Yang, Q., Kai-min, C., Jun-li, S., & Li, Y. (2010). Design Analysis and Implementation for Ontology Learning Model. *2nd International Conference on Computer Engineering and Technology.*

Yangarber, R., Grishman, R., Tapanainen, P., & Huttunen, S. (2000). Automatic acquisition of domain knowledge for information extraction. In *Proceedings of the 18th International Conference on Computational Linguistics.* doi:10.3115/992730.992782

Yuhuang, W., & Yuhuang, L. (2009). *Design and realization for ontology learning model based on web.* IEEE. doi:10.1109/ITCS.2009.234

Zhao, M., Wang, J., & Fan, G. (2008). Research on Application of Improved Text Cluster Algorithm in intelligent QA system. *Proceedings of the Second International Conference on Genetic and Evolutionary Computing.* IEEE Computer Society. doi:10.1109/WGEC.2008.49

Zhou, W., Liu, Z., Zhao, Y., Xu, L., Chen, G., Wu, Q., & Qiang, Y. et al. (2006). *A Semi-automatic Ontology Learning Based on WordNet and Event-based Natural Language Processing.* ICIA. doi:10.1109/ICINFA.2006.374119

KEY TERMS AND DEFINITIONS

Agents: Pieces of software that interpret the content of web server & present it to the user as a web page.

Conceptual Clustering: It is a machine learning paradigm for unsupervised classification. It is distinguished from ordinary data clustering by generating a concept description for each generated class.

Conceptualization: It is defined as a set of objects which an observer thinks exist in the world of interest and relation between them.

Information Extraction: It is the task of automatically extracting structured information from unstructured and/or semi-structured machine-readable documents.

Knowledge Acquisition: It is the process used to define the rules and ontologies required for a knowledge-based system.

Semantics: It is the study of meaning. It focuses on the relation between words, phrases, signs & symbols & their denotations.

Taxonomy: It is the science of naming, describing and classifying organisms and includes all plants, animals and microorganisms of the world.

Chapter 7
Semi–Automatic Ontology Design for Educational Purposes

Monica Sankat
Barkatullah University, India

R. S. Thakur
MANIT, India

Shailesh Jaloree
SATI, India

ABSTRACT

In this paper, we present a (semi) automatic framework that aims to produce a domain concept from text and to derive domain ontology from this concept. This paper details the steps that transform textual resources (and particularly textual learning objects) into a domain concept and explains how this abstract structure is transformed into more formal domain ontology. This methodology targets particularly the educational field because of the need of such structures (Ontologies and Knowledge Management). The paper also shows how these structures make it possible to bridge the gap between core concepts and Formal ontology.

INTRODUCTION

Ontology defines a common vocabulary for researchers who need to share information in a domain (Noy & McGuinness, 2000). The proposed method is to build a semi automatic ontology for educational data for various topics. Ontology can be treated as set of topics connected with different types of relations. Each topic includes a set of related documents. Construction of such ontology from a given corpus can be a very time consuming task for the user. In order to get a feeling on what the topics in the corpus are, what the relations between topics are and, at the end, to assign each document to some certain topics, the user has to go through all the documents. The proposed method will overcome this by building a semi automated ontology which helps the user by suggesting the possible new topics and visualizing the topic ontology created. The Semi-Automatic ontology building starts from small core ontology constructed by

DOI: 10.4018/978-1-5225-0536-5.ch007

domain experts and learn the new concepts and relationships between concepts. The proposed method aims at assisting the user in a fast semi-automatic construction of the ontology from a large document collection of educational data.

Introduction to Ontology

Ontology has been attracting a lot of attention recently since it has emerged as a very important discipline in the areas of knowledge representation (Sowa, 2000). Ontology refers to the shared understanding of a domain of interest and is represented by a set of domain relevant concepts, the relationships among the concepts, functions and instances (Bhowmick et al, 2010).Ontology is used for representing the knowledge of a domain in a formal and machine understandable form in areas like intelligent information processing. Thus it provides the platform for effective extraction of information and many other applications (Choudhary & Roy, 2012). It is very useful for expressing and sharing the knowledge of semantic web (Tiwari & Thakur, 2012). There exist many definitions of ontology in different areas by different people. In philosophy, Ontology means theory of existence. It tries to explain what is being and how the world is configured by introducing a system of critical categories to account things and their intrinsic relations.

One scenario of ontology is in Artificial Intelligence, where it is defined as *Ontology is a formal, explicit specification of shared conceptualization*. This definition is given by Gruber (Gruber, 1993) which is most commonly used by knowledge engineering community. Here Conceptualization is a *world view* that often present as a set of concepts and their relations. It is the abstract representation of a real world entity (view) with the help of domain relevant concepts (Bhowmick et al, 2010).Since the ontologist has huge amount of knowledge which is unstructured and it should be organized. Conceptualization helps to organize and structures the acquired knowledge using external representations that are independent of the implementation languages and environments (Aguado et al, 1998). Another scenario from compositional view of ontology is *Ontology is a hierarchical organization of concepts along with relationship between them*. From knowledge-based systems point of view, ontology is defined as *a theory (system) of concepts/vocabulary used as building blocks of an information processing system* by R. Mizoguchi (Mizoguchi, 1995). One thing that we should understand about ontology is Semantic web which requires semantic interoperability among metadata in which ontology is expected to fill the semantic gap between metadata (Mizoguchi, 1995). Ontologies act as a conceptual backbone for semantic document access by providing a common understanding and conceptualization of a domain (Kietz,2001).

Though essentially different, ontologies are closely related to knowledge bases and database schemas. An ontology can be distinguished from a knowledge base in the fact that it is a conceptual structure of a domain while a knowledge base is a particular state of domain. An ontology also separates itself from a database schema in that an ontology is sharable and reusable while a database schema tends to be specific to the domain and is context-dependent; therefore is unlikely to be shareable and reusable. For instance, an OWL DL ontology is essentially equal to a description logic knowledge base which contains both a TBox (elements of which constitute an ontology), and an ABox (which comprises instances of the ontology).

BACKGROUND

Domain Ontologies capture the knowledge of the domain where the task is performed. Several domain ontologies for different domains have been developed. CHEMICALS (Fernandez, 1999) are an ontology representing the domain of chemical elements and crystalline structures. This ontology is represented with Ontolingua. This has been used in the projects like OntoGeneration and ChamicalOntoAgent. The domain of pollutant chemical materials is represented by the ontology Environmental Pollutants. It captures the pollutant chemical materials in different media like water, air soil etc. Ontology representation language here is XML. These ontologies provide detailed description of the domain concepts from a restricted domain therefore sometimes referred as 'vertical' ontology. WebODE (Vega, 2000) is an advanced ontological engineering workbench that provides varied ontology related services, and gives support to most of the activities involved in the ontology development process. It has been developed using a three tier model having Client Tier, Middle Tier and Database Tier. The main components of WebODE ontology are concepts, groups of concepts, taxonomies (single and multiple inheritances) ad-hoc relations, constants, formulae, instances (of concepts and relations) and references. Ontology pruning is to build a domain ontology based on different heterogeneous sources. It has the following steps. First, generic core ontology is used as a top level structure for the domain-specific ontology. Second, a dictionary is used to acquire domain concepts. Third, domain specific and general corpora of texts are used to remove concepts that were not domain specific. This method can quickly construct aim ontology for a specific domain, but for the lack of domain generic core ontology and the efficient method of pruning still now, the effect of exist application is not so good (Kietz et al, 2001).

The purpose of Standard Upper Merged Ontology (Niles & Pease, 2001) is to make Computers utilize the ontology in the applications needing data interoperability, information search and retrieval, natural language processing. The knowledge representation language for the SUM0 is a version of KIF (Knowledge Interchange Format) called SUO-KIF. This is a somewhat simplified version of KIF, and it is itself a separate proposed standards effort. LinkFactory (Ceusters & Martens, 2001) is an ontology management system that provides a way to create and manage large scale, complex, multilingual and formal ontologies. It has been used to develop the medical linguistic knowledge base LinKBase. The LinKFactory Server and the LinKFactory Workbench (clientside component) are two major components of the system. The user can customize the tool to view and manage the ontology. Different views of the ontology like Concept tree, Concept criteria and full definitions, Linktype tree, Criteria list, Term list, Search pane, Properties panel, Reverse relations are managed through Java beans. The server is responsible for storing the ontology physically into a relational database implemented in Oracle. The access to the database is abstracted by some intuitive APIs like get-children, find-path, join concepts, get terms for concept X. Protégé (Gennari et al, 2002) is probably the most popular ontology development tool. Protege is a free, Java-based open source ontology editor. Protege offers two approaches for the modeling of ontologies: a traditional frame-based approach (via Protege-Frame) and a modeling approach using OWL (via Protege-OWL). Protege ontologies can be stored in a variety of different formats, including RDF/RDFS, OWL and XML Schema formats. Protege facilitates rapid prototype and application development, and has a very flexible architecture via a plug-and-play environment. Protege helps knowledge engineers and domain experts to perform knowledge management tasks. It includes support for class and class hierarchy with multiple inheritances, slots having cardinality restrictions, default values, inverse slots, metaclass and metaclass hierarchy. It supports easy navigation through the class hierarchy through tree controls. The knowledge model is OKBC compatible. The distinguishing features in Protege are the scalability and extensibility.

A standard upper ontology [SUO] has been being developed at IEEE P1600.1 [SUO]. This is one of the most comprehensive ontologies among those in AI community. Recently, SUMO (Standard Upper Merged Ontology) [SUMO] has been proposed as a candidate of SUO.SUMO is implemented in DAML+OIL. DAML+OIL evolved from a merger of DAMLONT, an earlier DAML ontology language. The goal of this merger was to integrate the formal foundations found in description logics into DAML and revise DAML-ONT in response to community comments. DAML+OIL's goal is to support the transformation of the Web from being a forum for information presentation to a resource for interoperability, understanding, and reasoning. Arabshian (Arabshian et al, 2012) in his paper propose LexOnt; a semi-automatic ontology creation tool for a high-level service classification ontology. LexOnt uses the Programmable Web directory as the corpus, although it can evolve to use other corpora as well. The main contribution of LexOnt is its novel algorithm which generates and ranks frequent terms and significant phrases within a PW category by comparing them to external domain knowledge such as Wikipedia, Wordnet and the current state of the ontology. LexOnt (Danielsen et al, 2013) is developed as a Protege plug-in .The GUI design and implementation of LexOnt is given in this paper. It uses the Programmable Web directory as its corpus. LexOnt is built specifically for those who are not experts within a domain, but want to understand the domain on a high-level and create an ontology that describes it. The LexOnt interface itself allows a user to easily find relevant terms and phrases within the original corpus as well as the already constructed ontology. The goal of LexOnt is to find high-level properties of a class that distinguish it from other classes. The process is semi-automate because it works by creating a tool that automatically analyzes a corpus of data within a domain to aid a user, unfamiliar with that field, to choose descriptive terms and then automate attribute creation within the ontology.

Boyce (Boyce & Pahl, 2007) presented a method for domain experts rather than ontology engineers to develop ontologies for use in the delivery of courseware content. They focused in particular on relationship types that allow us to model rich domains adequately. Since ontologies can be used for instructional design and the development of course content. They can be used to represent knowledge about content, supporting instructors in creating content or learners in accessing content in a knowledge-guided way (Tiwari et al., 2010) . Fortuna (Fortuna et al, 2006) proposed a semi-automatic and data-driven ontology editor called OntoGen, focusing on editing of topic ontologies (a set of topics connected with different types of relations).The system combines text-mining techniques with an efficient user interface to reduce both: the time spent and complexity for the user. In this way it bridges the gap between complex ontology editing tools and the domain experts who are constructing the ontology and do not necessarily have the skills of ontology engineering. Fortuna (Fortuna et al, 2007) presents a new version of OntoGen system. The system integrates machine learning and text mining algorithms into an efficient user interface lowering the entry barrier for users who are not professional ontology engineers. The main features of the systems include unsupervised and supervised methods for concept suggestion and concept naming, as well as ontology and concept visualization. Mei-ying Jia et al. (Jia et al, 2009) has proposed automated ontology construction method. The method is not pure auto-mated. It uses existing thesaurus and database of Military Intelligence. The thesaurus provides classes information for the ontology and the database provides the instances. Here, only three types of relationships are used between concepts of constructed ontology. Finally uses, Protégé, open source editing tool, to represent ontology that provides a friendly interface for users.

Bhowmick (Bhowmick et al, 2010) present a framework for manual ontology engineering in education domain for managing learning materials of the curriculum related requirements of school students. In this paper, a multilingual framework for management of knowledge structures of such domains in a participatory way. They used a three tier knowledge model to represent the domain knowledge in education domain. They provided a set of 11 relations is found to cover most types of relations between two concepts. The developed ontology has been utilized to index learning materials into different ontological levels. The framework also provides the ways to perform personalized search by consulting the user profiles and the created index structures.

To reduce the effort of manual ontology building, Choudhary propose a methodology for building ontology in semi-automatic manner. In his paper algorithms are developed for automatic discovery of concepts from Web for building domain ontology. Relationships among the concepts are assigned in semi-automated manner (Choudhary & Roy, 2012). Navigli (Navigli et al, 2003) In his paper, presented a methodology for automatic ontology enrichment and document annotation with concepts and relations of an existing domain core ontology. They defined Natural language definitions from available glossaries in a given domain are processed and regular expressions are applied to identify general-purpose and domain-specific relations. They evaluate the methodology performance in extracting hypernymy and nontaxonomic relations.

The main drawbacks in existing work in this area are:

1. There are not integrated methods and tools that combine different techniques and heterogeneous knowledge sources with existing ontologies to accelerate the development process and these methods are not generalized to other domains.
2. They only provide some specialized relationships among the concepts. Again these relationships are not sufficient to define knowledge structure of education domain.
3. Developing domain ontology is a difficult task because correct installation requires adequate domain knowledge and an efficient ontology can be built only by a domain expert.
4. They do not provide the facility of indexing contents with the entities present in ontology. This is important for efficient and automated content organization.
5. Multilingual framework: No system except Link Factory provides the platform where knowledge can be authored in multilingual environment.
6. Doesn't provide Easy interface for domain experts having little technological expertise.

More specifically, regarding ontology, these are the questions need to ask:

1. Is the usual hierarchical organization of concepts in ontologies sufficient?
2. If not, are there education-specific relationship types in addition to the more common subtype hierarchies?
3. Are these education-specific relationships, if any, transferable between subjects and Languages?

Motivation

The specific features of this domain are:

1. Every concept refers to a semantically distinct entity. The concepts in a domain are related to each other through different relationships.
2. Different types of relationships may exist.
3. The phenomenon of synonymy is very common. So the same concept may be referred to by several terms. For example, the terms DS and Data structures refers to the same concept.
4. The same concept can be represented by different words.
5. Analyzing the specific features of the domain, it is identified that requirements for representing the domain knowledge are as follows:-
6. Finding information at the concept level is very important to reduce the Redundancy occurring due to the synonymous ambiguity between the terms.
7. Different types of relationships may be used differently in systems that make use of the domain knowledge.

MAIN FOCUS OF THE CHAPTER

Feigenbaum (Feigenbaum, 1977) proposed concept of knowledge engineering, which is mainly utilization of rule base technology. The rule base technology was a key technology by which expertise is encoded in the form of if-then rule to develop a large rule base. Task ontology (Mizoguchi, 1995) was an achievement to overcome the problem of building ontology from the scratch.

Theories in AI fall into two broad categories: mechanism theories and content theories. Ontologies are content theories about the sorts of objects, properties of objects, and relations between objects that are possible in a specified domain of knowledge. They provide potential terms for describing our knowledge about the domain (Chandrasekaran et al, 1999). Similarly, there are two types of researches theory in AI history, one is *Form-oriented research* and the other is *Content-oriented research*. Form- oriented research investigates logic, knowledge representation, search, etc. and the Content-oriented research defines content of knowledge .The former has widely used AI research to date. But now days, to solve a lot of real-world problems such as knowledge systematization, knowledge sharing Content-oriented research has attracted considerable attention because, through understanding, large-scale knowledge bases, etc. The key factor of Content-oriented research is knowledge engineering. But still there is a problem of sharing and reuse of knowledge because in this type of research we don't have knowledge based system. This leads to development of Ontological Engineering. Ontological Engineering is a research methodology which gives us the design rationale of a knowledge base, conceptualization of the world of interest, semantic constraints of concepts together with sophisticated theories and technologies enabling accumulation of knowledge which is expendable for knowledge processing in the real world.

Why Develop Ontology?

According to Natalya F.Noy (Noy & McGuinness, 2000), An ontology defines a common vocabulary for researchers who need to share information in a domain. It includes machine-interpretable definitions of basic concepts in the domain and relations among them. There are many reasons that *Why would someone want to develop an ontology?* Some of the reasons are:

- To share common understanding of the structure of information among people or software agents.
- To enable reuse of domain knowledge i.e.to avoid "re-inventing the wheel" (Mike, 1996).
- To make domain assumptions explicit.
- To separate domain knowledge from the operational knowledge.
- To analyze domain knowledge.

Ontology Representation Languages

For ontologies to be understood, shared and executed, they need to be represented in some way. For human understanding, they can be expressed in high-level languages such as conceptual graphs, semantic networks, UML or even natural languages. However, for ontologies to be process able by computer, they must be represented in a computer-readable language (such as OWL). Ontology Representation Language is used to structure ontology hierarchy of concepts is used. Ontology representation language is also an important issue in developing ontology building tools, as one of the primary objectives of ontology is to enable shared communication and a set of standard ontology representation languages helps other domain experts to cross validates created ontology easily. Existing ontology specification languages fall into the following categories: traditional ontology languages and web ontology languages. In the following, this paper briefly introduces major ontology specification languages, starting with Ontolingua, one of the most traditional languages, and ending with OWL, the most popular web ontology language.

Traditional Ontology Languages

- Ontolingua is the language used by the Ontolingua Server (Farquhar et al, 1996). Ontolingua is implemented as a Frame Ontology, which is built on top of the knowledge interchange format KIF.
- CycL is a formal language that was first developed in the Cyc Project (Lenat & Guha, 1990).It is based on first-order predicate calculus.
- Open Knowledge Base Connectivity (OKBC) Protocol (Chaudhri et al, 1998) is a protocol for accessing knowledge in knowledge representation systems.
- Frame Logic (F-Logic) (Kifer et al, 1995) combines features from both frame-based languages and first-order predicate calculus. It has a sound and complete resolution-based proof theory.
- LOOM (MacGregor, 1991) is based on description logic. It facilitates knowledge representation and reasoning.

Web Ontology Languages

Web ontology languages include OIL, DAML+OIL, XOL, SHOE and OWL. To facilitate interoperability in the web environment, these languages are based on the web standards XML and RDF:

- **Extended Markup Language (XML)** (Bray et al, 2000): A markup language which aims to separate web content from web presentation. Although XML is extensively used as a web standard for representing information, its lack of semantics is often mentioned as one of its major drawbacks.
- **Resource Description Framework (RDF)** (Lassila & Swick, 1999): A W3C standard used to describe web resources. Each RDF statement is called a triple which consists of subject, predicate

and object. An RDF triple can be visualized as a directed graph where the subject and object are modeled as nodes, and the predicate is modeled as a link which is directed from the subject to the object. RDF aims to facilitate the exchange of machine-understandable information on the web.

- **RDF Schema (RDFS)** (Brickley & Guha, 2002): A layer built on top of the basic RDF models. RDFS serves as a set of ontological modeling primitives which allows developers to define vocabularies for RDF data.

- **Ontology Inference Layer (OIL)** (Horrocks et al, 2000): Developed in the On-To-Knowledge project. It is based on description logics, frame-based languages and web standards (e.g., XML, RDF and RDFS). It is designed for both describing and exchanging ontologies.

- **DAML+OIL** (Horrocks & Harmelen, 2001): The result of an effort to combine DARPA Agent Markup Language (DAML) and OIL. DAML+OIL is more efficient than OIL in that it includes more features from description logics. However, many frame-based features were removed from DAML+OIL, which makes it more difficult to use DAML+OIL with frame-based tools.

- **XML-based Ontology Exchange Language (XOL)** (Karp et al, 1999): Developed as a format for the exchange of ontology definitions.

- **Web Ontology Language (OWL)** (Dean et al, 2002): A standard for representing ontologies on the Semantic Web. It was developed in 2001 by the Web-Ontology (WebOnt) Working Group and became a W3C recommendation in 2004. The design of OWL is based on DAML+OIL and is therefore heavily influenced by description logics, the frame-based paradigm and RDF. OWL aims to give developers more power to express semantics, and to allow automated reasoners to carry out logical inferences and derive knowledge.

Types of Ontology

A variety of different types of ontologies are considered in the literature. There are a few types of ontologies which have different roles. Several ontologies have been developed in various domains and for varying purposes. They differ in the way:-

- The ontology is structured,
- The ontology representation language that has been used to represent the ontology,
- And the application domain they are targeted for.

These ontologies can be categorized into several groups as follows:

Top Level Ontologies

The portion of Philosophers work which includes higher level categories that explain what exist in the world, which is called upper ontology or Top level ontologies. This type of ontology defines the concepts from the universe like entity, event, feature, etc. It is articulated in the sense that distinction is made where it is necessary. In Sowa's Top Level Ontology (Sowa, 1995) the categories and distinctions are derived from the sources like logic, linguistics, artificial intelligence and philosophy. The ontology has a lattice structure where the top level concept is of universal type and the bottom level concepts are absurd type. The primitive concepts are taken from the set: independent, continuant, occur rent, concrete and abstract. A standard upper ontology (SUO) has been being developed at IEEE P1600.1 (SUO). This is one of the most comprehensive ontologies among those in AI community. Recently, SUMO (Standard Upper Merged Ontology) [SUMO] has been proposed as a candidate of SUO.

The purpose of Standard Upper Merged Ontology (Niles & Pease, 2001) is to make Computers utilize the ontology in the applications needing data interoperability, information search and retrieval, natural language processing. The knowledge representation language for the SUMO is a version of KIF (Knowledge Interchange Format) (Genesereth, 1991) called SUO-KIF. This is a somewhat simplified version of KIF, and it is itself a separate proposed standards effort. SUMO is implemented in DAML+OIL (McGuinness et al, 2002). As described above, DAML (DARPA Agent Markup Language) is a ontology language to support Semantic Web development and the Ontology Inference Layer (OIL) (Bechhofer et al, 2002) is a description logic .DAML+OIL evolved from a merger of DAMLONT (McGuinness et al, 2002), an earlier DAML ontology language. The goal of this merger was to integrate the formal foundations found in description logics into DAML and revise DAML-ONT in response to community comments. DAML+OIL's goal is to support the transformation of the Web from being a forum for information presentation to a resource for interoperability, understanding, and reasoning.

Task Ontologies and Domain Ontologies

In a context of problem solving, ontologies are divided into three types:

1. **Task Ontologies:** Characterize the computational architecture of a knowledge-based system which performs a task and domain ontology which characterizes knowledge of the domain (Mizoguchi, 1995). By a task, we mean a problem solving process like diagnosis, monitoring, scheduling, design, and so on. The idea of task ontology which serves as a system of the vocabulary/concepts used as building blocks for knowledge-based systems might provide us with an effective methodology and vocabulary for both analyzing and synthesizing knowledge-based systems.

2. **Domain Ontologies:** Capture the knowledge of the domain where the task is performed. Several domain ontologies for different domains have been developed. CHEMICALS (Fernandez, 1999) are an ontology representing the domain of chemical elements and crystalline structures. This ontology is represented with Ontolingua. This has been used in the projects like OntoGeneration and ChamicalOntoAgent. The domain of pollutant chemical materials is represented by the ontology Environmental Pollutants. It captures the pollutant chemical materials in different media like water, air soil etc. Ontology representation language here is XML. These ontologies provide detailed description of the domain concepts from a restricted domain therefore sometimes referred as 'vertical' ontology.

3. **Aguado** (Aguado et al, 1998): Organizes and converts an informally perceived view of a domain into a semiformal specification, using a set of intermediate representations that the domain expert and ontologist can understand. These IRs bridges the gap between how people think about a domain and the languages in which ontologies art formalized.

Natural Language Ontologies and Linguistic Ontologies

Natural Language Ontologies contain lexical relations between the language concepts; they are large in size and do not require frequent updates. Usually they represent the background knowledge. SENSUS (Knight, 1994) is a natural language based ontology developed for the machine translation project by

ISI. It is a hierarchically structured concept base. The Ontology Base at the upper level represents the generalization needed in the process of translation. The middle level represents the model of the world by storing English word senses and the bottom most level have concepts representing anchor points for different applications.

Linguistic Ontologies capture the semantics of the grammatical units.

Wordnet (Goerge, 1995) is the largest lexical database for English. It is categorized into synsets each representing one lexical concept. The synsets are related to each other by a set of linguistic relationships like hypernymy and hyponymy, meronymy and holonymy, hynonymy and antonymy. Wordnet represents lexical entries into five categories: nouns, verbs, adjectives, adverbs and functional words. It is used in natural language processing based applications.

Ontology Instances

Ontology instances represent the main piece of knowledge presented in the Semantic Web. The ontology instances will serve as the Web pages and will contain the links to other instances similar to the links to other Web pages (Omelayenko, 2001).Ontology should be formal so that it becomes machine understandable and enable to share knowledge across the communities (Bhowmick et al, 2010). Ontologies serve as metadata schemas, providing a controlled vocabulary of concepts, each with explicitly defined and machine-process able semantics. By defining shared and common domain theories, ontologies help people and machines to communicate concisely—supporting semantics exchange, not just syntax. Hence, the Semantic Web's success and proliferation depends on quickly and cheaply constructing domain-specific ontologies (Maedche & Staab, 2001).

SOLUTIONS AND RECOMMENDATIONS

Ontology has emerged as a very important discipline as its usefulness has been demonstrated in varying types of applications which include information organization and extraction, personalization, natural language processing, artificial intelligence, knowledge representation and acquisition. Ontology is going to play a major role in the evolution process of the WWW to the Semantic Web, the second generation web (Choudhary & Roy, 2012). The main benefits in using an ontology to describe services are that it provides structure and semantics to service metadata which allows it to be easily classified and shared (Arabshian et al, 2012).

Ontology Building Methods

For most of the aspects of ontologies mentioned so far in this report, software tools have been developed to assist developers and users in fulfilling their tasks. With ontologies being increasingly applied in many critically important applications, what is needed is a platform that serves as an integrated support environment for the whole ontology development. Ontology Development is area of knowledge of domain of interest (Danielsen & Arabshian, 2013). Ontology building tools provide framework for manual, semi automatic or automatic ontology engineering. Ontology building tools provide the facilities and environments to build a new ontology from scratch, modify existing ontologies, reuse other ontologies and also provide a visual interface for viewing ontology.

There are mainly three ways to develop Ontology:-

1. Manual Ontology Building
2. Semi-automated Ontology Building
3. Automated Ontology Building

Manual Ontology

Generally, ontologies are developed manually. Manual Ontology building tools provide the facilities and environments to build a new ontology manually e.g. Protégé, LinkFactory etc.

There are two approaches for Manual Ontology building:

1. Top down approach
2. Bottom up approach

In Top down approach first start with core concepts of ontology which are used as a top level structure for the domain-specific ontology. Then analyze the domain or some domains knowledge. Then we find the relationship between concepts. Add the concepts and relationship between concepts manually in ontology building tool. In Bottom up approach, using data dictionary or data source to extract all concepts, by use of domain corpus remove non domain related concepts, find the relationship between domains related concepts, then Add the concepts and relationship between concepts manually in ontology building tool.

Drawbacks of Manual Ontology

Manual ontology building requires lots of efforts by domain experts and hence time consuming and costly. Manual ontology building approach has many problems and some of them are mentioned below:

*   The manual ontology construction require lots of human efforts hence time consuming and costly.
*   It is a difficult task because correct installation requires adequate domain knowledge.
*   An efficient ontology can be built only by a domain expert.

In order to overcome the problems of manual ontology building, researchers are working on semi-automatic and also on automatic ontology building approaches.

Semi-Automatic Ontology

Semi-Automatic ontology building starts from small core ontology constructed by domain experts and learn the new concepts and relationships between concepts automatically using expert algorithms. Ontologies are often subjective descriptions of a given domain which require human evaluation. However, we can semi-automate this process by creating a tool that automatically analyzes a corpus of data within a domain to aid a user, unfamiliar with that field, to choose descriptive terms and then automate attribute creation within the ontology (Danielsen & Arabshian, 2013).

Ontology Building Method

Building domain-specific ontologies is a time-consuming and expensive manual construction task. This approach is to develop a domain ontology using semi automatic approach for educational data. The concepts will be generated automatically and the relations between concepts are assigning manually. Ontology is built in this step by linking concepts and relations extracted. The final ontology is presented in the form of a semantic network. The proposed work will focus in particular on relationship types that allow us to model rich domains adequately. The method used to build Ontology is shown in Figure 1.

Extraction of Candidate Terminology

Extraction refers to discovery of terms that are good candidates for the concepts in ontology. The Documents are collected from a large Corpus for the Extraction of Candidate Ontology. Then the documents are preprocessed for the extraction of main specific concepts.

Figure 1. Overview of ontology design process

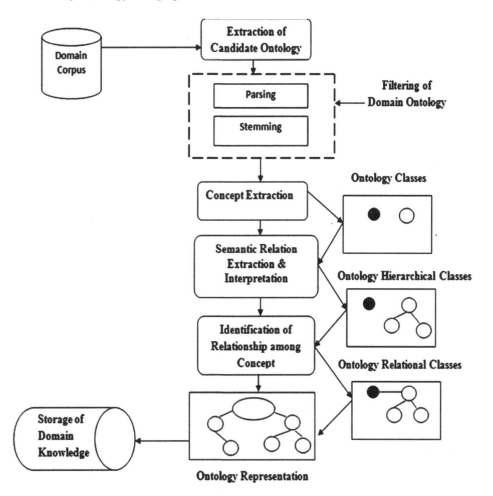

Filtering of Domain Ontology

This step consist of two components namely Parsing and Stemming. This system assumes that the input documents are in the plain text format. Text files in other formats are converted to plain text before processing & to individual words in the documents. In Parsing, Firstly it is needed to parse it to collect domain oriented concepts. In parsing, each line is scanned to find domain word first. Now, hierarchy words have been selected after from domain word. In Stemming, a group of words where words in the group are small syntactic variants of one another may share the same word stem. So, it is useful for the ontology learning system to identify such group of words and collect only the root word stem per group. For example, the groups of words: computation, computing, computes shares a common word stem, compute, and must be viewed as the same word for different occurrences.

Concept Extraction

Concepts are identified by a statistical algorithm from text. These concepts are called the key concepts of the target domain.Concept extraction are based on words. First, keywords were identified from the text. These words are typically single-word terms and will be seen as the concepts.

The event-based concept learning algorithm involves the following steps:-

1. Examine each input sentence one at a time; ignore sentences that do not contain at least two nouns, one of which should be ontology concept.
2. Extract all the possible pairs of nouns in the sentence. One of which should be an existing concept of the ontology. Preserve their order and all the words in between.
3. Infer a relationship R between two ontology concepts (or one ontology concept and one frequent noun) connected by a verb or an action denoting noun.
4. If both N1 and N2 are ontology concepts, the verb should be added into the ontology as the relation of N1 and N2. This relationship will be denoted by (N1, R, and N2).
5. The relation R as the relation between Nl and N2 into ontology.
6. The process can be cyclic in the sense that the resulting ontology can be enriched applying the method iteratively.

Semantic Relation Extraction

Semantic relations of the key concepts are extracted from the text. These include taxonomic and non-taxonomic relations. We extract semantic relations between multi-word terms as well as relations between multi-word terms and single-word terms from text collection.

Verbs are hypothesized to indicate semantic relations between concepts. A semantic relation of the (Concept, Relation, Concept) tuple thus has a lexical realization in text in the form of (Noun1, Verb, Noun2), where Noun1 and Noun2 are noun terms in text and concepts in the ontology, Verb is the verb term in text, Noun1 is the subject of Verb, and Noun2 is the object of Verb.

As texts have been fully parsed by the NLP component, syntactic are assigned to sentences. They represent the semantic relations between the concepts extracted. The Noun and Verb terms are identified by the regular expressions below:

Noun: (DT)+(JJ)+(NN|NNS|NNP|NNPS)+
Verb: (VB|VBD|VBN|VBZ)+

where JJ represents an adjective, NN, NNS, NNP, and NNPS represent nouns; DT represents an article, and VB, VBD, VBN and VBZ represent verbs.

Interpretation of Semantic Term for input files are then processed. Syntactic tags are assigned.

Semantic Interpretation

Semantic Interpretation is the process of first determining the right concept (sense) for each component of a complex term (this is known as semantic disambiguation) and then identifying the semantic relations holding among the concepts to build a complex concept. This system starts by hierarchically arranging the set of validated terms into sub trees according to simple string inclusion. Fig.2 is an example of a Data Structure Ontology tree T. In the absence of semantic interpretation, however, we cannot fully capture conceptual relationships between senses (for example, the 'Is-a' relation between item and node in Fig.2).

Identification of Relationship among Concept

For the topic of data Structures n the education domain, concepts are shown above in Figure 2. in which most relationships between the concepts within this data set could be catered for by the 'is-a' relationship, there were some relationships between concepts that were not generalization/specialization relationships and therefore would be misrepresented if the 'is-a' relationship was used. For this reason, a number of other relationship types were created and defined such as Part-of, Kind-of. All these words belong to education domain concepts. For example: List, Stack, Queue and so on. To identify Relationships among concept we use to type of mapping, first is Term-to-class relationship mapping, which is a process that finds out the relations between terms and classes and Term-to-term relationship mapping, which finds out the relations between all terms within a class.

Figure 2. Represenatation of data structure ontology using 'is_a' relationship

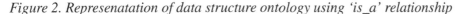
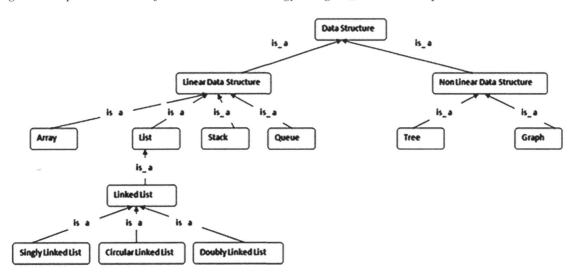

Ontology Creation

This is final process that generates ontology as the knowledge representation with more specific relationships as shown in Figure 3.

FURTHER RESEARCH DIRECTIONS

It is likely that, with increased development and availability of ontology, we would take up the challenge of developing ontologies in areas where as domain experts and would make these ontologies available to the public. Also would try handling more complex ontology and making use of existing ontology to avoid re-inventing the wheel.

CONCLUSION

In this paper, we presented a solution to semi-automatically generate ontology from domain documents. This paper details the steps that transform textual resources (and above all textual learning objects) into a domain concept and explains how this abstract structure is transformed into more formal domain ontology. We would like to realize the generation of more complex learning objects that exploit the semi automatic ontology concept as well as available ontologies to fulfill Educational objective.

Figure 3. Representation of data structure ontology with more relationship types

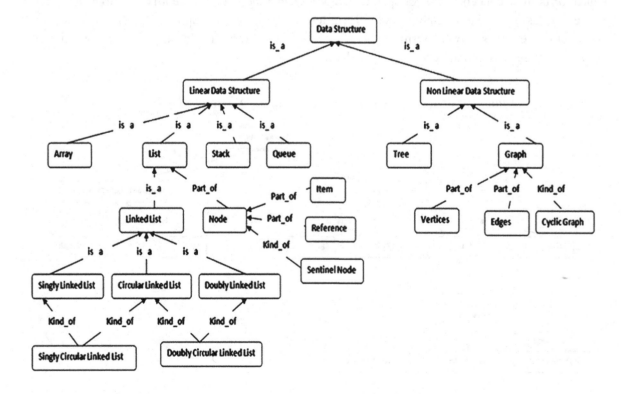

REFERENCES

Aguado, G., Banon, A., Bateman, J., Bernardos, M. S., Fernandez-Lopez, M., Gomez-Perez, A., … Sanchez, A. (1998). Ontogeneration: Reusing Domain and Linguistic Ontologies for Spanish Text Generation. *Workshop on Applications of Ontologies and Problem Solving Methods.*

Arabshian, K., Danielsen, P., & Afroz, S. (2012). Lexont: Semiautomatic ontology creation tool for programmable web. In *AAAI 2012 Spring Symposium on Intelligent Web Services Meet Social Computing.*

Bechhofer, S., Broekstra, J., Decker, S., Erdmann, M., Fensel, D., Goble, C., … Studer, R. (2002). *An Informal Description of OIL-Core and Standard OIL: A Layered Proposal for DAML-O.* Retrieved from: www.ontoknowledge.org/oil/downl/dialects.pdf.

Bhowmick, P.K., Roy, D., Sarkar, S., & Basu, A. (2010). *A Framework For Manual Ontology Engineering For Management Of Learning Material Repository.* Academic Press.

Blaz, F., Marko, G., & Dunja, M. (2006). Semi-automatic Data-driven Ontology Construction System. In *Proceedings of the 9th International multi-conference Information Society IS-2006.*

Blaz, F., Marko, G., & Dunja, M. (2007). OntoGen: Semi-automatic Ontology. In Human Interface, Part II, HCII 2007, (LNCS), (vol. 4558, pp. 309–318). Springer.

Boyce, S., & Pahl, C. (2007). Developing Domain Ontologies for Course Content. *Journal of Educational Technology & Society, 10*(3), 275–288.

Bray, T., Paoli, J., Sperberg-McQueen, C. M., & Maler, E. (2000). *Extensible MarkupLanguage (XML) 1.0, Second Edition, W3C Recommendation, 2000.* Retrieved from http://www.w3.org/TR/REC-xml

Brickley, D., & Guha, R. V. (2002). *RDF Vocabulary Description Language 1.0: RDF Schema, W3C Working Draft.* Retrieved from: http://www.w3.org/TR/PR-rdf-schema

Ceusters, W., & Martens, P. (2001). LinKFactory: an Advanced Formal Ontology Management System. *Proceedings of Interactive Tools for Knowledge Capture Workshop, KCAP 2001.*

Chandrasekaran, B., Josephson, J. R., & Benjamins, V. R. (1999). What are ontologies? Why do we need them? *IEEE Intelligent Systems.*

Chaudhri, V. K., Farquhar, A., Fikes, R., Karp, P. D. & Rice, J. P. (1998). *Open Knowledge Base Connectivity 2.0.3.* Technical Report.

Choudhary J. & Devshri, R. (2012). An Approach to Build Ontology in Semi-Automated way. *Journal of Information and Communication Technologies, 2*(5).

Danielsen, P. J., & Arabshian, K. (2013). User Interface Design in Semi-Automated Ontology Construction. *IEEE 20th International Conference on Web Services.*

Dean, M., Connolly, D., van Harmelen, F., Hendler, J., Horrocks, I., McGuinness, D. L., . . . Stein, L. A. (2002). *OWL Web Ontology Language 1.0Reference, W3C Working Draft.* Retrieved from: http://www.w3.org/TR/owl-ref/

Farquhar, A., Fikes, R., & Rice, J. (1996). The Ontolingua Server: a Tool for Collaborative Ontology Construction. In *Proceedings of the 10th Bank Knowledge Acquisition for Knowledge Based System Workshop* (KAW95). doi:10.1006/ijhc.1996.0121

Feigenbaum, E.A. (1977). The art of artificial intelligence – Themes and case studies of knowledge engineering. *Proc. of 5th IJCAI.*

Fernandez Lopez, M. (1999). Overview of Methodologies for Building Ontologies. In *Proceedings of the IJCAI99 Workshop on Ontologies and Problem-Solving Methods:Lessons Learned and Future Trends.*

Genesereth, M. (1991). Knowledge Interchange Format. *Proceedings of the Second International Conference on the Principles of Knowledge Representation and Reasoning* (KR-91). Morgan Kaufman Publishers.

Gennari, J. H., Musen, M. A., Fergerson, R. W., Grosso, W. E., Crubzy, M., Eriksson, H., & Tu, S. W. et al. (2002). The evolution of Protege: An Environment for Knowledgebased Systems Development. *International Journal of Human-Computer Studies, 58*(1), 89–123. doi:10.1016/S1071-5819(02)00127-1

Goerge, M. A. (1995). Wordnet: A Lexical Database for English. *Communications of the ACM, 38*(11), 39–41. doi:10.1145/219717.219748

Gruber T. R. (1993). A Translation Approach to Portable Ontology Specifications. *Knowledge Acquisition, 5,* 199–220.

Horrocks, I., Fensel, D., Harmelen, F., Decker, S., Erdmann, M., & Klein, M. (2000). OIL in a Nutshell. In *ECAI'00 Workshop on Application of Ontologies and PSMs.*

Horrocks, I., & van Harmelen, F. (2001). *Reference Description of the DAMLOIL Ontology Markup Language.* Technical report. Retrieved from http://www.daml.org/2001/03/reference.html

Jia, M., Yang, B., Zheng, D., Sun, W., Liu, L., & Yang, J. (2009). Automatic Ontology Construction Approaches and Its Application on Military Intelligence. *Asia-Pacific Conference on Information Processing* (APCIP).

Karp, R., Chaudhri, V., & Thomere, J. (1999). *XOL: An XML-Based Ontology Exchange Language.* Technical Report. Retrieved from http://www.ai.sri.com/pkarp/xol/xol.html

Kietz, J. U., Maedche, A., & Volz, R. (2001). A Method for Semi-Automatic Ontology Acquisition from a Corporate Intranet. In N. Aussenac-Gilles, B. Biebow, & S. Szulman (Eds.), *EKAW'00 Workshop on Ontologies and Texts.* Juan-Les-Pins, France: CEUR. Available: http://CEURWS.org/Vol-51

Kifer, M., Lausen, G., & Wu, J. (1995). Logical foundations of object-oriented and frame-based languages. *Journal of the ACM, 42*(4), 741–843. doi:10.1145/210332.210335

Knight, K., & Luk, S. K. (1994). Building a Large Knowledge Base for Machine Translation. *Proceedings of the American Association of Artificial Intelligence Conference.*

Lassila, O., & Swick, R. (1999). *Resource description framework (RDF) model and syntax specification, W3C Recommendation.* Retrieved from: http://www.w3.org/TR/REC-rdf-syntax/

Lenat, D. B., & Guha, R. V. (1990). *Building Large Knowledge-Based Systems: Representation and Inference in the Cyc Project*. Boston: Addison-Wesley.

MacGregor, R. (1991). Inside the LOOM classifier. *SIGART Bulletin, 2*(3), 70-76.

Maedche, A. & Staab, S. (2001). *Ontology Learning for the Semantic Web*. IEEE.

McGuinness, D. L., Fikes, R., Hendler, J., & Stein, L. A. (2002). DAML + OIL: An Ontology Language for the Semantic Web. *IEEE Intelligent Systems, 17*(5), 72–80. doi:10.1109/MIS.2002.1039835

Mizoguchi, R. (1995). *Tutorial on ontological engineering*. Academic Press.

Muschold, M. (1996). Ontologies: principle, methods and application. *The Knowledge Engineering Review, 1*(2), 93-136.

Navigli, R., Gangemi, A., & Velardi, P. (2003). *Ontology learning and its application*. Academic Press.

Niles, I., & Pease, A. (2001). Towards a Standard Upper Ontology.*Proceedings of the International Conference on Formal Ontology in Information Systems*.

Noy, N.F., & McGuinness, D.L. (2000). *Ontology Development 101: A Guide to Creating Your First Ontology*. Academic Press.

Omelayenko, B. (2001). Learning of Ontologies for the web: the analysis of existent Approaches. In *Proceedings of the international Workshop on web Dynamics, held in conj. withthe 8th International Conference on Database theory* (ICDT'01).

Sowa, J. F. (1995). Top-level Ontological Categories. *International Journal of Human-Computer Studies, 43*(5-6), 669–685. doi:10.1006/ijhc.1995.1068

Sowa, J. F. (2000). *Knowledge Representation – Logical, Philosophical, and Computational Foundations*. Pacific Grove, CA: Brooks/Cole.

SUO. (n.d.). *Standard Upper Ontology*. Retrieved from: http://suo.ieee.org/

Tiwari, V., & Thakur, R. S. (2012). A level wise Tree Based Approach for Ontology-Driven Association Rules Mining. *CiiT International Journal of Data Mining and Knowledge Engineering, 4*(5).

Tiwari, V., Tiwari, V., Gupta, S., & Mishra, R. (2010). Association Rule Mining- A Graph based approach for mining Frequent Itemsets.*IEEE International Conference on Networking and Information Technology (ICNIT)*. doi:10.1109/ICNIT.2010.5508505

Vega, J. C. A. (2000). *WebODE 1.0: User's Manual*. Laboratory of Artificial Intelligence, Technical University of Madrid.

KEY TERMS AND DEFINITIONS

Conceptualization: It is defined as a set of objects which an observer thinks exist in the world of interest and relation between them.

Data Properties: They describe relationship between two instances and data values.

Explicit: Unambiguous Terminology Definitions.

Formal Specification: Formal specification means machine readability with computational capability.

Object Properties: They describe relationship between two instances or two individual of classes.

Semantics: It is the study of meaning. It focuses on the relation between words, phrases, signs, symbols and their denotations.

Chapter 8
Improving Multimodality Image Fusion through Integrate AFL and Wavelet Transform

Girraj Prasad Rathor
AISECT University, India

Sanjeev Kumar Gupta
AISECT University, India

ABSTRACT

Image fusion based on different wavelet transform is the most commonly used image fusion method, which fuses the source pictures data in wavelet space as per some fusion rules. But, because of the uncertainties of the source images contributions to the fused image, to design a good fusion rule to incorporate however much data as could reasonably be expected into the fused picture turns into the most vital issue. On the other hand, adaptive fuzzy logic is the ideal approach to determine uncertain issues, yet it has not been utilized as a part of the outline of fusion rule. A new fusion technique based on wavelet transform and adaptive fuzzy logic is introduced in this chapter. After doing wavelet transform to source images, it computes the weight of each source images coefficients through adaptive fuzzy logic and then fuses the coefficients through weighted averaging with the processed weights to acquire a combined picture: Mutual Information, Peak Signal to Noise Ratio, and Mean Square Error as criterion.

INTRODUCTION

With the growing advancements in technology, it becomes possible to obtain information from multi-modality images. However, all the geometrical and physical details in need for full assessment might not be available by analyzing the multimodality images separately. In multisensory images, there is often a trade-off between spatial and spectral resolutions resulting in information loss. Image fusion combines perfectly registered multimodality images from multiple sources to provide a high quality fused image with high spatial and spectral information. It integrates complementary information from various modalities based on specific rules to give a better visual appearance of a scene, suitable for machine pro-

DOI: 10.4018/978-1-5225-0536-5.ch008

cessing. An image can be expressed either by its original spatial representation or in frequency domain. By Heisenberg's uncertainty, information cannot be compact in both spatial and frequency domains simultaneously. This motivates the use of wavelet transform which gives a multi-resolution solution based on time-scale analysis. Each sub-band is processed at a different resolution, capturing localized time-frequency data of image to provide unique directional information useful for image representation and feature extraction across different scales.

BACKGROUND

Multimodalities data fusion has become a discipline to which more and more general formal solutions to a number of application cases are required. Several situations in image processing simultaneously require high spatial and high spectral information in a single composite image. This is important in medical diagnosis, remote sensing. However, the multimodalities are not capable of providing such information either by design or because of observational constraints. One possible solution for this is data fusion. Image fusion is the process of combining information from two or more multimodalities images of a scene into a single composite image that is more informative and is more suitable for visual perception or computer processing. The aim of multimodalities image fusion is to integrate complementary information of multi-sensor, multi-temporal and/or multitier into one new image. The goal is to reduce uncertainty and minimize redundancy in the output while maximizing relevant information particular to an specific application or task. An area based maximum selection rule, and consistency verification steps are used for feature selection. The algorithms are checked for multi sensor as well as multi focus image fusion.

In Medical Image Fusion Based on Discrete Wavelet Transform Using Java Technology (Ligia & Vaida, 2009), authors discus the importance of information offered by the medical images for diagnosis support can be increased by combining images from different compatible medical devices. The fusion process allows combination of salient feature of these images. In this paper different techniques of image fusion, Author's work for medical image fusion based on discrete wavelet transform and how to understand to integrate this process into a distributed application. The dedicated application considers Java technology for using its facilities as a future development, regarding a remote access mechanism. In Novel Masks for Multimodality Image Fusion using DTCWT (Shahid & Gupta, 2006), authors present an image fusion technique using the Dual tree complex wavelet transform (DTCWT). We they proposed novel masks to extract information from the decomposed structure using DTCWT. The main goal of this paper is to introduce a new approach to fuse multimodality images using dual tree complex wavelet transform. Experiment results show that the proposed fusion method based on complex wavelet transform is remarkably better than the fusion method based on classical discrete wavelet transform. This method is relevant to visual sensitivity and tested by merging multisensor, multispectral and defoucused images apart from medical images (CTand MR images). Fusion is achieved through the formation of a fused pyramid using the DTCWT coefficients from the decomposed pyramids of the source images. The fused image is obtained through conventional inverse dual tree complex wavelet transform reconstruction process. Results obtained using the proposed method show a significant reduction of distortion. In A Novel Wavelet Medical Image Fusion Method (Zhang H. et al, 2007), authors propose a novel global energy merging scheme that is a region-based analysis approach. At first, multi-resolution wavelet decomposition on each source image is performed, and then the energy of the each 3*3 matrix region is calculated. The match measure can produce using wavelet decomposition coefficient and the energy. The three high frequency coefficients of the merging image produce through comparing match measure of several source images and the low frequency coefficient lies on the choice of the three high frequency coefficient. Finally by applying the inverse wavelet transform the final fused image is obtained. The composite images can preserve more relevant information about the edges. Experiments showed that the proposed wavelet image fusion method can have better performance than existing medical image fusion methods. In Information Fusion and Wavelet Based Segment Detection with Applications to the Identification of 3D Target T-ray CT Imaging (Yin X. et al, 2006) Author investigatets segmentation techniques depending on T-ray CT functional imaging. A set of linear image fusion and novel wavelet scale correlation segmentation techniques are adopted in order to achieve classification within 3D objects. The methods are applied to a T-ray CT image dataset of a glass vial containing a plastic tube. His experiment simulates the imaging of a simple nested organic structure, which will provide an indication of the potential for using T-ray CT imaging to achieve T-ray pulsed signal classification of heterogeneous layers.

In Biomedical Image Fusion Using Wavelet Transform and SOFM Neural Network (Patnaik D.2009),Use of Computer Tomography (CT), Magnetic Resonance (MR), Single Photon Emission Computed Tomography (SPECT) techniques in biomedical imaging has revolutionized the process of medical diagnosis in recent years. Further advancements in biomedical imaging are being done by development of new tools of image processing. One of tools is image fusion .The fusion of CT scan, MR and SPECT images can make medical diagnosis much easier and accurate. On the basis of review of research papers published earlier in the area of image fusion, author presents a method of image fusion based on Discrete Wavelet Transform(DWT) and Self Organizing Feature Mapping(SOFM) neural network. The proposed method is a feature level fusion method 2-dimensional DWT is used to decompose the images into various details at different levels to extract useful features and SOFM neural network is used to recognize complementary features. These features are then integrated using criteria based on activity level. Final fused image is constructed from fused feature set. The proposed method of fusion has been applied to MR, SPECT and CT scan images, and results obtained are presented in this paper. In Terahertz Computed Tomographic Reconstruction and its Wavelet-based Segmentation by Fusion (Yin et al,2007) terahertz (T-ray) computed tomographic (CT) imaging and segmentation techniques are investigated. The traditional filtered back projection is applied for the reconstruction of terahertz coherent tomography. A set of linear image fusion and novel wavelet scale correlation segmentation techniques is adopted to achieve material discrimination within a three dimensional (3D) object. The methods are applied to a T-ray CT image dataset taken from a plastic vial containing a plastic tube. This setup simulates the imaging of a simple nested organic structure, which provides an indication of the potential for using T-ray CT imaging to achieve T-ray pulsed signal classification of heterogeneous layers. The wavelet based fusion scheme enjoys the additional benefit that it does not require the calculation ofa single threshold and there is only a segment parameter to adjust.

IN Image Fusion Based on Wedgelet And Wavelet (Liu F. et al,2007) Wavelet transform has been widely used in image fusion; it can well represent smooth regions and regular textures. However, wavelet is unable to provide a good representation of 2D edges. Wedgelet transform has good performance in approximation to edges. In this paper, we propose a new fusion method; it makes good approximation to edges in original images by using wedgelet and retains texture features in residual images with wavelet. Through combining wedgelet with wavelet, we develop a detector of edges and texture features in residual images. So the respective superiorities of wedgelet and wavelet can be combined by adding the fusion results using wavelet on the fusion results using wedgelet respectively. The experiments show that this novel method provides improved qualitative results compared to previous wavelet and dual tree complex wavelet (DT-CWT) fusion methods. In Medical Image Fusion Based on Wavelet Packet Transform and Self-adaptive Operator (Licai Y. et al, 2008) auther combining wavelet packet transform with self adaptive operator together, a medical image fusion algorithm is put forward. In this algorithm, the medical imagines that have been matched are firstly decomposed using wavelet packet transform, and the wavelet coefficients as well as the sub-images decomposed are processed with self-adaptive operators. Then the fusion imagines are gained by the wavelet packet reconstruction for the decomposed imagines. The simulation results show that this algorithm is feasible and effective for the clinical applications of medical fusion imagines.

Medical Image Fusion Based on Wavelet Transform and Independent Component Analysis (Cui Z.et al, 2009) Author proposes a novel method for this particular image fusion, which is using discrete wavelet transform and independent component analysis. Firstly, each of CT images was decomposed by 2-D discrete wavelet transform. Then independent component analysis was used to analyze the wavelet coefficients in different level for acquiring independent component. At last, we use wavelet reconstruction to synthesize one CT medical image which could contain more integrated accurate detail information of different soft tissue such as muscles and blood vessels. By contrast, the efficiency of our method is better than weighted average, laplacian pyramid method in medical image fusion field. In Wavelet based Approach for Fusing Computed Tomography and Magnetic Resonance Images (Yang Y et al,2009) The multimodality medical image fusion plays an important role in clinical applications which can support more accurate information for physicians to diagnose diseases. In this paper, a new fusion scheme for computed tomography and magnetic resonance images based on wavelet analysis is proposed. After the images are decomposed by wavelet transform, the low frequency coefficients are performed with the maximal absolute values followed by verifying their consistency, and the high frequency coefficients are selected by a maximal local variance rule. The resultant image is then reconstructed by using the inverse wavelet transform with the combined wavelet coefficients. The performance of their method is qualitatively and quantitatively compared with some existing fusion approaches. Experimental results show that the proposed method can preserve more useful information and with higher spatial resolution. In Fusion Algorithm of Functional Images and Anatomical Images Based on Wavelet Transform (Zhang J. et al, 2009), Fusion problem of medical functional images and anatomical images is studied in author paper. Based on wavelet multi-scale decomposition the fusion algorithm of functional images and anatomical images is advanced and elaborated, and the method of fusion rule selection is summarized in detail. Using the algorithm, a PET image and a MRI image of a brain are merged. With the index integrating entropy and cross entropy, the fusion result is assessed indicating the validity of the algorithm and the method.

In PET/CT Medical Image Fusion Algorithm Based on Multiwavelet Transform (Liu & Yang, 2010) PET/CT medical image fusion has important clinical significance. As the multiwavelet transform has several particular advantages in comparison with scalar wavelets on image processing, author proposes a medical image fusion algorithm based on multiwavelet transform after in-depth study of wavelet theory. The algorithm achieves PET/CT fusion with wavelet coefficients fusion method. Experimental results show that fusion image combines information of the source images, adds more details and texture information, and achieves a good fusion result. Based on the proposed algorithm we can obtain the best result when using gradient fusion in the low-frequency part and classification fusion in the high frequency part. In Multimodal Medical Image Fusion Based on Integer Wavelet Transform and Neuro-Fuzzy (Kavitha & Chellamuthu, 2010),Medical image fusion is used to derive useful information from multimodality medical image data. The idea is to improve the image content by fusing images like computer tomography

(CT) and magnetic resonance imaging (MRI) images, so as to provide precise information to the doctor and clinical treatment planning system. This paper proposes image fusion based on Integer Wavelet Transform (IWT) and Neuro-Fuzzy. The anatomical and functional images are decomposed using Integer Wavelet Transform. The wavelet coefficients are then fused using neuro-fuzzy algorithm. Then Inverse Integer Wavelet Transform (IIWT) is applied to the fused coefficients to get the fused Image. The performance of this algorithm is compared with image fusion based on Discrete Wavelet Transform (DWT) and neuro-fuzzy using entropy metric. Fusion Symmetry (FS) which quantifies the relative distance in terms of mutual information of the fused image with respect to input images is measured. Fusion Factor (FF) the criterion of maximizing the joint mutual information is also quantified.

Image Fusion using ComplexWavelets (Hill et al,2002)

The fusion of images is the process of combining two or more images into a single image retaining important features from each. Fusion is an important technique within many disparate fields such as remote sensing, robotics and medical applications. Wavelet based fusion techniques have been reasonably effective in combining perceptually important image features. Shift invariance of the wavelet transform is important in ensuring robust subband fusion. Therefore, the novel application of the shift invariant and directionally selective Dual Tree Complex Wavelet Transform (DT-CWT) to image fusion is now introduced. This novel technique provides improved qualitative and quantitative results compared to previous wavelet fusion methods. In Image Fusion Using an Improved Max-lifting Scheme(Yang &Chen E,2009), author presents a novel image fusion algorithm using an improved nonlinear wavelet-decomposition-scheme. The scheme is obtained by introducing redundancy in the max-lifting scheme. Experimental results based on real-world images show that the proposed algorithm produces good results in medical image fusion and visual infra-red image fusion; moreover, it is computationally efficient as a shift-invariant scheme. In Image Fusion Using A 3-D Wavelet Transform (Nikolov et al,1999) Author describe the successful fusion of images acquired from different modalities or instruments is of great importance in many applications, such as medical imaging, microscopic imaging, remote sensing, computer vision, and robotics. With 3-D imaging and image processing becoming widely used, there is a growing need for new 3-D image fusion algorithms capable of combining 3-D multimodality or multisource images. Such algorithms can be used in areas such as 3-D medical imaging (e.g. fusion of Magnetic Resonance (MR) and Computed Tomography (CT) images, fusion of MR and ultrasound (US) images),or 3-D microscopic imaging (e.g. fusion of Co focal Laser Scanning Microscopy (CLSM) and Scanning Acoustic Microscopy (SAM) images, fusion of MR and CLSM images. In Image Fusion Using Multi Decomposition Levels of Discrete Wavelet Transform (Berbar et al,2003) Many researchers are concerning with using powerful image processing tools to achieve high quality images for their applications. Recently, great interest has been arisen on using wavelet transforms to analysis multi-resolution images and to fuse remote sensing images. Image fusion especially in remote sensing applications is one of the fields that growing continuously. Many methods have been proposed to fuse panchromatic and multi-spectral images. This work presents a proposed scheme to fuse the Landsat-7 low-resolution (30m) multi-spectral images and its high- resolution panchromatic images. The proposed image fusion method is based on Two Dimensional Discrete Wavelet Transform (2D-DWT). The method aims to fuse two images in order to produce high resolution (15m) multi-spectral image. It also presents a comparison between the implemented 2D-DWT method and other conventional methods of image fusion using correlation between the output image and the two input images to ascertain the best possible technique that can result in better results of multi-sensor image fusion. The output image of the 2D-DWT technique contains 86.6% of spectral content of the multi-spectral image and 97.08% of the spatial content of panchromatic image.

In Image Fusion: Using A New Framework For Complex Wavelet Transforms (Hill & Canagarajah, 2005)

Image fusion is the process of extracting meaningful visual information from two or more images and combinining them to form one fused image. Image fusion is important within many different image processing fields from remote sensing to medical applications. Previously, real valued wavelet transforms have been used for image fusion. Although this technique has provided improvements over more naive methods, this transform suffers from the shift variance and lack of directionality associated with its wavelet bases. These problems have been overcome by the use of a reversible and discrete complex wavelet transform (the Dual Tree Complex Wavelet Transform DT-CWT). However, the existing structure of this complex wavelet decomposition enforces a very strict choice of filters in order to achieve a necessary quarter shift in coefficient output. This paper therefore introduces an alternative structure to the DTCWT that is more flexible in its potential choice of filters and can be implemented by the combination of four normally structured wavelet transforms. The use of these more common wavelet transforms enables this method to make use of existing optimized wavelet decomposition and recomposition methods, code and filter choice. Image Enhancement using Artificial Neural Network and Fuzzy Logic(Narnaware & Khedgaonkar,2005) Author describe that Digital images are important source of information used for analysis and interpretation. During image acquisition image is degraded up to some extent. Thus we have to go through the process called image enhancement. It improves the visual appearance of an image. This paper presents a technique for image enhancement using artificial neural network and fuzzy logic. It denoise and enhance an image when it is corrupted by different noises such as salt and pepper, gaussian and non gaussian noises. In Image analysis, denoising and enhancing are most important pre-processing and post-processing steps. Several filters have been illustrated till date but have many limitations. In his proposed technique, artificial neural network determines type of noises whereas Fuzzy logic used for denoising and enhancement purpose. Experimental results show the effectiveness of the proposed method by quantitative analysis and visual illustration. Several parameters like PSNR, MSE, AD,NAE are used for performance evaluation. In Medical Ultrasound Image Denoising based on Fuzzy ogic (Shi S. et al,2014), An effective image denoising algorithm based on fuzzy logic is proposed. This algorithm combines the fuzzy logic with the Perona-Malik method. This algorithm builds a new diffusion coefficient in partial derivative equation with the fuzzy membership between the image gradient and the corresponding smooth regions. By defining reasonable fuzzy membership function, the algorithm based on a selective and improved diffusion coefficient and performs adaptively towards different gradients. Simulated experiments show the algorithm can effectively reduce the noise of the image, and its results need not to be adjusted, which can enhance the precision of edge orientation. In Edge Detection Technique by Fuzzy Logic and Cellular Learning Automata using Fuzzy Image (Patel & More, 2013) Edge is the boundary between an object and the background, and identifies the boundary between overlapping and non-over lapping objects. This means that if the edges in an image can be identified accurately, all of the objects can be located and basic properties such as area, perimeter, and shape can be measured. Here fuzzy logic based image processing is used for accurate and noise free edge detection and Cellular Learning Automata (CLA) is used for enhance the previously-detected edges with the help of the repeatable and neighborhood considering nature of CLA. The different result of edge detection technique is compared with fuzzy edge detected and resulting edge is enhanced using CLA. In this paper, all the algorithms and result are prepared in MATLAB.

MAIN FOCUS OF THE CHAPTER

Produce a single image from a set of input images. The fused image should have more complete information which is more useful for human or machine perception (Ligia & Vaida, 2009)

Advantages of Image Fusion

- Improve reliability (by reducing redundant information)
- Improve capability (by enhancing complementary information)[Zhang H. et al, 2007]

Objectives of Image Fusion Schemes

- Extract all the useful information from the source images
- Do not introduce artifacts or inconsistencies which will distract human observers or the following processing.
- Reliable and robust to imperfections such as mis-registration. [Yin X. et al, 2006]

Research Domain Area Where Image Fusion Technique Can Apply

- Computer Vision
- Automatic object detection
- Image processing

Figure 1. Basic idea of image fusion

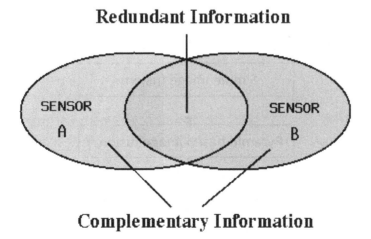

- Parallel and distributed processing
- Robotics Remote sensing

The Evolution of Image Fusion Research

The evolution of image fusion research is shown in Figure 2.

SOLUTIONS AND RECOMMENDATIONS

For that research we choose a technique as a Wavelet Transformation with Adaptive Fuzzy Logic(AFL).

Wavelet Transformation

The wavelet transform is a powerful tool for multiresolution analysis. The multiresolution analysis requires a set of nested multiresolotion sub-spaces as illustrated in the following Figure1 Wavelet theory.

The original space $V0$ can be decomposed into a lower resolution sub-space $V1$, the difference between $V0$ and $V1$ can be represented by the complementary sub-space $W1$. Similarly, we can continue to decompose $V1$ into $V2$ and $W2$. The above graph shows 3-level decomposition. For an N-level decomposition, we will obtain N+1 sub-spaces with one coarsest resolution sub-space Vn and N difference sub-space Wi, i is from 1 to N. Each digital signal in the space $V0$ can be decomposed into some components in each sub-space. In many cases, it's much easier to analyze these components rather than analyze the original signal itself.

2D: Discrete Wavelet Transform (2D-DWT)

Since image is 2-D signal, we will mainly focus on the 2-D wavelet transforms. The following figures show the structures of 2-D DWT with 3 decomposition levels:

After one level of decomposition, there will be four frequency bands, namely Low-Low (LL), Low-High (LH), High-Low (HL) and High-High (HH). The next level decomposition is just apply to the LL band of the current decomposition stage, which forms a recursive decomposition procedure. Thus, an N-

Figure 2. Evolution of image fusion

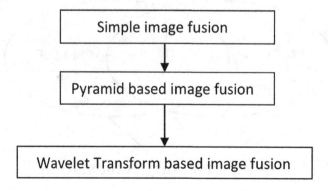

Figure 3. Methodology of image fusion

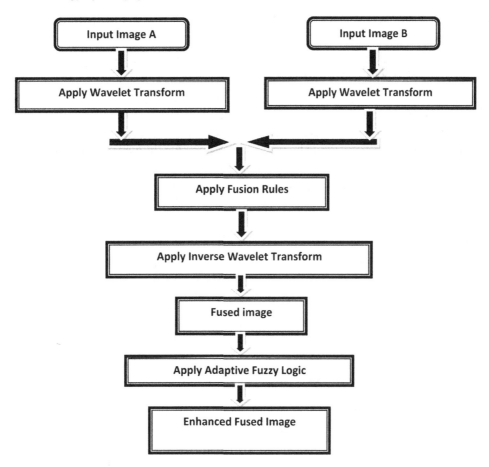

Figure 4. Nested multiresolution space

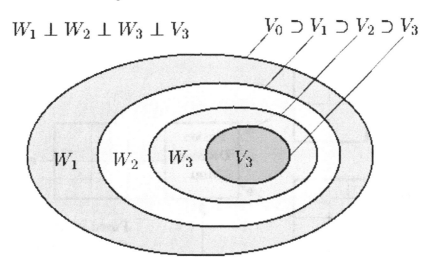

level decomposition will finally have *3N+1* different frequency bands, which include *3N* high frequency bands and just one LL frequency band. The 2-D DWT will have a pyramid structure shown in the above figure. The frequency bands in higher decomposition levels will have smaller size.

Image Fusion Using Wavelet Transform

- The block diagram of a generic wavelet-based image fusion scheme is shown in Figure 6.
- Wavelet transform is first performed on each source images, then a fusion decision map is generated based on a set of fusion rules. The fused wavelet coefficient map can be constructed from the wavelet coefficients of the source images according to the fusion decision map. Finally the fused image is obtained by performing the inverse wavelet transform.

Figure 5. Frequency decomposition

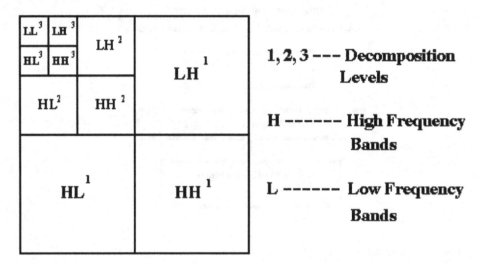

Figure 6. Block diagram for wavelet based image fusion

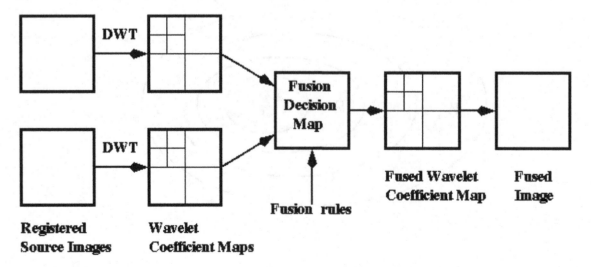

- From the above diagram, we can see that the fusion rules are playing a very important role during the fusion process. Here are some frequently used fusion rules in the previous work

FUZZY SET THEORY AND FUZZY LOGIC

Fuzzy set theory and fuzzy logic offer us powerful tools to represent and process human knowledge represented as fuzzy if-then rules (Narnaware & Khedgaonkar, 2005).

Fuzzy Set Theory

If a certain wavelet coefficient and its neighbouring coefficients are small enough we know that this coefficient is noisy for almost sure and should be put equal to zero. Coefficients above a certain threshold contain the most important image structures and should not be reduced, but coefficients with values around the threshold contain both noise and signals of interest. A good threshold is generally chosen so that most coefficients below the threshold are noise and values above the threshold are signals of interest. In such situation it can be advantageous to use fuzzy set theory as kind of soft-threshold method. Fuzzy set theory is a mathematical extension of the binary set theory.

Fuzzy Logic

Fuzzy image processing consists of fuzzy sets which is the collection of all approaches that understand, represent and process the images, their segments and features (Shi S. et al,2014). It has a human like reasoning ability. If image features are interpreted as linguistic variable then fuzzy if-then rules are used to segment the image.

Fuzzy image processing consisting of three main steps:

Figure 7. Basic fusion rule

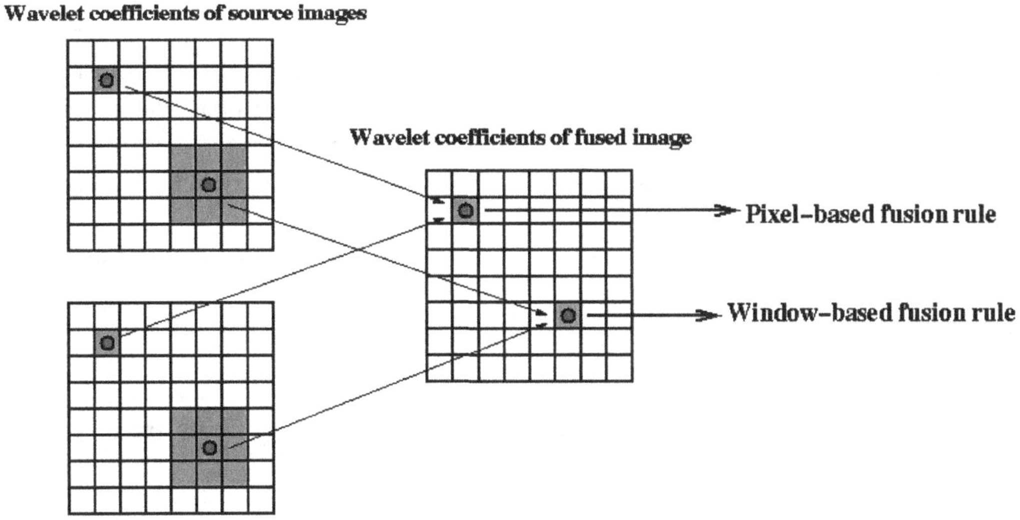

Figure 8. Fusion enhancement

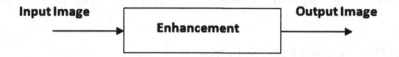

1. Image fuzzification,
2. Membership modification and image
3. Defuzzification as shown in Fig

Fuzzy if-then rules are used to segment the image into different regions, when we interpret the image features as linguistic variables. A simple fuzzy segmentation rule is given as follows: IF the pixel is dark AND its neighborhood is also dark AND homogeneous THEN it belongs to the background. The fuzzification and defuzzification steps are due to the fact that we do not yet possess fuzzy hardware. Therefore, the coding of image data (fuzzification) and decoding of the results (defuzzification) are steps that make it possible to process images with fuzzy techniques. The main power of fuzzy image processing lies in the second step (modification of membership values). After the image data is transformed from input plane to the membership plane (fuzzification), appropriate fuzzy techniques modify the membership values. This can be a fuzzy clustering, a fuzzy rule-based approach, a fuzzy integration approach etc(Patel & More, 2013)

SOLUTION AND RECOMMENDATION

The integration of 2D DWT image fusion with adaptive fuzzy logic in the broader framework of 2D DWT image processing and visualization is the ultimate goal of this study. We would see that the proposed method clearly reduces the complexies in terms of execution time. A future advantage of the method is the ability of incorporate more information (e.g. interscale and/or colour information) by adding other fuzzy rules to improve the noise reduction performance. Future work should be done on this promising issue.

Along this research, some image fusion approaches have been studied. Some of them were found reliable fusion methods, and in conjunction they gave acceptable results in multimodality fusion schemes. But our research would proposed a new hybrid technique for enhancing of image fusion, especially in the area of medical, remote sensing applications. The wellknown DWT Technique combine with adaptive fuzzy logic to reduce uncertainity & redundancy and improve reliability & Capability. The main advantages of the new method are:

Figure 9. The main principle of fuzzy image enhancement

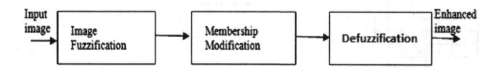

1. The complexity of the method is much lower than the probabilistic one (which results in a lower execution time),
2. Do not lose any noise reduction performance and
3. By adding new fuzzy rules it should be easily extendable to incorporate other information as well (e.g. interscale or interband information).

FUTURE RESEARCH DIRECTION

In the future, we want to integrate other techniques for fusion and testing it for different types of complementary images. Our application is intended to be useful for users who need to fusion multi-modality images for support in useful applications.

REFERENCES

Berbar, M. A., Gahe, S. F., & Ismail, N. A. (2003). *Image Fusion Using Multi Decomposition Levels Of Discrete Wavelet Transform,The Institution of Electrical Engineers*. Stevenage: Michael Faraday House, Six Hills Way.

Cui, Z., Zhang, G., & Wu, J. (2009). Medical Image Fusion Based on Wavelet Transform and Independent Component Analysis.*International Joint Conference on Artificial Intelligence*. IEEE.

Hill, P., Canagarajah, N., & Bull, D. (2002). *Image Fusion using Complex Wavelets*. BMVC-2002.

Hill, P., Canagarajah, N., & Bull, D. (2005). Image Fusion Using A New Framework For Complex Wavelet Transform. IEEE.

Hinal, M. M., & Chavan, P. V. (2015). Fuzzy Logic Based Image Encryption For Confidential Data Transfer Using (2, 2) Secret Sharing Scheme. *International Conference on Advances in Computer Engineering and Applications*. ICACEA.

Kashyap, S. K. (2015). *IR and Color Image Fusion Using Interval Type 2 Fuzzy Logic System*. IEEE. doi:10.1109/CCIP.2015.7100732

Kavitha, C. T., & Chellamuthu, C. (2010). *Multimodal Medical Image Fusion Based on Integer Wavelet Transform and Neuro-Fuzzy*. IEEE.

Licai, Y., Xin, L., & Yucui, Y. (2008). *Medical Image Fusion Based on Wavelet Packet Transform and Self-adaptive Operator*. IEEE.

Ligia, C., & Vaida, M. F. (2009). Medical Image Fusion Based on Discrete Wavelet Transform Using Java Technology. *Proceedings of the ITI 2009 31st Int.Conf. on Information Technology Interfaces*.

Liu, F., Liu, J., & Gao, Y. (2007). Image Fusion Based On Wedgelet And Wavelet.*Proceedings of 2007 International Symposium on Intelligent Signal Processing and Communication Systems*. IEEE.

Liu, Y., & Yang, J. (2010). *PET/CT Medical Image Fusion Algorithm Based on Multiwavelet Transform*. IEEE.

Narnaware, S., & Khedgaonkar, R. (2005). Image Enhancement using Artificial Neural Network and Fuzzy Logic. *IEEE Sponsored 2nd International Conference on Innovations in Information Embedded and Communication Systems ICIIECS'15*. IEEE. doi:10.1109/ICIIECS.2015.7193203

Nikolov, S. G., Bull, D. R., Canagarajah, C. N., Halliwell, M., & Wells, P. N. T. (1999). *Image Fusion Using A 3-D Wavelet Transform. Image Processing And Its Applications*. IEEE.

Patel, D. K., & More, S. A. (2013). Edge Detection Technique by Fuzzy Logic and Cellular Learning Automata using Fuzzy Image Processing. *International Conference on Computer Communication and Informatics*. ICCCI. doi:10.1109/ICCCI.2013.6466130

Ranamuka, N. G., Gayan, R., & Meegama, N. (2013). Detection of hard exudates from diabetic retinopathy images using fuzzy logic. IET.

Shahid, M., & Gupta, S. (2006). Novel Masks for Multimodality Image Fusion using DTCWT. IEEE International Conference on Image Fusion.

Shi, S., Ying, S. Y., & Li, W. Y. (2014). *Medical Ultrasound Image Denoising based on Fuzzy Logic*. IEEE. doi:10.1109/ISDEA.2014.143

Yang, B., & Chen, E. (2009). *Image Fusion Using an Improved Max-lifting Scheme*. IEEE.

Yang, Y., Park, D.S., Huang, S., Fang, Z., & Wang, Z. (2009). Wavelet based Approach for Fusing Computed Tomography and Magnetic Resonance Images. IEEE.

Yin, F. Mickan, & Abbott. (2007). Terahertz Computed Tomographic Reconstruction and its Wavelet-based Segmentation by Fusion. IEEE.

Yin, X., Ferguson, H., Mickan, S. P., & Fischer, B. M. (2006). Information Fusion and Wavelet Based Segment Detection with Applications to the Identification of 3D Target T-ray CT Imaging. *Biomedical Image Fusion Using Wavelet Transform and SOFM Neural Network, 1*, 1189–1194.

Zhang, H., Liu, L., & Nan Lin, N. (2007). A Novel Wavelet Medical Image Fusion Method. *International Conference on Multimedia and Ubiquitous Engineering*.

Zhang, J., Zhou, Z., Jionghua, T., & Ting, L. (2009). *Miao Zhiping Fusion Algorithm of Functional Images and Anatomical Images Based on Wavelet Transform*. IEEE.

KEY TERMS AND DEFINITIONS

Adaptive Fuzzy Logic (AFL): This approach provides us a powerful and flexible image enhancement technique. Image enhancement based on adaptive fuzzy logic that indicates the removing impulse noise, smoothing out non-impulse noise, and enhancing (or preserving) edges and certain other salient structures.

Discrete Wavelet Transform (DFT): This wavelet transform is a very effective signal analysis tool for many problems for which Fourier based methods have been inappropriate.

Enhancement: An increase or improvement in quality of entity.

Fusion: The process of combining two or more things together to form a single composite entity.

Fuzzy Interference System (FIS): A Fuzzy Inference System is a manner of mapping an input space to an output space using fuzzy logic A fuzzy inference system uses fuzzy set theory to map inputs to outputs.

Mutual Information (MI): The mutual information (MI) of two random variables is a measure of the mutual dependence between the two variables.

Peak Signal to Noise Ratio (PSNR): This ratio is often used as a quality measurement between the original and an enhanced image. Better the quality of the enhanced image means the higher the PSNR.

Chapter 9
Big Data:
Techniques, Tools, and Technologies – NoSQL Database

Vinod Kumar
Maulana Azad National Institute of Technology, India

Ramjeevan Singh Thakur
Maulana Azad National Institute of Technology, India

ABSTRACT

With every passing day, data generation is increasing exponentially, its volume, variety, velocity are making it quite challenging to analyze, interpret, visualize for gaining the greater insights from the available data. Billions of networked sensors are being embedded in devices such as smart phones, automobiles, social media sites, laptop, PC's and industrial machines etc. that operates, generate and communicate data. Thus, the data obtained from various resources exists in structured, semi-structured and unstructured form. The traditional database system is not suitable to handle these data formats. Therefore, new tools and techniques are developed to work with these data. NoSQL is one of them. Currently, many NoSQL database are available in the market, each one of them specially designed to solve specific type of data handling problems, most of the NoSQL databases are developed with special attention to problem of business organizations and enterprises. The chapter focuses various aspects of NoSQL as tool for handling the big data.

INTRODUCTION

Big Data analysis involves making "sense" (Oracle White Paper, 2013) out of huge amount of varied data that are in its raw format. Today, technologies of storage devices have attained a great height in storage capacity. The organizations are capable to store the data of big data Category. But only storage of big data is not enough for any organization. The benefit lies in getting the valuable insights from the stored data to help in making planning, decisions and other organization's strategies. The valuable information can only be obtained by analysis of big data (Katal A., et al, 2013). Moreover, the data comes from variety

DOI: 10.4018/978-1-5225-0536-5.ch009

of resources such as smart phones, sensor embedded machines, social media sights, IT log Files, Web servers, email servers etc. Due to the large volume, Variety, Velocity, Variability and Complexity (Katal A., et al, 2013) of Big Data, the analysis task becomes very challenging and difficult. Thus, it requires advanced tools, techniques and specialized data analysis skills over the traditional tools and methods.

It has been obviously noticed that Relational Data Base Management Systems (RDBMS) can no longer handle all the data management issues posed by many currently running application software. It is mostly because of:

1. The large, and constantly increasing, amount of data needed to be stored by many companies/enterprises/diverse organizations.
2. The tremendous query workload needed to access and analyze these data.
3. The need of flexibility in the database schema.

With the arrival of Web 2.0 service, the amount of data managed by large-scale web services has grown exponentially, posing new challenges and infrastructure requirements. This has led to new programming paradigms and architectural choices, such as map-reduce and NoSQL databases/data stores, which make up two of the key peculiarities of the specialized extremely, distributed systems well-known as Big Data architectures. The basic computer infrastructures generally encounter complexity requirements, resulting from the need for efficiency and speed in processing over vast surfacing data sets. This is made possible by taking benefits from the features of new technologies, such as the automatic scaling and replica provisioning of Cloud environments. Although performance is the main issue for the considered applications. Precisely, NoSQL (Olivier Cure, et al. 2011) databases are the next generation databases mostly dealt with some of the points: being non-relational, distributed, open-source and horizontally scalable.

HADOOP DISTRIBUTED FILE SYSTEM (HDFS)

- **Hadoop:** Hadoop (White, 2010) is an Apache Open Source software framework for working with big data. It was created by Doug cutting and Michael J. Cafarella. Doug who was working at yahoo at that time, it named after his son's toy elephant. It was derived from Google technology and put to practice by yahoo and others. But big data is too varied and complex for a one-size-fits-all solution. While Hadoop has surely captured the greatest name, recognition, it is just one of three classes of technologies well suited to storing and managing big data. Hadoop is software framework which means it includes a number of components that were specifically designed to solve large-scale distributed data storage, analysis and retrieval tasks.

Basic Key and Important Terms Related to the Hadoop

- **Open-Source Software:** Open source software is dissimilar from commercial and proprietary software due to the wide and open network of developers that form and handle the programs. Usually, it's free to download, use and contribute to, though more and more commercial versions of Hadoop are making available for use.
- **Framework:** Framework provides users everything needed to develop and run software applications – programs, tool sets, connections, etc.

Figure 1. High level Hadoop architecture
(White, 2010)

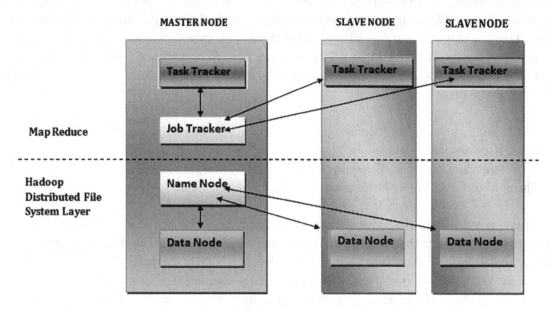

- **Distributed:** Its simply mean, the data is divided and stored across several machines, and computations can be run in parallel across multiple connected machines.
- **Massive storage:** The Hadoop framework can store huge amounts of data by breaking the data into blocks and storing it on clusters of lower-cost commodity hardware.
- **Faster processing:** Hadoop processes large amounts of data in parallel across clusters of tightly connected low-cost computers for quick results.

The Apache Hadoop framework is basically composed of the following modules:

- **Hadoop Common:** It holds libraries and utilities required by other Hadoop modules;
- **Hadoop Distributed File System (HDFS):** When the amount of data outflows the storage capability of a single physical machine, it becomes essential to divide it across a number of distinct machines. Distributed file system manages the storage across a network of machines. because they are network-based, all the complexities of network programming creeps in, thus it make distributed file systems(DFS) more complex than regular disk file systems. For example, one of the biggest challenges is making the file system bear node failure without suffering loss in data. Hadoop comes with a distributed file system called HDFS (Katal A., et al, 2013; Tom White, 2010) which stands for Hadoop Distributed File System. Hadoop integrates with other storage machines such as the local file system. The distributed file-system (DFS) keeps data on commodity hardware (machines) provides very large collective bandwidth across the cluster.
- **YARN:** It is a resource-management platform accountable for managing computing resources in clusters and using them for scheduling of users applications.
- **Map Reduce:** It is a programming paradigm for processing large scale data.

MAP REDUCE: A PROGRAMMING PARADIGM

MapReduce published in 2004 by Google. It is a parallel programming model for processing the huge amount data. Hadoop can run MapReduce (Katal A., et al, 2013) programs written in various languages like Java, Ruby, Python and C++. Applications processing data on Hadoop are written using the Map Reduce (Palit I & Reddy CK, 2012) paradigm. A map Reduce job usually splits the input data-set into independent chunks, which are processed by the map tasks in a completely parallel manner. The framework sorts the outputs of the maps, which are then input to the reduce tasks. Typically, both the input and the output of the jobs are stored in a file system. The framework takes care of scheduling tasks, monitoring them and re-executes the failed tasks.

Map Reduce applications specify the inputs/output locations and supply map and reduce functions via implementation of appropriate Hadoop interfaces such as Mapper and Reducer. These and other parameters comprise the job configuration. The Hadoop job client then submits the job(Jar/executable, etc.) and configuration to the job tracker, which then assumes the responsibility of distributing the software/configuration to the slaves, scheduling tasks and m0onitoring them, provide status and diagnostic information to the job client.

The Map/Reduce framework (White, 2010; Dean et al, 2015) operates exclusively on <Key, Value> i.e., the framework views the input to the job as a set of <Key, Value> pairs and produces a set of <Key, Value> pairs as the out of the job, conceivably of different types.

Map Reduce Limitations

It can't control the order in which the maps or reductions are run in the system. For maximum parallelization, you need maps and reducer do not depend on data generated in the same MapReduce job (i.e. Stateless). A database with an index will always be faster than a map reduce job on un-indexed data. The Reduce operations do not take place until all maps are complete. General assumption that the output of reduce is smaller than the input to map; large data source used to generate smaller final values.

Figure 2. Map reduce, a programming model

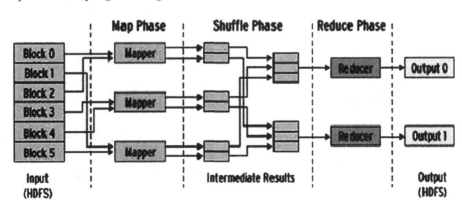

THE DAWN OF NOSQL AS A SOLUTION FOR HANDLING BIG DATA

The word "NoSQL" (Strozzi & Carlo, 2010) was in initially used in 1998 by Carlo Strozzi for the Relational Database Management System, Strozzi NoSQL. Although, Strozzi coined the term mainly to differentiate to his solution from other Relational Database Management

System solutions which make use of Structured Query Language. He used the term NoSQL just for the reason that his database did not expose a SQL interface. Now, the word NoSQL (Not Only SQL) has come to express a large set of databases which do not have characteristics of conventional relational databases and which are usually not queried with SQL. The term revitalized in the current years with giant enterprises and companies like Google, Amazon, Apache by their own data storage centers to amass and process large amounts of data as they emerge in their applications and stirring up other vendors to take part in it. The main characteristics of NoSQL databases are horizontal scaling, replicating and partitioning data over several servers. In recent years, different kinds of NoSQL databases have been produced mainly by practitioners and web enterprise to fulfill their particular requirements regarding performance, maintenance, scalability and feature-set. In the present scenario, our need has changed unlike the some years later we were need. Therefore, currently NoSQL has emerged as a solution for today's data store requirements and has been a subject of talk and research.

- **CAP Theorem:** The NoSQL database follows the concept of CAP (Strozzi & Carlo 2010) (Consistency, Availability, and Partition-Tolerance) Theorem in contrast to ACID (Atomicity, Consistency, Isolation, and Durability) property in relational database management system.
- The CAP theorem, also known as Brewer's Theorem says that you can provide only two out of the following three characteristics: consistency, availability, and partition tolerance. Diverse datasets and different runtime rules cause you to make different trade-offs. The complexity of the data and the scalability of the system also come into play." These three terms states -
- **Consistency:** Every read would get you the most recent write and it is achieved by updating several nodes before allowing further reads.
- **Availability:** Every node (if not failed) always executes queries and availability is achieved by replicating the data across different machines.
- **Partition-Tolerance:** Even if the connections between nodes are down, the other two (Availability & Consistency) promises are kept. The system continues to operate as a whole even if individual servers fail or can't be reached.

HOW NOSQL DATABASES DIFFER FROM TRADITIONAL RELATIONAL DATABASE?

NoSQL database (Stonebraker, 2010) is designed unlike the traditional Relational database management system. NoSQL works going beyond the RDBMS. It solves the problem of limitation of Relational database management system. In today's world to information the variety of the data and its size has grown exponentially. NoSQL is a completely new way of thinking about a database storage system in the modern era of ocean of data. NoSQL (Olivier Cure, et al. 2011) is different in a number of ways from traditional database management system. NoSQL database also tries to handle the unstructured data to a great extent unlike the relational database management system which can handle only structured data.

Future development in database design is greatly focused towards such data storage and management system which will not be only for structured data. It will be able to deal with structured, semi-structured and unstructured data too. Table 1 describes briefly some basics differences (M. Stonebraker, 2010) that make distinction between RDBMS and NoSQL databases-

NEED OF NOSQL DATABASES

The reality is that a relational database model may not be the best solution for all situations. The easiest way to think of NoSQL (Olivier Cure, et al. 2011; Jing Han et al., 2011) is that of a database which does not adhering to the traditional relational database management system (RDMS) structure.

To improve programmer productivity by using a database that better matches an application's needs.

To improve data access performance via some combination of handling larger data volumes, reducing latency, and improving throughput.

WHAT NoSQL DATABASES CAN DO?

It will not be wrong to say that the NoSQL (Olivier Cure, et al. 2011) is the inevitable demand of today's completive world of business. NoSQL solves many problems existing in the traditional database systems. All four types of NoSQL database helps in the manner as follows:

1. The Key-value databases/data stores are usually useful for storing session information, user profiles, preferences, shopping cart data. It should be avoided using Key-value databases when there is need to query by data, have relationships between the data being stored or need to operate on multiple keys at the same time.

Table 1. Comparison of NoSQL database and RDBMS

SL	NoSQL Database	Traditional Relational Database Management System
1.	NoSQL is unstructured way of storing the data.	RDBMS database completely structured way storing of data.
2.	The amount of data stored does not depend on the Physical memory of the system. It can be scaled horizontally as per the requirement.	The amount of data stored mainly depends on the Physical memory of the system.
3.	It can effectively handle million and billions of records	It can Effectively handle few thousands of records
4.	It is never advised for transaction management	It is best suited for transaction management
5.	Processing time depends upon number of cluster machines	The processing time depends on the server machine's configuration
6.	Availability is preferred over consistency.	Consistency is preferred over availability
7.	It follows CAP theorem.	It follows ACID property of transaction
8.	It scales horizontally as well as vertically.	It scales better vertically
9.	There is no need of normalization.	Tables must be normalized.
10.	Most of the NoSQL Databases are schema less	Traditional databases use the strict schema of database design.

2. The document databases are basically helpful for ecommerce-applications, content management systems (CMS), blogging platforms, web analytics; real-time analytics. It should be avoided using document databases for systems that need complex transactions spanning multiple operations or queries against varying aggregate structures.

3. The Column based databases are normally useful for content management systems, blogging platforms, maintaining counters, expiring usage, heavy write volume such as log aggregation. It should be avoided using column databases for systems that are in early development, changing query patterns.

4. The Graph databases are properly suitable for problem spaces where there exists data, such as social networks, spatial data, routing information for goods and money, recommendation engines

AVAILABLE NoSQL DATABASES IN THE MARKET

NoSQL databases have gained great popularity in the market as solution in the substitution traditional databases. NoSQL databases are more or less able to solve the big data problem for handling the mass of data that is being generated each and every moment from various data sources. All big and small companies like Google, Yahoo, Twitter, LinkedIn, Facebook, etc. are not only utilizing the NoSQL Databases but also putting their great efforts in improving it for meeting the company's current needs of handling the huge amount of data for getting the greater insights. Currently, there exist more than 150 NoSQL databases in the present market and catering the facilities with diverse demands in the world of data. The NoSQL databases are broadly classified into four types:

1. Key-Value Store
2. Document Oriented
3. Column Store
4. Graph database

Some popular NoSQL Databases available in the market

KEY-VALUE STORES

In the paper, Bajpayee, Priya and kumar (2015) and DeCandia (2007) stores use the associative array as their fundamental data model. In this model, data is represented as a collection of key-value pairs, such that each possible key appears at most once in the collection. The key-value model is one of the simplest non-trivial data models, and richer data models are often implemented on top of it.

- **Redis:** Redis is a data structure server. It is open-source, networked, in-memory, and stores keys with optional durability.
- **Riak:** Riak is a distributed NoSQL key-value data store that offers extremely high availability, fault tolerance, operational simplicity and scalability. In addition to the open-source version, it comes in a supported enterprise version and a cloud storage version that is ideal for cloud computing environments.

- **Oracle NOSQL Database:** It is a distributed key-value database and designed to provide highly reliable, scalable and available data storage across a configurable set of systems that function as storage nodes. NoSQL and the Enterprise Data is stored as key-value pairs, which are written to particular storage node(s), based on the hashed value of the primary key. Storage nodes are replicated to ensure high availability, rapid failover in the event of a node failure and optimal load balancing of queries.
- **TreodeDB:** It is written in Scala and replicas vote on writes and reads also Hashes keys onto array of replica cohorts. It provides multi version concurrency Control and provides multi-row atomic writes.
- **Sophia:** It is a modern embeddable key-value NoSQL database developed for a high load environment. It is implemented as a small C-written, BSD-licensed library. It is equipped with unique architecture that was created as a result of research and rethinking of primary algorithmical constraints, associated with a getting popular Log-file based data structures.

DOCUMENT-ORIENTED DATABASES

Document-oriented databases are one of the main categories of NoSQL databases. Document oriented database is developed for storing, retrieving and managing the document-oriented information. The central concept of a document-oriented database is that Documents. In contrast to relational database in which tuple (Row) is the central concept. Document oriented database system is designed around the abstract notion of "Document".

- **MongoDB:** MongoDB is a document database that provides high performance, high availability, and easy scalability. A MongoDB deployment hosts a number of databases. A manual: database holds a set of collections. . Documents have dynamic schema. Dynamic schema means that documents in the same collection do not need to have the same set of fields or structure, and common fields in a collection's documents may hold different types of data.
- **Couchbase Server:** Couchbase Server, originally known as Membase, is an open source, distributed (shared-nothing architecture) NoSQL document-oriented database that is optimized for interactive applications.
- **FatDB:** FatDB is the next generation NoSQL database for Windows that extends database functionality by integrating Map Reduce, a work queue, file management system, high-speed cache, and application services
- **ArangoDB:** ArangoDB is an open source, multi model database that combines a document store with a graph database. This combination allows you to model your data with a lot of flexibility. I will show you how ArangoDB is different from other NoSQL database – from its support for transactions to the powerful query language AQL.
- **RavenDB:** RavenDB is a transactional, open-source Document Database written in .NET, and offering a flexible data model designed to address requirements coming from real-world systems. RavenDB allows you to build high-performance, low-latency applications quickly and efficiently.
- **OrientDB:** OrientDB is an open source NoSQL database management system written in Java. It is a document-based database, but the relationships are managed as in graph databases with direct connections between records. It supports schema-less, schema-full and schema-mixed modes.

- **BaseX:** BaseX is a native and light-weight XML database management system and XQuery processor, developed as a community project on GitHub.It is specialized in storing, querying, and visualizing large XML documents and collections. BaseX is platform-independent and distributed under a permissive free software license.

COLUMN STORE

In the paper, R. Bajpayee, S. Priya and Vinod kumar (2015), the column of a distributed database is a NoSQL object of the lowest rank in a key space. It is a row (a key-value pair) comprising of three elements.

Unique Name: Column is referenced by it.
Value: The substance of the column. It can contain diverse types, like AsciiType, LongType, TimeUUID-Type, and UTF8Type among others.
Timestamp: The system timestamp used to resolve the valid content.

- ○ **Cassandra:** Apache Cassandra is an open source distributed database management system designed to handle large amounts of data across many commodity servers, providing high availability with no single point of failure. It is being used by facebook and twiter for handling the huge query generated in social media. Initially, it is released in Year 2008. It is open source and supports windows, Linux and OSX.
- ○ **Big Table:** BigTable is designed with semi-structured data storage in mind. It is a large map that is indexed by a row key, column key, and a timestamp. Each value within the map is an array of bytes that is interpreted by the application. Every read or write of data to a row is atomic, regardless of how many different columns are read or written within that row.
- ○ **HBase:** HBase is an open source, non-relational, distributed database modeled after Google's BigTable and written in Java. It is developed as part of Apache Software Foundation's Apache Hadoop project and runs on top of HDFS (Hadoop Distributed File system), providing BigTable-like capabilities for Hadoop.
- ○ **BangDB:** BangDB is a multi-flavored distributed key value nosql data store. The goal of BangDB is to be fast, reliable, robust, scalable and easy to use data store for various data management services required by applications.
- ○ **Sedna Xml:** Sedna is an open source database management system that provides native storage for XML data. The distinctive design decisions employed in Sedna are:
    - ▪ Schema-based clustering storage strategy for XML data and
    - ▪ Memory management based on layered address space.

GRAPH DATABASE

R. Bajpayee, S. Priya and Vinod kumar (2015) discusses, the graph database is one of the abstract types of data store. It is based on the graph theory and uses the nodes along with edges to represent and store the data. In graph database each and every element contains a direct to its adjacent elements and no index lookups are necessary.

- **Neo4j:** It is most popular Database in Graph.Neo4j is an open-source graph database, implemented in Java. Neo4j is ACID compliant. Its Java based but has bindings for other languages, including Ruby and Python.
- **WhiteDB:** WhiteDB is a fast lightweight graph/N-tuples shared memory database library written in C with focus on speed, portability and ease of use. Both for Linux and Windows, dual licensed with GPLv3 and a free nonrestrictive royalty-free commercial license.

COMPARATIVE STUDY OF NOSQL DATABASES

Since, it is already discussed that there are four types of NoSQL databases name Key-Value, Document Oriented, Column Store and Graph Database. The authors R. Bajpayee, S. Priya and Vinod kumar (2015), in the following given tables summarized information of various NoSQL Databases are put together.

Key-Value Stores

Summary of key-value stores type databases is shown in Table 2.

Document-Oriented Databases

Summary of document-oriented databases is shown in Table 3.

Column Store

Summary of Column Store type databases is shown in Table 4.

Graph Database

Summary of Graph Type Databases is shown in Table 5.

INTEGRATION OF NOSQL DATABASE

Simple NOSQL Integration Overview

Implementation and integration of NOSQL database for making it functional to obtain the desired result is a very important and inevitable task. It is a little complex task because of diverse data model used in the NoSQL databases. Here, Olivier Cure, Robin Hecht, Chan Le Duc & Myriam Lamolle (2011) focuses on a simple integration overview of integration has been discussed for the sake of convenience to understand the role of NoSQL database.

To facilitate the querying of NoSQL databases within a data integration (Segev et al, 2013) framework. Following step will take place:

Table 2. Summary of key-value stores type databases

SL	Name	Initial/Stable Release	License	Language	Developer	Characteristic
1	Redis	2009/2014	BSD Open Source	C	Salvatore Sanfilippo	Consistency Partition Tolerance Persistence
2	Riak	2009/2014	Apache Open Source Proprietary	Erlang	Basho Technologies	High Availability Partition Tolerance Persistence
3	Aerospike	2012/2014	AGPL Proprietary	C	Aerospike	Persistence
4	Voldemort	2009/2014	Apache Open Source	Java	LinkedIn	Consistency High Availability Partition Tolerance
5	MemcacheDB	2008/2014	BSD	C	Danga Interactive	Consistency Partition Tolerance Persistence
6	Hypertable	2010/2013	GPL Open Source	C++	Hypertable Inc	Consistency Partition Tolerance Persistence
7	Hibari	2010/2013	Apache Open Source	Erlang	Hibari developers	Strongly Consistent Highly available
8	STSdb W4.0	2011/2014	GPL Open Source	C#	STS Soft SC	Consistency High Availability
9	FoundationDB	2013/2014	Proprietary	Flow, C++	FoundationDB	Consistency High Availability Partition Tolerance Persistence
10	DynamoDB	2012/2013	Proprietary	Java, .NET	Amazon.com	Consistency High Availability
11	Tokyo Cabinet	2007/2009	GPL	C	FAL Labs	Robust High Availability
12	Berkeley DB	1994/2014	AGPLv3	C	Sleepycat Software, later Oracle Corporation	Multi Version Concurrency ACID
13	Scalaris	/2014	Apache License 2.0	Erlang	Apache	Concurrency Replication ACID
14	hamsterdb	2005/2014	Apache	C/C++	RockSolid SQL, Tony Bain	ACID

1. Define a mapping language between the target and the sources which takes into account the denormalization part of NoSQL databases. This is realized by storing preferred access paths for a given mapping affirmation. Moreover, this mapping language incorporates features dealing with conflicting data.
2. Take the help of Bridge Query Language (BQL) that enables a transformation from an SQL query defined over the target to the query executed over a given source.
3. Prototype example of implementation which generates query programs for a popular document oriented database, namely MongoDB.

Table 3. Summary of Document-Oriented Databases (R. Bajpayee et al, 2015)

SL	Name	Initial/Stable Release	License	Language	Developer	Characteristic
1	MongoDB	2009/2014	1AGPL Open Source	C++,	MongoDB Inc.	Consistency Partition Tolerance Persistence
2	Couchbase Server	2011/2014	Apache	C/C++	Couchbase, Inc.	Consistency High Availability Persistence
3	Apache Jackrabbit	2004/2014	Apache Open Source	Java	Apache Software Foundation	Consistency High Availability Persistence
4	CouchDB	2005/2014	Apache Open Source	Erlang	Apache Software Foundation	High Availability Partition Tolerance Persistence
5	FatDB	2012/2013	Proprietary	C#	Free Community	Consistency High Availability Partition Tolerance Persistence
6	SimpleDB	2007/2013	Proprietary	Python, Perl	Amazon	High Availability
8	ArangoDB	2012/2014	Apache	C#, D, ruby, python, Java, Python	Apache	Consistency Persistence
9	RavenDB	2010/2014	AGPL Open Source Proprietary	.NET	RavenDB	Consistency High Availability Partition Tolerance Persistence
10	MarkLogic	2003/2011	Proprietary	C++	Mark Logic Community	Consistency High Availability Partition Tolerance Persistence
11	OrientDB	2001/2010	Apache	Java	Orient Technologies LTD	Consistency High Availability Partition Tolerance Persistence
12	BaseX	1983/2012	BSD Open Source	Java	BaseX Team	High Availability
13	Solr	2004/2014	Apache	Java	Apache Software Foundation	High Availability
14	djondb	2012/2014	GPL LGPL Open Source Proprietary	C++	Community	Consistency
15	iBoxDB	2012/2014	Persistence	Java,c#	Community	Concurrency Transaction support

Example

In the following document oriented database (MongoDB) stores information of drug aimed at an application targeting the general public. According to features proposed by the application software, two

Table 4. Summary of Column Store type databases (R. Bajpayee et al, 2015)

SL	Name	Initial/Stable Release	License	Language	Developer	Characteristic
1	Cassandra	2008/2014	Apache Open Source	Java	Apache Software Foundation	High Availability Partition Tolerance Persistence
2	Big Table	2005/2010	Proprietary GPLv2	C,C++, JAVA	AGPL Open Source Proprietary	Consistency High Availability Partition Tolerance Persistence
3	HBase	2012/2014	Apache Open Source	Java	Apache Software Foundation	Consistency Partition Tolerance Persistence
4	BangDB	2008/2014	BSD	C++	IQLECT	Consistency High Availability Partition Tolerance Persistence
5	Hazelcast	2003/2014	Open Source	Java	Apache 2	Consistency High Availability Partition Tolerance
6	Sedna Xml	2003/2014	Apache Open Source	C, C++	Apache License 2.0	Durability Consistency
7	Accumulo	2013/2014	Apache License 2.0	Java	Apache Software Foundation	Consistency High Availability Partition Tolerance Persistence
8	cloudera	2004/2014	Apache Softw are Foundation	Java, C, C++, Python, and Ruby	Cloudera, Inc.	High Availability
10	MonetDB	2004/2014	MonetDB License (based on the MPL 1.1)	MonetDB License	MonetDB Developer Team	Consistency Concurrency
12	Apache Flink (incubating)	2013/2014	Apache License, Version 2.0	Java,scale	incubator-flink development	Scalable Reliable Fast Hadoop Compatible
13	Hypertable	2009/2013	GNU General Public License 2.0	C++	Hypertable Inc.	Concurrency Consistency Replication

so-called collections are taken:

drugD and *therapD*. drugD keeps documents revealing drug related information whereas therapD contains documents with information about therapeutic classes and drugs used for it.

Each *drugD* document is recognized by a drug identifier. In this example, its attributes are limited to the name of the product, its price, pharmaceutical lab and a list of therapeutic classes. The key for *therapD* documents is a string corresponding to the therapeutic class name. It contains a single attribute corresponding to the list of drug identifiers treating this therapeutic class. Figure presents an extract of this database. Finally, in order to ensure an efficient search to patients an index on the attribute name of the *drugD* document is defined.

Table 5. Summary of Graph Type Databases(R. Bajpayee et al, 2015)

SL	Name	Initial/Stable Release	License	Language	Developer	Characteristic
1	Neo4j	2007 2007/2014s	AGPL GPL Open Source	Java	Neo Technology	High Availability Partition Tolerance Persistence
2.	FlockDB	2010/2012	Apache License	Scala, Java, Ruby	Twitter	Multi versioning Concurrency Consistency
3	Meronymy	1996/2012	Open Source	C++	Community Development	High Performance ACID Transation
4.	Filament	2012/2014	BSD	Java	Filament Inc.	High Availabity Multi version Concurrency
5	BrightstarDB	2001/2014	MIT License	C#	GitHub	Flexibility Scalability Performance
6	WhiteDB	#731642/2013	GPLv3 and a free commercial licence	C	WhiteDB Team	Protability Prtsistence Concurrency
7	Bigdata	2012/2014	GPLv2, evaluation license, or commercial license.	Java	Systap Software Company	High Performance High availabity
9	AllegroGraph	2004/2014	Proprietary commercial software	C#, C, Common Lisp, Java, Python	Franz, Inc.	Atomicity Consistency Isolation Durability
10	Trinity	2010/2014	Proprietary	C#, C, X64 Assembly	Microsoft	Highly concurrency Concsistency
11	HyperGraphDB	2001/2010	LGPL	Java	Kobrix Inc.	High scalability
12	InfoGrid	2008/2011/	AGPLv3, free for small entities	Java	Netmesh Inc.	Light Weight
13	TITAN	2012/2014	Open Source with liberal Apache 2	Java, Blueprints, REST,	Community	Consistency High availability Fault tolerance
14	DEX	2008/2014	Dual-licensed	Java, .NET, C++, Blueprints Interface	Sparsity Technologies	High Performance
15	Infinite Graph	2010/2014	Evaluation (EULA), and commercial	Java	Objectivity, Inc.	Highly Scalable

ORACLE NOSQL DATABASE INTEGRATION

Although some of near the beginning NoSQL solutions built their systems atop existing relational database engines, they speedily came at conclusion that such systems were developed for SQL -based access patterns and latency demands that are reasonably different from those of NoSQL databases, so these same organizations started to develop new storage layers. On the contrary, Oracle's Berkeley DB artifact row was the original key and value store; Edition of Oracle Berkeley DB Java has been in com-

Figure 3. Data integration overview architecture
(Olivier Cure et al, 2011)

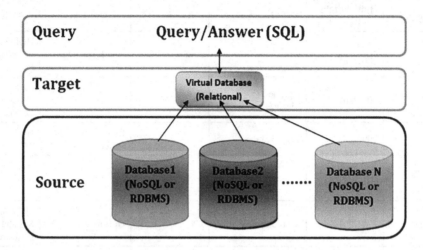

Figure 4. Example of document oriented NoSQL database
Olivier Cure et al (2011)

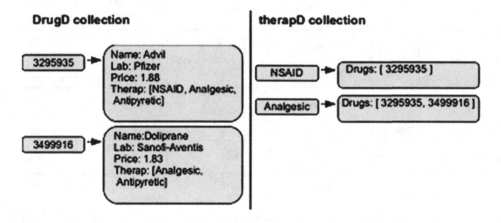

mercial use for more than many years. By using Oracle Berkeley DB Java as the fundamental storage engine beneath a NoSQL database system, Oracle brought enterprise stability, High Availability and robustness, to the NoSQL landscape.

In addition, until newly, integrating NoSQL solutions with an enterprise application architecture required physical integration and configurable/custom development; Oracle's NoSQL Database/data store provides all the needed features of NoSQL solutions necessary for seamless integration into an enterprise application architecture.

Figure 5 depicts how Oracle's NoSQL data stores fits into a canonical *Acquire-Organize-Analyze* (*Oracle White Paper, 2013*) Data-Cycle Ecosystem. The Adapters provided by Oracle allows the Oracle NoSQL Database/Data stores to integrate with a Hadoop and MapReduce framework. Moreover it can also be integrated with Oracle Database in -database MapReduce, R-based analytics, Data Mining, or whatever business needs demand.

Figure 5. Oracle NoSQL Database integrates seamlessly into the data management (Dean et al, 2015)

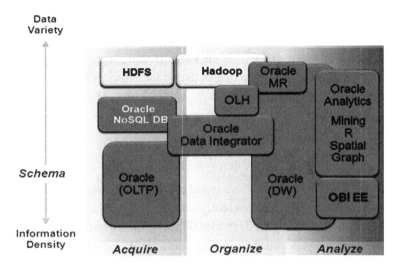

Acquire Big Data

This is the initial step in any analysis system. Hereafter the next phases came into play for processing of Data. The acquisition stage (Oracle White Paper, 2013) is one of the most important changes in infrastructure from the days before big data. Because big data addresses to data streams of higher variety and higher velocity, the infrastructure essential to support the acquisition of big data must show low, expected latency in both acquiring data and in processing brief and easy queries; be able to handle very large transaction size, often in a distributed environment; and support flexible, dynamic data structures. NoSQL databases are frequently used to acquire and store big data. They are fit for highly scalable and dynamic data structures. The data stored in a NoSQL database is normally of a high diversity because the systems are planned to simply acquire all data without categorizing and parsing the data into a fixed schema.

For instance, NoSQL databases/data stores are often applied to gather and store social media data. While customer utilizing applications often modify, underlying storage structures are kept simple and convenient.

Instead of designing a schema with relationships between entities, these simple structures frequently just contain a main key to identify the data point, and then a content container keeping the relevant data (such as a customer id and a customer profile). This simple and dynamic structure permits modifications to take place without costly reorganizations at the storage.

Organize Big Data

The second step in big data processing involves the organization of data in the storage system. In traditional data warehousing words, organizing data (Oracle White Paper, 2013) is said data integration. Because there is such a lofty size of data, there is a probability to organize data at its primary destination, thus saving both time and money by not going around huge volumes of data. The infrastructure necessary for managing big data must be capable to process and operate data in the original storage position; support very high throughput to deal with large data sets processing steps; and handle a large variety of data formats, from unstructured to structure. Hadoop is a latest technology that permits huge data volumes to be controlled and processed while keeping the data on the original data storage location. Hadoop Distributed File System (HDFS) is the long-standing storage arrangement for web logs for instance. These web logs are turned into browsing behavior (sessions) by running MapReduce programs on the cluster and generating aggregated results on the same cluster. These accumulated results are then loaded into a Relational DBMS system.

Analyze Big Data

The analysis task (*Oracle White Paper, 2013*) is carried out in a distributed platform, where some datasets will reside where it was originally kept and be clearly accessed from a data warehouse. The infrastructure need for the task of analyzing (Ekanayake J, et al. 2008) big data must be capable to maintain deeper analytics such as statistical analysis and data mining, on a wider variety of data types kept in diverse systems; extend to extreme data volumes; provide faster response times driven by changes in behavior; and automate decisions based on analytical models. Most importantly, the infrastructure must be able to integrate analysis on the combination of big data and traditional enterprise data. New insight comes not just from analyzing new data, but from analyzing it within the context of the old to provide new perspectives on old problems.

For example, analyzing inventory data from a smart vending machine in combination with the events calendar for the venue in which the vending machine is located, will dictate the optimal product mix and replenishment schedule for the vending machine.

APPLICATIONS OF NOSQL DATABASES

Day By day, the use of NoSQL in different small and large organization is gaining momentum. In this section, some key areas and their subareas are pointed out to put light on the importance and use of NoSQL Databases. Hugh J. Watson (2014) describes areas in which NoSQL databases are useful for dealing with huge amount and diverse data generated from different application (C.L. Philip Chen & Chun-Yang Zhang, 2014) in the organizations. These are as follows

Marketing

- Campaign management and optimization
- Micro segmentation of Consumers and markets
- Location-based marketing
- Cross-selling and up-selling
- Sentiment Analysis
- One-to-one Marketing
- 360 –degree customer view

Finance

- Risk Management
- Fraud Detection and Prevention
- Wealth Management
- Anti- Money Laundering
- Credit risk, scoring and analysis

Government

- Fraud and Threat prediction and detection
- Cyber Security
- Compliance and Regulatory Analysis

Health Care

- Patient care quality and Outcomes Analysis
- Reimbursement modeling
- Public Health Reporting
- Clinical data Transparency
- Public Health Surveillance and Response
- Clinical Trial Design and analysis

Insurance

- Risk Assessment and avoidance
- Claims fraud detection
- Call center workload analysis
- Telematics-optimized underwriting
- Customer value management
- Catastrophic planning

Retail

- Merchandizing and market basket Analysis
- Supply chain Management and analytics
- Loyalty program management
- Event/Behavior based targeting
- Cross-Channel Customer service optimization

Telecommunications

- Customer churn Prevention
- Call detail record analysis
- Network planning and optimization
- Mobile user location analysis
- New product research and Development

FUTURE RESEARCH DIRECTIONS

The future work will focus on benchmarking and performance evaluation of various NoSQL databases available with respect to the size of datasets as well as the different type of the data sets.

CONCLUSION

This chapter concludes with the brief discussion of different aspects of NoSQL databases as a good alternative of traditional databases. It is found that NoSQL Database brings enterprise quality storage and performance to the highly-available, widely distributed NoSQL environment. Its commercial system delivers outstanding performance as well as robustness and reliability, and no single point of failure. Today, the use of and demand of NoSQL is in high. With whole discussion, it is now obvious that Most of the company's requirement is to utilize and development such as system which can handle the growing amount of unstructured data. The NoSQL database research area engraves a huge opportunity to make it mature and robust and economic.

REFERENCES

Bajpayee, Priya, & Kumar. (2015). Big Data: A Brief investigation on NoSQL Databases. *International Journal of Innovations & Advancement in Computer Science, 4*(1).

Big Data Analytics Advanced Analytics in Oracle Database. (2013). Oracle White Paper.

Chen, C. L. P., & Zhang, C.-Y. (2014). Data-intensive applications, challenges, techniques and technologies: A survey on Big Data. *Information Sciences, 275*, 314–347. doi:10.1016/j.ins.2014.01.015

Cure, O., Hecht, R., Le Duc, C., & Lamolle, M. (2011). Data Integration over NoSQL Stores Using Access Path Based Mappings. DEXA 2012.

Davenport, T. H., & Patil, D. J. (2012). Data Scientist: The Sexiest Job of the 21st Century. *Harvard Business Review, 90*(10), 70–76. PMID:23074866

Dean & Ghemawat. (2004). *MapReduce: Simplified Data Processing on Large Clusters.* Academic Press.

Dean & Ghemawat. (2015). *Map Reduce: Simplified Data Processing on Large Clusters.* Google, Inc.

DeCandia, G. (2007). Dynamo: Amazon's Highly Available Key-Value Store.*Proc. 21st ACM SIGOPS Symp. Operating Systems Principles (SOSP 07)*. doi:10.1145/1294261.1294281

Ekanayake, J., Pallickara, S., & Fox, G. (2008). Mapreduce for data intensive scientific analyses. *Proceedings of IEEE Fourth International Conference on eScience*.

Frank, L. (2011). Countermeasures against consistency anomalies in distributed integrated databases with relaxed ACID properties. *Innovations in Information Technology (IIT),International Conference*.

Gilbert & Lynch. (2002). *Brewer's conjecture and the feasibility of consistent, available, partition-tolerant web services*. SigAct News.

Gottfrid, D. (2007). *Self-service, Prorated Super Computing Fun!* Retrieved from: http://open.blogs.nytimes.com/2007/11/01/self-service-prorated-super-computing-fun/

Han, J., Haihong, E., Le, G., & Du, J. (2011). Survey on NoSQL database. *Pervasive Computing and Applications (ICPCA). 2011 6th International Conference*.

Herodotou, H., Lim, H., Luo, G., Borisov, N., & Dong, L. (2014). Starfish: a self-tuning system for big data analytics.*The Biennial Conference on Innovative Data Systems Research*.

Kaisler, S., & Armour, F., Espinosa, & Money. (2013). Big data: issues and challenges moving forward. *IEEE,46th Hawaii International Conference on System Sciences*.

Kambatla, K., Kollias, G., Kumar, V., & Grama, A. (2014). Trends in big data analytics. *Journal of Parallel and Distributed Computing, 74*(7), 2561–2573. doi:10.1016/j.jpdc.2014.01.003

Katal, A., Wazid, M., & Goudar, R. H. (2013). Big data: issues, challenges, tools and good practices. *Contemporary Computing (IC3), 2013 Sixth International Conference*.

Manyika, J., Chui, M., Brown, B., Bughin, J., Dobbs, R., Roxburgh, C., & Byers, A. H. (2011). *Big data: The next frontier for innovation, competition, and productivity*. McKinsey Global Institute. Retrieved from: http://www.mckinsey.com/insights/business_technology/big_data_the_next_frontier_for_innovation

Masudianpour, A. (2013). *An Introduction to Redis Server, an Advanced Key Value Database*. SlideShare. Retrieved from: www.slideshare.net/masudianpour/redis-25088079

McCreadie, R., Macdonald, C., & Ounis, I. (2012). MapReduce indexing strategies: Studying scalability and efficiency. *Journal of Information Processing and Management: An International Journal, 48*(5), 873-888.

Oracle NoSQL Database. (2012). Oracle White Paper.

Palit, I., & Reddy, C. K. (2012). Scalable and parallel boosting with MapReduce. *IEEE Transactions on Knowledge and Data Engineering, 24*(10), 1904–1916. doi:10.1109/TKDE.2011.208

Pillar Global. (n.d.). Retrieved from: http://www.3pillarglobal.com/insights/exploring-the-different-types-of-nosql-databases

Saecker, M., & Markl, V. (2013). Big Data Analytics on Modern Hardware Architectures: A Technology Survey. *Springer Lecture Notes in Business Information Processing*, *138*, 125–149. doi:10.1007/978-3-642-36318-4_6

Sagiroglu, S., & Sinanc, D. (2013). Big Data: A review. *Collaboration Technologies and Systems (CTS), 2013 International Conference.*

Segev, A., Jung, & Jung. (2013). Analysis of technology trends based on big data. *Big Data (BigData Congress), 2013 IEEE International Congress.*

Sheth & Amit. (2014). Transforming big data into smart data: deriving value via harnessing volume, variety, and velocity using semantic techniques and technologies. *Data Engineering (ICDE). IEEE 30th International Conference.*

Shukla, Pandey, & Kumar. (2015). Big Data Framework: At a Glance. *International Journal of Innovations & Advancement in Computer Science, 4.*

Singh, S., & Singh, N. (2012). Big data analytics. *IEEE, International Conference on Communication, Information & Computing Technology (ICCICT).*

Srivastava & Divesh. (2014). Data quality: the other face of big data. *Data Engineering (ICDE). IEEE 30th International Conference.*

Stonebraker, M. (2010). Sql databases vs. nosql databases. *Communications of the ACM*, *53*(4), 10–11. doi:10.1145/1721654.1721659

Strozzi & Carlo. (2010). *NoSQL – A relational database management system.* Retrieved from: http://www.strozzi.it/cgibin/CSA/tw7/I/en_US/nosql/Home%20Page

Watson. (2014). Big Data Tutorial: Concepts, Technologies and Applications. *Communications of the Association for Information Systems*, *34.*

White. (2010). *Hadoop: The Definitive Guide* (3rd ed.). O'Reilly Media.

White, T. (2012). *Hadoop: The Definitive Guide* (3rd ed.). O'Reilly.

Wielki, J. (2013). Implementation of the big data concept in organizations - possibilities, impediments and challenges. *Computer Science and Information Systems (FedCSIS), 2013 Federated Conference.*

Xiang, P., Hou, R., & Zhou, Z. (2010). Cache and consistency in nosql. *Computer Science and Information Technology (ICCSIT).3rd IEEE International Conference.*

Yahoo Launches World's Largest Hadoop Production Application. (2008). Retrieved from http://developer.yahoo.net/blogs/hadoop/2008/02/yahoo-worlds-largest-production-hadoop.html

KEY TERMS AND DEFINITIONS

CAP Theorem: The NoSQL database follows the concept of CAP (Consistency, Availability, and Partition-Tolerance).

Hadoop Distributed File System (HDFS): Distributed file system manages the storage across a network of machines.

Hadoop: Hadoop is an Apache Open Source software framework for dealing with big data.

MapReduce: MapReduce is the programming framework that works upon the HDFS for processing on data in distributed environment.

NoSQL: NoSQL stores are an alternative and appropriate solution against the limitations of relational database management system.

Section 3
Data Mining: Utilization and Application

Chapter 10
Bombay Stock Exchange of India:
Patterns and Trends Prediction Using Data Mining Techniques

Sachin Kamley
SATI, India

Shailesh Jaloree
SATI, India

R. S. Thakur
MANIT, India

ABSTRACT

Stock market nature is considered to be dynamic and susceptible to quick changes because it depends on various factors like share price, fundamental variables like P/E ratio, dividend yield etc. election results, rumors etc. Now a day's prediction is an important process which determines the future worth of a company. The successful prediction brings motivation and awareness in stock community as well as economic growth of the country. In past various theories and methods like Efficient Market Hypothesis (EMH), Random Walk Theory, fundamental and technical analyses have been proposed. These methods or combination of methods have not got as much success even yet because these methods are very complex and time consuming and performed well on short data. These days stock market users mostly rely on intelligent trading system which would be help them to predict share prices based on various situations and conditions. Data mining is a broad area and also supports various business intelligence techniques. It has mastery to raise various financial issues like buying/selling security, bond analysis, contract analyses etc. in this study various prediction techniques like linear regression, multiple regression, association rule mining, clustering, neural network have been proposed and their significant performances will be compared by Bombay Stock Exchange (BSE) data.

DOI: 10.4018/978-1-5225-0536-5.ch010

INTRODUCTION

In these days stock market index prediction is an important concern in finance and business but over the years we have been seen it fluctuating over time and most important affects the stock user's mentality. So determining more effective ways and adopting more and more profitable tools and techniques for stock market index prediction in order to make more accurate decision will be challenging for stock user's community (Abdoh & Jouhare, 1996). There are several stock exchanges are available in India due to their increasing profit and growing user's. Bombay Stock Exchange (BSE) is one of the fastest (speed 200 micro seconds) and more prominent stock exchange over the world. It is established in 1875. and has total 5500 companies listed making it world's no. one exchange in terms of listed companies (Abdulsalam et al., 2011; Ghezelbash, 2012). Over 140 years BSE has become eye witness of growth of Indian corporate sector by providing it an efficient capital raising platform. At the March 2015 end the total market capitalization calculated 1.68 USD Trillion which make it fifth largest leading exchange in the world (Ankerst, 2001). Data mining is a branch of computer science which is designated for finding hidden patterns (previously unknown) from large amount of data (Han & Kamber, 2006). It is one of important step of Knowledge Discovery in Databases (KDD). In today's competitive world huge amount of information stored in databases. The retrieval and analysis of this information makes data mining important and necessary technique. Financial institution such as stock market produces a vast amount of data throughout the year that provides a road map for data mining tools and techniques and helps to handle complex problems (Fayyad et al., 1996). Over the years various researchers has paid attention of solving these problems and gained a large profit. Obviously this will help the enhancing the data mining research in future. At a time research in data mining is increasing day by day due to the it's applicability in various fields and increasing information. Data mining in finance specifies various criteria like profit maximization, multi -resolution forecast (days, weekly and yearly) so it will be big challenge to data mining community to predict useful trends and patterns with reasonable cost and short span of time (Fayyad et al., 1996; Han & Kamber, 2006). Since many years stock price prediction is an interesting task for stock users. In the literature number of methods is applied to accomplish this task. There are various approaches of prediction like informal ways (like chart analysis) to formal ways (like regression methods). The only aim of prediction is to reduce uncertainty associated to investment decision making (Boston, 1998).

BACKGROUND

Data mining is the systematic process of searching hidden patterns and finding relationship between variables and item sets of data. The ultimate goal of data mining process is prediction and prediction data mining plays important role in financial applications (Hong Se & Weiss M., 2001; Tiwari & Thakur, 2015). Since three decades various researcher have contributed in stock market field. Here we have presented some significant research work. Beaver (1966) has proposed a comprehensive study on various financial ratios for bankruptcy prediction model. He concluded that cash flow to debt ratio was the best predictor for bankruptcy among the financial variables. Chih-fong and Yu-Chieh (2010) have proposed multiple feature selection methods with combination of more representative variables for stock market prediction. They used well known feature selection methods like Principal Component Analysis (PCA), Genetic Algorithms (GA) and Decision Trees (CART). In their study they followed various mathematical operations like union, intersection, and multi-intersection strategies to filter-out unrepresentative variables. The back propagation prediction model is proposed and finally experimental results shows that intersection between PCA and GA and multi-intersection between PCA, GA, and CART are best. The prediction accuracy of above analysis is estimated 7% and 78.98%.

Hadavandi et al. (2010) have proposed integrated approach based on Genetic Fuzzy System (GFS) and Artificial Neural Network (ANN) for stock market forecasting expert system. They divide their analysis in two steps:

1. At first step they used stepwise regression analysis method to identify most important factors which frequently affect the stock prices.
2. In the second step they used Self Organizing Map (SOM) neural network method by partitioning the raw data in to K-clusters. Finally all clusters were fed into Independent GFS models with the ability of rule base extraction and data base tuning.

They applied the proposed methods on IT sectors and Airline sector and compared the performance with previous methods. Finally proposed methods provided more promising results. Chen et al. (2003) have presented the significant study on application of neural networks on Taiwan Stock Exchange (TSE). The proposed model was used to forecast the direction of daily return on TSE. The Probabilistic Neural Network (PNN) model was used to forecast the stock prices. Finally results are compared with other investment strategies and it is shown by study PNN based investment strategy yielding high profit. Peter et al. (2012) has developed Artificial Neural Network (ANN) method for prediction of daily stock prices of Nigeria Stock Exchange (NSE). They used various banks of NSE index for the study. The Multilayer Feed-Forward Neural Network is used and finally they concluded that it is better method of stock market prediction.

Abdulsalam et al. (2011) have proposed a linear regression method of analyzing coupled behavior of stocks in the market. The method successfully predicts stock prices based on two variables. The results were more promising than traditional stock market analysis. Mcculloch et al. (1943) have proposed the first model of an artificial neuron. They developed neuron model based on the fact that the output of the neuron is unity if the weighted sum of its inputs is greater than. Hebb (1949) suggested that the strength of connections among neurons in brain changes dynamically. He suggested a physiological learning rule for the synaptic modification. Rosenblatt (1958) used Mcculloch and Pitts model and Hebb's proposition to developed perceptrons, the first neural network architecture that was capable of learning. Ankerst (2001) used data visualization techniques to analyze the stock prices for Dow Jones, Gold, and IBM etc. The individual vertical bars in the images corresponded to different years and the subdivision of the bars to the 12 months within each year. The coloring mapped high stock prices to light colors and low stock prices to dark colors, enabling the user to see the price change of a particular stock in a year easily.

Jie et al. (2008) presented a decision tree classification model which is suitable for forecasting financial data. They also studied behavior and accuracy of stock prices at extensive level. Srisawat (2011) has proposed an application of stock rules in stock market. He applied Association Rule Mining technique for discovering the relationships between individual stocks and used the transactional dataset consists of 242 trading days from 4 January 2010 to 30 December 2010. The more promising rules were generated from dataset. Argiddi et al. (2012) have proposed the FITI (First Intratransaction Then Intertransaction) algorithm which is adaptive to intertransaction association mining. It focuses on the two stages of mining frequent intertransaction item sets and rule generation. The experimental results show that the method is better for real world applications when compared to the high running time of EH-Apriori. Ugwu and Uzochukwu (2014) have proposed the combine approach i.e. machine learning and object oriented approach for prediction of 100, 200, and 300 trading days. The proposed system was implemented with java language and Neurograph software. The experimental results show that higher prediction accuracy with minimum error. Tsanga (2007) has developed NN5 model for Hong Kong stock price forecasting. The data are considered for study is divided in two parts i.e. training and testing. The system achieved the great performance in terms of overall hit rate of over 70%. Zhang et al. (2015) have proposed novel data mining techniques for financial time series forecasting. In their study they used Back Propagation Neural Network (BPNN) and Empirical Mode Decomposition (EMD) based neural network learning approaches over the three Asian stock exchanges. The various experiments are done by proposed model. Finally they found that BPNN with EMD models had great performance as compared to other models.

Zuo and Kita (2012) have proposed for analyzing the up-down movements of stock market. In this study they have selected three major stock indexes which are Dow Jones Industrial Average (Dow 30), Financial Times Stock Exchange (FTSE 100), and Nikkei Stock Average (Nikkei 225). They proposed Bayesian network approach for prediction of next day up-down movements of stock indexes. The experimental results show that proposed algorithm has better accuracy than traditional time series algorithms. Olatunji et al. (2013) have developed Artificial Neural Network (ANN) model for performance prediction of Saudi Arabia stock exchange. The only past days close prices is selected as input variable and next day's close prices are considered as output variable. In the experimental results high correlation coefficient was up to 99.9% and RMSE down to 1.8174, MAD down to 18.2835, and MAPE down to 1.6476. Finally they concluded that proposed system has positive impact on performance of Saudi stock market. Bola et al. (2013) have proposed Artificial Neural Network (ANN) and Bayesian Network (BN) model for Nigerian stock market price prediction. The proposed NN model has derived the relationship between input and output variables. The proposed BN model also discrediting the numeric attributes into distinct ranges from where the conditional probability was calculated which is stored in Conditional Probability Table (CPT). The final performance of ANN and BN models had respectively 59.38% and 78.13% in terms of prediction accuracy. Kamley et al. (2014) have proposed Back Propagation Neural Network (BPNN) method for predating the performance of Bombay Stock Exchange (BSE) of India. They employed the last nine years data for training and testing purpose. In their study three input variables open price, low price, high price and one output variable close price is considered. One hidden layer with eleven nodes is also considered for improving the performance of BSE index. Finally they got the best prediction accuracy with proposed architecture. Kamley et al. (2015) have proposed rule based approach for stock market expert system. In their study forward reasoning approach of expert system is carried out and found the output in terms of various productive and useful rules.

This study inspired by various data mining techniques like Linear Regression (LR), Multiple Regression (MR), Clustering, Association Rule Mining (ARM), and Back Propagation Neural Network (BPNN) approaches.

MAIN FOCUS OF THE CHAPTER

Stock market data collects huge amount of data throughout the year that is vague, uncertain, and incomplete in nature. To make prediction from such data is very difficult task. A data preprocessing step removes inconsistency from data set and prepares the data for prediction (Han & Kamber, 2006). This study considered last 10 years of data (Data Source: Bombay Stock Exchange of India, 2004- 2013) of Infosys index. The Data set contains various variables like Open Price, High Price, Low Price, and Close Price (Data Source: Bombay Stock Exchange of India, 2004- 2013). The Table 1 shows sample of data set.

Table 1. Sample of stock data set

Open	High	Low	Close
1198.7	1198.7	979	987.95
992	997	975.3	979
982.4	982.4	958.55	962.65
969.9	990	965	986.75
986.5	990	976	988.1
990	995	983.6	987.9
989.9	1004.6	986	993.65
1006	1100	990.35	997.85
1039.9	1039.9	992.9	994.85
1035	1035	995	995.6
996	1000.8	991.1	993.7
997	997.9	978.45	979.95
247.5	247.5	244	247.2
991	1015.5	991	1003.5
1005	1018.8	1002.95	1015.65
1018	1020	1001.2	1006.1
1007	1015	1002.5	1008.45
1012	1029.9	1010.3	1024.5
1032.4	1036.9	1020.15	1022.9
1024.85	1048.5	1022	1045.8
1048.4	1056	1037.1	1052.05
1048	1049	1027	1030.25
1029.1	1040	1026	1028.8
1027.5	1032.5	1015	1020.75
1016	1027.4	1012.5	1015.55
1019.25	1033	1016.15	1031
1035.6	1040.9	1020.65	1027.1
1029	1056.45	1026.35	1047.7
1057	1081	1054.45	1076.5
1080.3	1089	1075.5	1080.7
1081	1102.8	1075.05	1081.6
1083	1100	1083	1097.1
274.5	277.75	273.75	274.52

continued in next column

Table 1. Continued

Open	High	Low	Close
1100	1111.5	1085	1089.3
1110	1115	1077.65	1084.45
280.42	285.25	279.32	281.5
1134	1142	1125.25	1137.25
1140.15	1148.7	1136.1	1143.2
1144.8	1149.9	1129	1133.25
1137.25	1139	1122	1125.55
1125	1127	1110.75	1117.35
1115.6	1140.95	1115.6	1137.2
1142.25	1148	1135.2	1139.9
1145	1174.8	1145	1165.95
291.99	291.99	286.29	289.07
1150	1174.45	1142.3	1170.65
1130	1179.75	1125	1159.7
1161	1184	1161	1175.2
1181.75	1187.9	1167.7	1170.4
1173.95	1180	1160	1165.45
1165	1188.9	1156	1184.15
1187	1197.9	1177	1188.4
1191	1199	1190.1	1194.35
1199	1203.4	1191.1	1196.25
1204	1208	1190.2	1196.75
1198	1198	1184	1190.9
1191.5	1209.9	1191.5	1205.4
1209.45	1234.55	1206.5	1231
308.25	309.25	302.77	304.27
1207.8	1226	1195	1222.45
1230.6	1242	1224.15	1235.55
1239	1245	1230.15	1233.9
1234	1244	1208.65	1216.85
1216	1247.7	1205.55	1243.9
1248.15	1286	1245	1274.65
1281	1281	1257	1261.55

continued on following page

Table 1. Continued

Open	High	Low	Close
1265	1277	1239.1	1242.6
1249.25	1255.9	1221.55	1236.75
1240	1250	1208.5	1214.55
1216	1232.9	1215	1218.25
1218	1226.6	1196.05	1200.8
1204.95	1217	1204.85	1211.45
1220	1235.5	1214	1225.65
306.5	310.42	306.32	309.04
1242	1244.7	1230.3	1233.15

continued in next column

Table 1. Continued

Open	High	Low	Close
1248.45	1265	1238	1262.65
1260	1274.8	1252.1	1256.5
1260	1268.5	1256.5	1262.55
1264.95	1277	1263.15	1272.7
1275.1	1275.1	1230	1240.15
1247.7	1247.7	1225	1227.85
1232.95	1272	1221.55	1267.95
1270	1285	1262.2	1270.55

The stock prices employed in this study is too much large and not feasible for computation (Data Source: Bombay Stock Exchange of India, 2004- 2013). So data set has been normalized. Data normalization process changes the large magnitude values in to small scale values i.e. 0 to 1. The process is needed to eliminate the effects of certain gross influences of data and makes data more feasible so that our algorithms can be easily and efficiently perform on that data. Before applying data normalization process first decimal points are removed from data set. After that data normalization process are applied to overall data (input variables to output variables). The Algorithm 1 describes the data normalization process.

Algorithm 1. Data normalization process

Step 1: Find out the Min and Max value in the data set.
Step 2: Decide the Min SP (Minimum Stock Price) and Max SP (Maximum Stock Price) for normalized scale.
Step 3: Consider a price (New Price) from the data set.
Step 4: The normalized value for the number (A) is given by the formula no. (1.1) (Han & Kamber, 2006).

$$\frac{(NP - MINSP)}{(MAXSP - MINSP)} \tag{1.1}$$

The Table 2 shows sample of normalized data set.

SOLUTIONS AND RECOMMENDATIONS

Linear Regression

Regression analysis is a technique that can be used to model the relationship between one or more independent or predictor variables and a dependent or response variable i.e. continuous valued. Linear

Table 2. Normalized data sample

Table 2. Continued

Open	High	Low	Close
0.48	0.46	0.51	0.48
0.48	0.51	0.49	0.41
0.41	0.4	0.44	0.38
0.37	0.38	0.42	0.4
0.39	0.36	0.41	0.34
0.34	0.33	0.42	0.34
0.34	0.34	0.42	0.36
0.32	0.29	0.34	0.33
0.33	0.38	0.34	0.3
0.31	0.28	0.22	0.2
0.21	0.24	0.26	0.27
0.27	0.22	0.083	0.16
0.16	0.17	0.21	0.18
0.17	0.11	0.12	0.13
0.13	0.23	0.18	0.27
0.27	0.3	0.32	0.36
0.35	0.32	0.31	0.26
0.26	0.26	0.21	0.2
0.18	0.2	0.24	0.27

Open	High	Low	Close
0.27	0.23	0.12	0.12
0.12	0.077	0	0.11
0.12	0.071	0.031	0.052
0.075	0	0.012	0
0	0.008	0.029	0.08
0.072	0.011	0.051	0.048
0.037	0.044	0.062	0.088
0.086	0.097	0.11	0.16
0.16	0.24	0.21	0.2
0.2	0.25	0.27	0.28
0.28	0.35	0.29	0.4
0.4	0.41	0.43	0.43
0.43	0.5	0.52	0.51
0.5	0.47	0.53	0.46
0.46	0.52	0.52	0.54
0.54	0.59	0.64	0.63
0.63	0.64	0.66	0.58
0.57	0.6	0.63	0.63

continued in next column

regression analysis is used for predictions which are based on the relationship that exists between two variables (Armstrong J., 2012, Pujari, 2006). A process that allows you to make predictions about variable "Y" based on knowledge you have about variable "X" as shown by straight line in equation no. (1.2).

$$Y = a + bX \tag{1.2}$$

Where variable Y is response or predictor variable and X is independent variable. a and b are line or regression coefficients specifying the Y intercept and slope of line, respectively. The regression coefficients a and b can be thought of as weights. The equation no. (1.3) can be used to show in terms of weights.

$$Y = a_1 + b_1 X \tag{1.3}$$

The method of least squares is used to solve for these coefficients which estimates the best-fitting line i.e. minimizing the error between actual data and predicted data. The value of b_1 is given by equation no. (1.4).

$$b_1 = \frac{\sum\limits_{i=1}^{D} (X_i - \overline{X})(Y_i - \overline{Y})}{\sum\limits_{i=1}^{D} (X_i - \overline{X})^2} \tag{1.4}$$

where, D is training set consists the value of predictor variable. X_i and Y_i shows data items and Thus equation no. (1.5) used to calculate the value of coefficient a_1

$$a_1 = \overline{Y} - b_1 \overline{X} \tag{1.5}$$

$\overline{X}$ and $\overline{Y}$ shows mean occurrence of X_i and Y_i items.

In this study four stock variables like open price, high price, low price, and close price are considered but we know very clearly the linear regression approach works on two variables. Therefore, we selected two variables open price and high price for study based on correlation factor. The equation no. (1.6) shows correlation formula between two variables.

$$r_{(X,Y)} = \sqrt{\frac{(\sqrt{XY})}{(\sqrt{XX}) * (\sqrt{YY})}} \tag{1.6}$$

The value of correlation is calculated 0.99 which shows very strong relationship between respective variables.

In this study open price denotes X sample and close price denotes Y samples. Here equation no. (1.4) & (1.5) used to calculate the coefficient of linear regression equation. Using this equation we calculated the value of variables a_1 & b_1 which are given below:

$$b_1 = 0.60, \, a_1 = 0.24$$

The equation no. (1.3) is used to get the final resultant linear regression equation.

$$Y = 0.24 + 0.6X \tag{1.7}$$

Experimental Results

In this study the database is built for a data mining software tool using the information obtained from the daily activity summary (equities) published by Bombay Stock Exchange of India spanning through last 10 years (Data Source: Bombay Stock Exchange of India, 2004- 2013). The obtained data firstly were analyzed and summarized as shown in above Table 2. The discovered data are used to generate new knowledge about the data in the database and identified patterns are depicted in the Figure 1, which shows the market trends of stock prices (2004-2007).

The proposed system predicts daily movement of stock prices using regression analysis. The method of least square is used to calculate the value of dependent variable Y on putting the values of X in equation (1.3). The Table 3 shows the 1 year (2008) (Data Source: Bombay Stock Exchange of India, 2004- 2013) forecasted value which have been drawn from proposed prediction system, which predicts the value of dependent variable Y (close price) based on independent variable X (open price).

Figure 1. Day wise open and close price of the stock market against the year 2004-2007

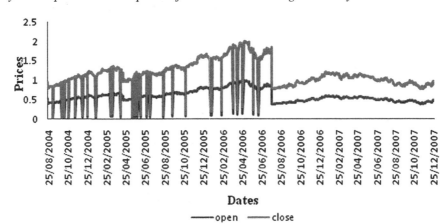

Table 3. Sample of stock forecasted price

Date	Open Price (X)	Predicted Close Price (Y)
01/01/2008	1.00	0.84
02/01/2008	0.96	0.82
03/01/2008	0.90	0.78
04/01/2008	0.86	0.76
07/01/2008	0.84	0.74
08/01/2008	0.80	0.72
09/01/2008	0.83	0.74
10/01/2008	0.84	0.74
11/01/2008	0.67	0.64
01/01/2008	0.84	0.74
02/01/2008	0.77	0.70
03/01/2008	0.72	0.67
04/01/2008	0.77	0.70
07/01/2008	0.70	0.66
08/01/2008	0.64	0.63

continued in next column

Table 3. Continued

Date	Open Price (X)	Predicted Close Price (Y)
09/01/2008	0.46	0.52
10/01/2008	0.55	0.57
14/01/2008	0.57	0.58
15/01/2008	0.54	0.56
16/01/2008	1.00	0.84
17/01/2008	0.96	0.82
18/01/2008	0.90	0.78
21/01/2008	0.86	0.76
22/01/2008	0.84	0.74
23/01/2008	0.80	0.72
24/01/2008	0.83	0.74
25/01/2008	0.84	0.74
14/01/2008	0.67	0.64
15/01/2008	0.84	0.74
16/01/2008	0.77	0.70

The Figure 2 shows the relationship between variables dates and price, the red line shows the predicted close price w.r.t. blue line (open price). When open price of variable changes than close price of variable also changes.

Standard Error Estimation

Every prediction has an associated error that indicates how close the predicted value comes to the observed value, which is shown in Table 4.

The last column of Table 4 shows that the sum of the squared errors of the prediction is 0.23 . For calculation of standard error the following formula is used which is shown by equation no. (1.8) (Gupta & Kapoor, 2000). For calculation of standard error the following formula is used which is shown by equation no. (1.8).

Figure 2. A line graph showing the predicted patterns of stock prices

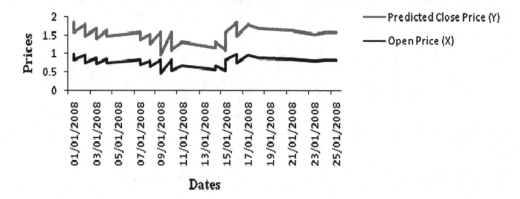

Table 4. Standard error estimation

Close Price (Y)	Predicted Close Price $(\overline{Y})$	Residual $(Y - \overline{Y})$	Residual $(Y - \overline{Y})^2$
1.00	0.84	0.16	0.03
0.99	0.82	0.17	0.03
0.92	0.78	0.14	0.02
0.89	0.76	0.13	0.02
0.82	0.74	0.08	0.01
0.85	0.72	0.13	0.02
0.87	0.74	0.13	0.02
0.83	0.74	0.09	0.01
0.86	0.64	0.22	0.05
0.79	0.74	0.05	0.00
0.74	0.70	0.04	0.00

continued in next column

Table 4. Continued

Close Price (Y)	Predicted Close Price $(\overline{Y})$	Residual $(Y - \overline{Y})$	Residual $(Y - \overline{Y})^2$
0.75	0.67	0.08	0.01
0.70	0.70	0	0.00
0.66	0.66	0	0.00
0.50	0.63	-0.13	0.02
0.42	0.52	-0.1	0.01
0.54	0.57	-0.03	0.00
0.52	0.58	-0.06	0.00
0.63	0.56	0.07	0.00
0.56	0.58	-0.02	0.00

$$\Sigma \left(Y\text{-}\overline{Y}\right)^2 = 0.23$$

$$SE = \sqrt{\frac{\text{Sum of Residual}(Y - \overline{Y})^2}{N}} \qquad (1.8)$$

where,

SE = Standard Error of the Estimate,

Y = Sample Values of the dependent variable,

$\overline{Y}$ = Corresponding estimated value from the regression equation,

N = No. of data points in the sample.

So, the standard error of estimate is 0.10 that means accuracy of prediction is 90% which may be acceptable. The bar graph in Figure 3 showing the trends of actual and predicted price.

Multiple Regression

Multiple regression is the most common data mining technique for predicting the future value of variable based on the linear relationship it has with other variables. The most basic use of the regression equation is to make predictions (Gupta & Kapoor, 2000, Han & Kamber, 2006). We can predict the value of Y for any particular combination of values of $X_1, X_2, ..., X_n$ into the regression equation and seeing we get the result $\overline{Y}$. The equation (1.9) is basic multiple regression equation used to obtain the value of Y (dependent variable) corresponding to independent variables $X_1, X_2, ..., X_n$.

$$\overline{Y} = W_0 + W_1 X_1 + W_2 X_2 + ... + W_n X_n \qquad (1.9)$$

Figure 3. A bar graph for trends of actual and predicted price

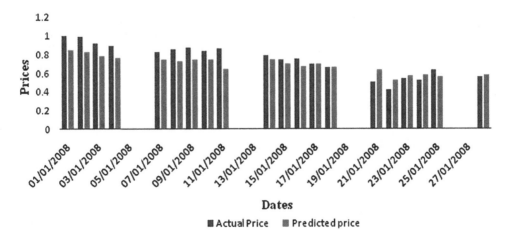

In this study multiple regression equation based on three variables proposed where, Y denotes close price and X_1, X_2 are values of corresponding attribute open and low price.

The method of least square is used to obtain the coefficient values W_0, W_1 and W_2. Here some statistical formulas are used to obtain the values which is shown by equation no. (1.10), (1.11) & (1.12) (Gupta & Kapoor, 2000).

$$W_1 = \frac{\left(\sum X_2^2\right)\left(\sum X_1 Y\right) - \left(\sum X_1 X_2\right)\left(\sum X_2 Y\right)}{\left(\sum X_1^2\right)\left(\sum X_2^2\right) - \left(\sum X_1 X_2\right)^2} \tag{1.10}$$

$$W_2 = \frac{\left(\sum X_1^2\right)\left(\sum X_2 Y\right) - \left(\sum X_1 X_2\right)\left(\sum X_1 Y\right)}{\left(\sum X_1^2\right)\left(\sum X_2^2\right) - \left(\sum X_1 X_2\right)^2} \tag{1.11}$$

$$W_0 = \bar{Y} - W_1 X_1 - W_2 X_2 \tag{1.12}$$

Using these equations we calculate the value of variables W_0, W_1 and W_2 which are given below:

$$W_0 = 0.01, W_1 = 0.79, \text{and } W_2 = 0.2$$

Finally resultant multiple regression equation is given by equation no. (1.13)

$$\bar{Y} = 0.01 + 0.79 X_1 + 0.2 X_2 \tag{1.13}$$

Experimental Results

The proposed system predicts daily movement of stock prices using regression analysis. Here method of least square is used, where value of dependent variable is calculated putting the values of X in equation no. (1.13). The Table 5 (Data Source: Bombay Stock Exchange of India, 2004- 2013) shows the twenty days forecasted values which have been drawn from proposed prediction system, which predicts the value of dependent variable $\bar{Y}$ (close price) based on independent variables X_1 and X_2 (i.e. open price and low price).

The Figure 4 shows the line graph for predicted patterns of stock prices against the dates.

Standard Error Estimation for Multiple Regression

The Table 6 shows standard error calculation between actual stock prices and predicted stock prices.

Table 5. Sample of stock forecasted price

Date	Open (X_1)	Low (X_2)	Close (Y)	$\bar{Y}$
01/01/2008	0.84	0.71	0.79	0.82
02/01/2008	0.77	0.64	0.74	0.75
03/01/2008	0.72	0.61	0.75	0.70
04/01/2008	0.77	0.59	0.70	0.74
07/01/2008	0.7	0.53	0.66	0.67
08/01/2008	0.64	0.25	0.50	0.57
09/01/2008	0.46	0.00	0.42	0.37
10/01/2008	0.55	1.00	1.00	1.00

continued in next column

Table 5. Continued

Date	Open (X_1)	Low (X_2)	Close (Y)	$\bar{Y}$
11/01/2008	0.67	0.58	0.86	0.65
14/01/2008	0.57	0.94	0.99	0.96
15/01/2008	0.54	0.86	0.92	0.90
16/01/2008	1	0.85	0.89	0.86
17/01/2008	0.96	0.76	0.82	0.83
18/01/2008	0.9	0.75	0.85	0.79
21/01/2008	0.86	0.81	0.87	0.83
22/01/2008	0.84	0.72	0.83	0.82

Figure 4. Line graph for predicted patterns of stock prices

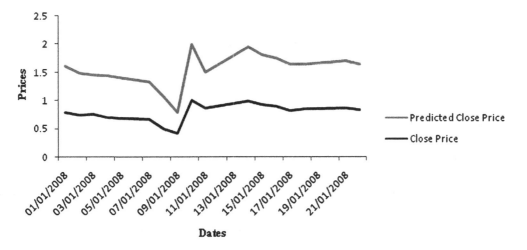

Table 6. Standard error estimation

Close Price (Y)	Predicted Close Price $(\bar{Y})$	Residual $(Y - \bar{Y})$	Residual $(Y - \bar{Y})^2$
1	1	0	0
0.99	0.96	0.03	0.0009
0.92	0.9	0.02	0.0004
0.89	0.86	0.03	0.0009
.	.	.	.
.	.	.	.
.	.	.	.
0.42	0.37	0.05	0.0025

continued in next column

Table 6. Continued

Close Price (Y)	Predicted Close Price $(\bar{Y})$	Residual $(Y - \bar{Y})$	Residual $(Y - \bar{Y})^2$
1	1	0	0
0.99	0.96	0.03	0.0009
0.92	0.9	0.02	0.0004
0.89	0.86	0.03	0.0009
0.82	0.83	-0.01	0.0001
0.85	0.79	0.06	0.0036

$$\Sigma \left(Y - \bar{Y} \right)^2 = 0.0719$$

The last column of Table 6 shows that the sum of the squared errors of the prediction is 0.0719. Therefore, for the calculation of standard error above formula no. (1.8) is used (Gupta & Kapoor, 2000). The calculated standard error of estimate is 0.054 and prediction accuracy is 99.94% which is better. The following Figure 5 shows the bar graph of the actual and predicted stock price patterns.

ASSOCIATION RULE MINING

The Association Rule Mining (ARM) model is proposed for prediction task on stock market data set. Association Rule mining is one of the most important and well define technique for extract correlations, sequential item set, and associations among set of items in the transactional database or other repositories (Han & Kamber, 2006; Tiwari et al., 2010). The proposed ARM model is used to generate some significant rules from stock market data that will show that whether to purchase or sell the stock, so that stock users can earn maximum profit.

Association rule generation process mainly consists steps:

1. Firstly, minimum support is applied to find all frequent item sets in a database.
2. Second phase is most important to find rules based on these frequent item sets and the minimum confidence constraint (Han & Kamber, 2006, Pujari, 2006).

In this study, we apply Association Rule Mining (ARM) algorithm on stock data set, finding the relationship among stock variables open price, high price, low price, and close price and generating the rules with these variables.

Proposed Methodology: Apriori Algorithm

Apriori algorithm Developed by Agarwal and Srikant (1994) (Han & Kamber, 2006), which is innovative way to find association rules on large scale dataset. The algorithm attempts to find subsets which are common to at least a minimum number c (the cutoff, or confidence threshold) of the item-sets. Apriori uses a "bottom up" approach, where frequent subsets are extended one item at a time a step known as candidate generation, and groups of candidates are tested against the data (Han & Kamber, 2006). The

Figure 5. A bar graph for trends of actual and predicted price

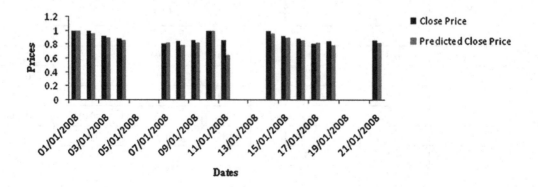

algorithm terminates when no further successful extensions are found. Apriori uses breadth-first search and a hash tree structure count candidate item sets efficiently (Pujari, 2006). The Figure 6 shows flow-chart of Apriori algorithm.

EXPERIMENTAL RESULTS

The SAS (Statistical Analysis Software) 9.2 is used to generate association rules from stock market data. The preprocessed data is shown in Figure 7.

The next task to apply mining algorithm and to predict stock prices. Stock prices are highly correlated with each other i.e. change in one price value may affect other price value. The ARM algorithm easily finding the association between items set (variables) and finds the frequent item set based on support and confidence value (Toivonen, 1996). For this purpose different experiments conducted on stock data set. The different support value 2%, 4%, & 6% are considered for different size rule generation, which are shown through the Tables 7, 8, & 9.

The above results show the interesting measure when confidence (%) increases than number of rules decreases and the rules are generated with different combinations like length-2 {open, close}, length-3 {open, high, close}, length-4 {open, high, low, close} etc., the graph is shown by Figure 8. To find interesting rules confidence value is fixed on above 90% and considered only 10 rules, which are shown in Table 10.

The Table 10 shows the extracted rule in the following manner. According to Id-1 when open price and high price of share increases then close price of share also increases. If market opens high from that position so investing money will be fruitful. In the same manner (Id-8) if low price and close price of share increase then open prices of share also increases so selling of share may be beneficial.

Figure 6. Flowchart of Apriori Algorithm
(Han & Kamber, 2006)

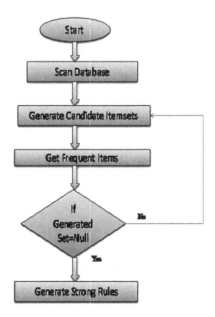

Figure 7. Pre-processed data for association rule mining process

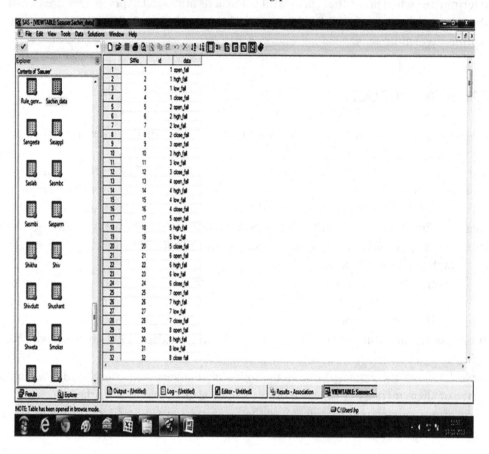

Table 7. Maximum no. of rule generated with support= 2%

Confidence (%)	Max Length 2	Max Length 3	Max Length 4
10%	32	108	176
20%	32	108	176
40%	32	108	159
60%	32	102	135
80%	32	100	128
100%	06	45	75

Table 8. Maximum no. of rule generated with support= 4%

Confidence (%)	Max Length 2	Max Length 3	Max Length 4
10%	32	108	100
20%	32	108	100
40%	32	108	100
60%	32	108	100
80%	32	100	100
100%	06	45	75

Clustering

Clustering is the process of grouping the data objects into classes or clusters. However the objects within a cluster have high similarity in comparison to one another but are very dissimilar to objects in other clusters (Pujari, 2006). Dissimilarities are access based on attribute values describing that objects. Mostly

Table 9. Maximum no. of rule generated with Support=6%

Confidence (%)	Max Length 2	Max Length 3	Max Length 4
10%	32	108	176
20%	32	108	176
40%	32	108	159
60%	32	102	135
80%	32	100	128
100%	06	45	75

Figure 8. Total no. of rules generated with different values of confidence (%)

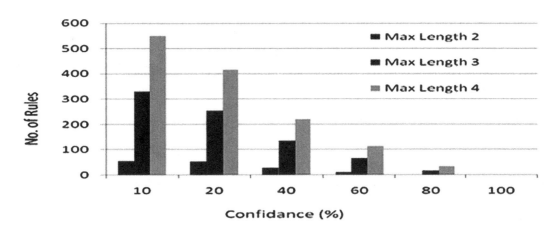

Table 10. Association rules with confidence > 90%

Id	Rules	Confidence (%)
1	Open_rise & High_rise=>Close_rise	100
2	Open_rise & Low_rise=>High_rise	100
3	Low_rise & High_rise=>Open_rise	100
4	Open_rise=>Low_rise & Close_rise	97.44
5	Close_rise & Low_rise =>Open_rise	97.37
6	Open_rise & Low_rise=>Close_rise	97.37
7	Open_rise & Close_rise=>Low_rise	94.87
8	Low_rise & Close_rise=>Open_rise	94.87
9	Open_rise=>High_rise & Close_rise	94.87
10	Close_rise=>Open_rise & High_rise	92.5

distance measure is used to find the distance between two objects. It is one of the most important data mining techniques and can be used in many areas like statistics, biology, and machine learning (Han & Kamber, 2006).

Proposed Methodology: K-Means Algorithm

The K-means algorithm proposed by MacQueen in 1967 is one of the well known unsupervised learning algorithms (Fayyad et al., 1996). The process takes the input parameter, K, and partitions a set of n objects into K clusters so that the resulting intracluster similarity is high but the intercluster similarity is low. The cluster similarity is measured w.r.t. to mean value of the objects in a cluster, which can be viewed as the centroid of the cluster (Pujari, 2006). The following algorithm shows K-means clustering algorithm.

Step 1: D is a dataset representing n objects and set the initial K clusters value.
Step 2: Assign each object to the group that has the closest centroid.
Step 3: When all objects have been assigned recalculate the positions of the K centroids.
Step 4: Steps 2 and 3 repeated until the centroids no longer move i.e. this produces a separation of the objects into groups from which the metric to be minimized can be calculated.
Step 5: End.

Experimental Results

In this study K-means clustering algorithm is proposed for stock price prediction. The maximum value of k is set is 5 i.e. objects are classified into these clusters based on similarity measure. The Figure 9 shows output of K-means algorithm.

The Figure 9 shows the maximum distance from cluster seed 236.92.

The next task is to calculate the proximities between the dimensions. The following figure shows cluster proximities.

The Figure 10 shows the cluster 4 and 3 have interclustered similarity. In the same manner cluster 2 and 5 have similarity. The cluster 1 is separate alone i.e. no cluster has joined to 1.it is representing as outliers. The Table 11 and Table 12 shows summary of clustering process.

The Figure 11 shows code window generated during clustering process.

ARTIFICIAL NEURAL NETWORK (ANN)

Artificial Neural Networks, one of the most promising research area over the last few years and have been successfully applied for the diversified range of problem domains such as Medical, Finance, Engineering, Geology and Physics (Han & Kamber, 2006). Artificial Neural Networks (ANNs) model consist of many nodes, i.e. processing units as similar to neurons in the human brain. Artificial Neural Network works like an information processing system. In this information processing system, the elements called neurons, process the information (Sivanandam et al., 2006). The Figure 12 shows the structure of neural cell in the human brain.

Figure 9. Clusters for stock market dataset

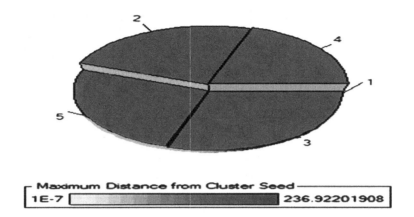

Figure 10. Cluster proximities against the Dimensions.

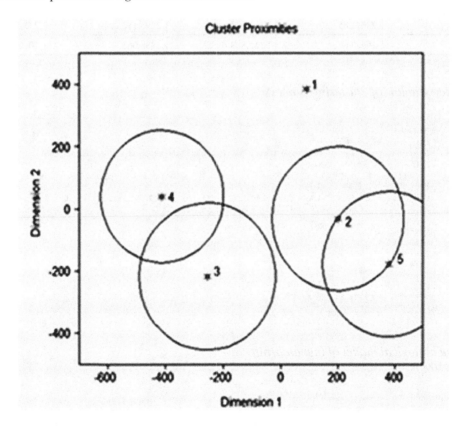

Figure 12 shows the neurons consists of a core, dendrites for incoming information and axon with dendrites for outgoing information that is passed from one neuron to another neuron in the form of electrical stimulations along the dendrites. The information is incoming from the neuron's dendrites is added up and then delivered along the neuron's axon to the other dendrites end, where the information is passed to other neurons if the stimulation has been exceeded a certain predefine threshold.

Table 11. Summary of clustering process one

Cluster	Frequency of Cluster	Root-Mean-Square Standard Deviation	Maximum Distance from Cluster Seed	Nearest Cluster
1	1	55.13346.	0	2
2	9	69.15549	231.5648	5
3	3	85.96486	236.922	4
4	10	57.25441	212.8944	3
5	4	74.45691	233.2591	2

Table 12. Summary of clustering process two

Distance to Nearest Cluster	Open	High	Low	Close
438.0827	2325.75	2361.08	2253.99	2256.48
247.7661	2149.489	2202.218	2020.149	2085.516
302.6103	2196.457	2344.537	2089.823	2252.49
302.6103	2361.285	2431.377	2295.173	2354.006
247.7661	1964.965	2115.888	1886.063	2060.628

Figure 11. Code window of clustering process

```
Title;
Options nodate;
Proc     fastclus     data=clusfi     (label="clustered     seeds     for
EDATA.VIEW_LM6);
Outstate=EMPROJ.CLSX63U     (label="clustered     statistics     for
EDATA.VIEW.LM6);
CLUSTER=SEGMANT_RADIOUS=0,          REPLACED=FULL,
MAX=1, CORV=0.0001, DISTANCE STD=NONE;
VAR;
OPEN;
CLOSE;
LOW;
HIGH;
RUN;
QUIT;
***END OF FILE***
```

Figure 12. The biological model of human brain
(Han & Kamber, 2006)

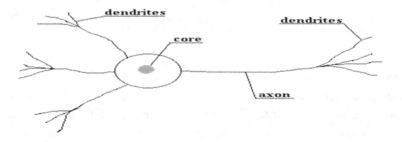

The concept is adopted from human brain and applied in neural network model where model consists of input unit, processing of that input and output unit (Pujari, 2006). The Figure 13 shows simple structure of neuron in a neural net.

Figure 13. show an artificial neuron looks similar to a biological neural cell. And it works in the same way. The input (information) is sent to the neuron with incoming weights and this input is processed by a propagation function that adds up the values of all incoming weights. The resulting value is compared with a certain threshold value by the neuron's activation function (Sivanandam et al., 2006). If the input exceeding the certain threshold value, then neurons will be activated, otherwise it will be inhibited. If activated, the neuron sends an output on its outgoing weights to all connected neurons and so on (Han & Kamber, 2006, Sivanandam et al., 2006).

Proposed Methodology: Feed- Forward Back Propagation Neural Network

A Feed-Forward Artificial Neural Network (FFANN) consists of layers of processing units; each layer feeding input to the next layer in a feed-forward manner through a set of connecting weights (Sutheebanjard & Premchaiswadi, 2010). The Back-Propagation Neural Network (BPNN) is supervised method for training artificial neural network. It is a Multi-Layer Feed-Forward Neural Network with no backward loop but it back propagates the error so that it is named as "Back Propagation Neural Network". This algorithm is divided into three main parts which are feed forward, error calculation and the last part is updating the weight (Sivanandam et al., 2006, Han & Kamber, 2006). The Figure 14 shows step by step procedure of the back propagation learning algorithm.

Experimental Results

In this study last 10 years data from Infosys Company of BSE index is considered for study (Data Source: Bombay Stock Exchange of India, 2004- 2013). The 3-15-1 architecture i.e. 3 input variables (open, high, and low), 1 hidden layer (15 neurons in the hidden layer), and 1 neuron in output layer is used to create the required Feed Forward Neural Network model for predicting stock prices. The 70% data considered for training (i.e. 1685 samples), 15% data for validation purpose (i.e. 361 samples), and 15% data for testing purpose (i.e. 361 samples). The Levenberg-Marquardt back propagation algorithm has been used. It is the most commonly used training algorithm for time series prediction. The Figure 15 shows network training performance.

Figure 13. Structure of a neuron in a neural network
(Sivanandam et al., 2006)

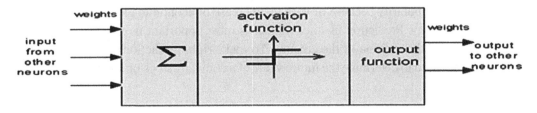

Figure 14. Back Propagation (BP) learning algorithm
(Sivanandam et al., 2006)

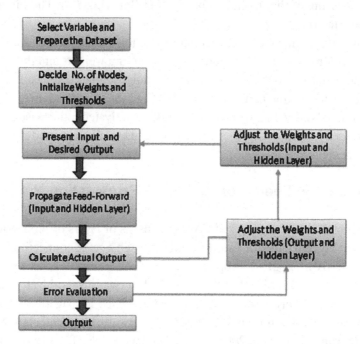

The Graph 16 shows the performance measure in the form of Mean Squared Error (MSE) against number of epochs. The numbers of epochs are set to 1000 and got the best validation performance at epoch number 12 which is 144.7982. The training state of network is shown in Figure 16.

The Figure 17 shows training state of network.

The Figure 18 shows the regression plot of network performance based on training, testing and validation which depend linearly on their unknown parameters are easier to fit than models which are non-linearly related to their parameters and because the statistical properties of the resulting estimators are easier to determine.

The Figure 19 shows comparison between actual prices and predicted prices.

The Table 13 gives the target close price, predicted close price and error in prediction i.e. the difference between actual close price and predicted close price.

The Figure 20 shows error plot between actual and predicted prices

CONCLUSION

Data mining in stock market is one of the fascinating issues in stock market research field and this area of research is gaining popularity because of with the increase of economic globalization and evolution of information technology. Prediction in stock market is most important issue because its impacts on economical and financial condition of the country. To make right predictions from stock data is very challenging task. It is used to determine the future value of a company stock or other financial instrument

Figure 15. Training of network

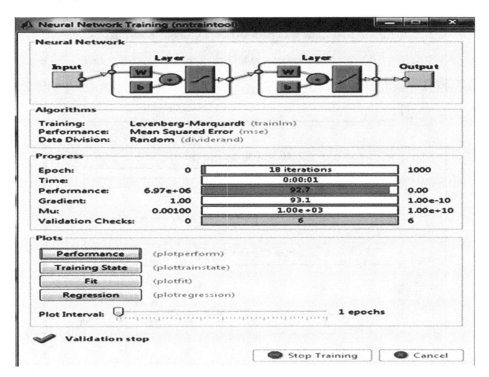

Figure 16. Performance plot of network

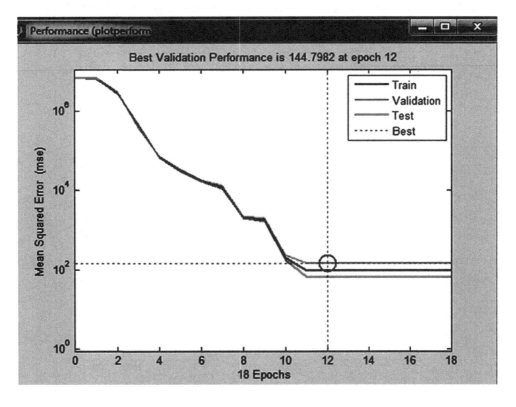

Figure 17. Training state of network

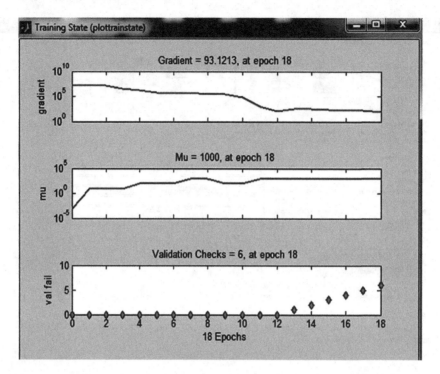

Figure 18. Regression plot of network

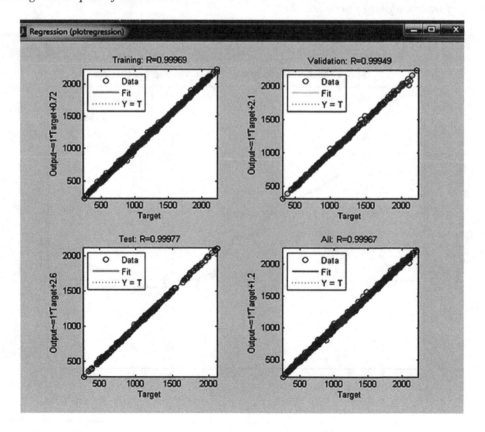

Figure 19. Comparison between actual price and predicted price

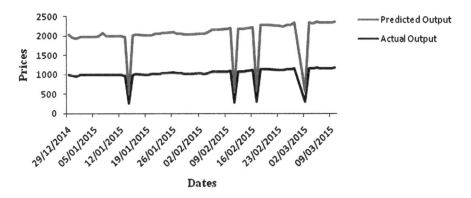

Table 13. Sample of actual price, predicted price and error in prediction

Actual Price (AP)	Predicted Price (PP)	Error (AP-PP)
988	1043	-55
979	983	-4
963	966	-3
987	979	8
988	980	8
988	987	1
994	995	-1
998	1068	-70
995	1005	-10
996	1006	-10
994	993	1
980	984	-4
247	237	10
1004	1006	-2
1016	1011	5
1006	1007	-1
1008	1007	1
1025	1021	4
1023	1026	-3
1046	1038	8
1052	1045	7
1030	1034	-4

continued in next column

Table 13. Continued

Actual Price (AP)	Predicted Price (PP)	Error (AP-PP)
1029	1032	-3
1021	1021	0
1048	1046	2
1077	1071	6
1081	1081	0
1082	1092	-10
1097	1093	4
275	273	2
1089	1098	-9
1084	1091	-7
1116	1109	7
1117	1116	1
1137	1133	4
1140	1140	0
1166	1166	0
289	285	4
1171	1163	8
1160	1166	-6
1175	1176	-1
1170	1176	-6
1165	1169	-4
1184	1177	7

Figure 20. Error plot between actual and predicted prices

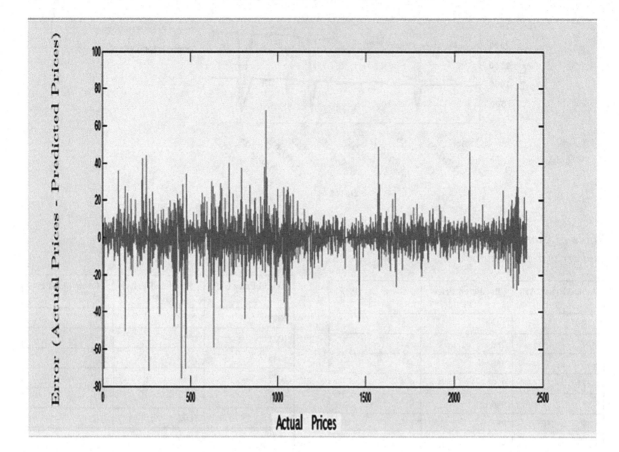

traded on a financial exchange. The successful prediction of a stock future price could yield significant profit for stock brokers and investors in decision making.

The aim of our research study was finding the best prediction model for investors who can take the decision of buying or selling using the model. Based on the findings of this study it can be concluded that:

Statistical methods linear regression and multiple regression are used to find the relationship between two or more variables, but methods are unable to find the complex relationship when number of variable increases. But we got the accuracy of linear regression based approach is 90%.

The proposed system predicts the stock prices based on multiple regression approach using three variables and found the accuracy of system is 99%, which is more accurate than linear regression approach. In this research study we applied Association Rule Mining algorithm, which hepls to learn investment plan and understanding the market conditions. Aassociation Rule Mining has wide range of applicabilty in stock market research. In this research work, a real time dataset is used for analysis purpose and a group of association rules and frequent itemsets are obtained. First itemsets are mined for a given minimum support and based on these itemsets obtained; the association rules are computed for a given minimum confidence. The generated pattern helps investors to make investment strategies may be planned. It is observed that associations rules for stock data set is generated which will definitely give better returns in long term.

The K-means clustering algorithm is proposed for stock market prediction. This helps to groping the object (i.e. prices) on specified clusters based on similarity measure. Finally it is shown by experimental results it is better approach than traditional tools and techniques.

Finally Neural Network (NN) approach is applied on stock data set. The NN method has ability to extract useful information from the data and it is widely play very important role in stock market prediction. It is used to control and monitor the entire stock market price behavior and fluctuation. Artificial Neural Network (ANN) forecasting method has the ability to overcome problems of non-linear data through learning and recognition of the pattern in the data, which cannot be done by statistical methods.

FUTURE RESEARCH DIRECTIONS

No research work is complete without suggesting the directions for future research. This research work has primarily focused on empirically testing of BSE stock exchanges and their characteristics. In The integrate neural networks and other techniques such as genetic techniques, wavelet analysis, fuzzy inference, pattern recognition and time series models can be used for finance and economic forecasting.

In future, for improving prediction results more data variables such as moving indices, volume trend, exchange rate, price/earnings ratio can be considered for study. A better neural network (different no. of neurons, layers etc.) can be found using trial and error. As growing number of investor, the stock data is growing fast. To study this incremented data there is need to design a good predictor model that can predict correct trends. The soft computing techniques can also useful to handle current situation of stock market data. Since from beginning researchers have been put more effort for numeric stock price prediction. No researchers have been attempted symbolic stock price prediction. There may be good opportunity to explore the area of stock market especially for symbolic forecast. However, this research covers only one sector of Indian economy. Accordingly, further research is needed to explore the issues surrounding payout policy more fully by extending the study to other sectors of Indian economy as well as more emerging world markets. Every possible effort has been made to make the study more intensive and practicable but the time and resources have been the limiting factors due to which there may exist some gaps in the present study. Hence future research may be directed to bridge the gap so as to enhance the scope of analysis.

REFERENCES

Abdoh Tabrizi, H., & Jouhare, H. (1996). The Investigation of Efficiency of Stock Price Index of T.S.E. *Journal of Financial Research*, *13*, 11–12.

Abdulsalam Sulaiman Olaniyi, S., Adewole Kayode, S., & Jimoh, R. G. (2011). Stock Trend Prediction Using Regression Analysis – A Data Mining Approach. *ARPN Journal of Systems and Software*, *1*(4), 651–656.

Adetunji, , & Aderounmu, , Olusayo, & Adigun. (2013). Forecasting Movement of the Nigerian Stock Exchange All Share Index Using Artificial Neural and Bayesian Networks. *Journal of Finance and Investment Analysis*, *2*(1), 41–59.

Alam, , Napitupulu, & Yohanes Budiman. (2013). Prediction of Stock Price Using Artificial Neural Network: A Case of Indonesia. *Journal of Theoretical and Applied Information Technology*, *54*(1), 104–109.

Ankerst, M. (2001). *Visual Data Mining with Pixel-Oriented Visualization Techniques.ACM SIGKDD Workshop on Visual Data Mining*, San Francisco, CA.

Armstrong Scott, J. (2012). Illusions in Regression Analysis. *Journal of Forecasting, 28*(3), 689-695.

Avrma. (2004). Stock Return Predictability and Asset Pricing Models. *The Review of Financial Studies, 17*(3).

Beaver, W. H. (1966). Financial Ratios, as Predictors of Failure. *Journal of Accounting Research, 4*, 71–111. doi:10.2307/2490171

Boston, R. (1998). *A Measure of Uncertainty for Stock Performance.IEEE/IAFE/INFORMS Conference Computational Intelligence for Financial Engineering (CIFEr)*, New York, NY. doi:10.1109/CIFER.1998.690072

Brown, D. P., & Jennings, R. H. (1989). On Technical Analysis. *Review of Financial Studies, 2*(4), 527–551. doi:10.1093/rfs/2.4.527

Chen, A. S., Leung, M. T., & Daouk, H. (2003). Application of Neural Networks to an Emerging Financial Market: Forecasting and Trading the Taiwan Stock Index. *Computers & Operations Research, 30*(6), 901–923. doi:10.1016/S0305-0548(02)00037-0

Chih-Fong, T. (2010). Combining Multiple Feature Selection Methods for Stock Prediction: Union, Intersection, and Multi-Intersection Approaches. *Decision Support Systems, 50*(1), 258–269. doi:10.1016/j.dss.2010.08.028

Das, A. P. (2008). *Security Analysis and Portfolio Management* (3rd ed.). New Delhi, India: I.K. International Publication.

Dutta, A. (2001). Investors Reaction to the Good and Bad News in Secondary Market. A Study Relating to Investors Behavior. *Finance India, 15*(2), 567–576.

Fadai Nejad, M. I. (1994). Stock Market Efficiency: Some Misconceptions. *Journal of Financial Research, 1*(2), 227–236.

Fama Eugene, F. (1965). The Behavior of Stock Market Prices. *The Journal of Business, 38*(1), 34–105. doi:10.1086/294743

Fayyad, U. M., Piatetsky, Shapiro, G., Smith, P., & Uthurusamy, R. (Eds.). (1996). Advances in Knowledge Discovery and Data Mining. AAAI Press/MIT Press.

Freedman David, A. (2005). *Statistical Models: Theory and Practice*. Cambridge University Press. doi:10.1017/CBO9781139165495

Ghezelbash. (2012). Predicting Changes in Stock Index and Gold Prices to Neural Network Approach. *The Journal of Mathematics and Computer Science, 4*(2), 227 – 236.

Gupta, S. C., & Kapoor, V. K. (2000). *Fundamentals of Mathematical Statistics* (10th ed.). New Delhi, India: Sultan Chand and Sons.

Hadavandi, E., Shavandi, H., & Ghanbari, A. (2010). Integration of Genetic Fuzzy Systems and Artificial Neural Networks for Stock Price Forecasting. *Knowledge-Based Systems*, *23*(8), 800–808. doi:10.1016/j.knosys.2010.05.004

Han, J., & Kamber, M. (2006). *Data Mining: Concepts and Techniques* (2nd ed.). San Francisco, CA: Morgan Kaufmann.

Hebb, D. O. (1949). *The Organization of Behavior: A Neuropsychological Theory*. New York: Wiley.

Hirji, K. K. (2001). Exploring Data Mining Implementation. *Communications of the ACM*, *44*(7), 87–93. doi:10.1145/379300.379323

Hong, T.-P., Horng, C.-Y., Wu, C.-H., & Wang, S.-L. (2009). An Improved Data Mining Approach Using Predictive Item sets. *Expert Systems with Applications*, *36*(1), 72–80. doi:10.1016/j.eswa.2007.09.009

Jie, S., & Hui, L. (2008). Data Mining Method for Listed Companies Financial Distress Prediction. *Knowledge-BasedSystemsJournal*, *21*(1), 1–5.

Kamley, S., & Jaloree, S. (2014). Stock Market Behavior Prediction Using NN based Model. *British Journal of Mathematics and Computer Science*, *4*(17), 2502–2515. doi:10.9734/BJMCS/2014/9819

Kamley, S., & Jaloree, S., & Thakur, R.S. (2015). Rule Based Approach for Stock Selection: An Expert System. *International Journal of Computing Algorithm*, *4*(Special Issue), 1142–1146.

Mcculloch, W. S., & Pitts, W. H. (1943). A Logical Calculus of the Ideas Immanent in Nervous Activity. *Bull. Math. Biopsy*, *5*(4), 115–133. doi:10.1007/BF02478259

Nandagopal, S., Arunachalam, V. P., & Karthik, S. (2012). A Novel Approach for Mining Inter-Transaction Itemsets. *European Scientific Journal*, *8*, 14–22.

Olatunji, S. O. (2013). Forecasting the Saudi Arabia Stock Prices based on Artificial Neural Networks Model. *International Journal of Intelligent Information Systems*, *2*(5), 77–86. doi:10.11648/j.ijiis.20130205.12

Peter, I., Osakwe, C., Kayode, A.A., & Adagunodo, E.R. (2012). Prediction of Stock Market in Nigeria Using Artificial Neural Network. *International Journal of Intelligent Systems and Applications*, *11*, 68–74.

Philip, M. T., Paul, K., Choy, S. O., Reggie, K., Ng, S. C., Mak, J., & Tak-Lam, W. et al. (2007). Design and Implementation of NN5 for Hong Stock Price Forecasting. *Journal of Engineering Applications of Artificial Intelligence*, *20*(4), 453–461. doi:10.1016/j.engappai.2006.10.002

Pujari, A. K. (2006). Data Mining Techniques (10th ed.). Hyderabad, India: Universites (India) Press Private Limited.

Rajesh, , & Sulabha. (2012). Fragment Based Approach to Forecast Association Rules from Indian IT Stock Transaction Data. *International Journal of Computer Science and Information Technologies*, *3*(2), 3493–349.

Ray, M., Sharma, H. S., & Choudhary, S. (2006). A Reference book on Mathematical Statistics (4th ed.). Agra, India: Ram Prakash and Sons.

Rosenblatt, F. (1958). The Perceptron: A Probabilistic Model for Information Storage and Organization in the Brain. *Psychological Review*, *65*(6), 386–408. doi:10.1037/h0042519 PMID:13602029

Saeedmanesh, M., Izadi, T., & Ahvar, E. (2002). *A Hybrid Data Mining Technique for Stock Exchange Prediction*. International Multi Conference, China.

Se, H. (2001). Advances in Predictive Models for Data Mining. *Pattern Recognition Letters*, *22*(1), 55–61. doi:10.1016/S0167-8655(00)00099-4

Sim, K., Gopalkrishnan, V., Phua, C., & Cong, G. (2012). 3D Subspace Clustering for Value Investing. *IEEE Intelligent Systems*, *99*(1), 1–8.

Sivanandam, S. N., Sumathi, S., & Deepa, S. N. (2006). *Introduction to Neural Networks Using Matlab 6.0* (7th ed.). New Delhi, India: Tata McGraw Hill Publishing Company Limited.

Srisawat. (2011). An Application of Association Rule Mining Based on Stock Market. *3rd International Conference on Data Mining and Intelligent Information Technology Applications* (ICMIA).

Stock Market Data Source. (n.d.). Retrieved from http://www.bseindia.com

Sutheebanjard, P., & Premchaiswadi, W. (2010). Stock Exchange of Thailand Index Prediction Using Back Propagation Neural Networks.*2nd International Conference on Computer and Network Technology (IEEE)*. doi:10.1109/ICCNT.2010.21

Tan, P., Kumar, V., & Shrivastava, J. (2004). Selecting the Right Interesting Measure for Association Patterns. *Information Systems*, *29*(4), 293–331. doi:10.1016/S0306-4379(03)00072-3

Tiwari, V., & Thakur, R. S. (2015). Contextual Snowflake Modeling for Pattern Warehouse Logical Design. Sadhana - Academy Proceedings in Engineering Science, 40(1), 15-33.

Tiwari, V., Tiwari, V., Gupta, S., & Mishra, R. (2010). Association Rule Mining- A Graph based approach for mining Frequent Itemsets.*IEEE International Conference on Networking and Information Technology (ICNIT)*. doi:10.1109/ICNIT.2010.5508505

Toivonen, H. (1996). Sampling Large Databases for Association Rules. In *Proc. 22nd VLDB*.

Tsanga, K. M. P. (2007). Desing and Implementation of NN5for Hong Kong Stock Price Forecasting. *Engineering Applications of Artificial Intelligence*, *15*(4), 453–461. doi:10.1016/j.engappai.2006.10.002

Tuzhilin, A., & Silberschatz, A. (1996). What Makes Patterns Interesting in Knowledge Discovery Systems. *IEEE Transactions on Knowledge and Data Engineering*, *8*(6), 970–974. doi:10.1109/69.553165

Ugwu, C., & Onwuachu, C. (2014). Machine Learning Application for Stock Market Price Prediction. *The Pacefic Journal of Science and Technology*, *15*(2), 155–166.

Vaisla, , & Bhatt, . (2010). An Analysis of the Performance of Artificial Neural Network Technique for Stock Market Forecasting.*International Journal on Computer Science and Engineering*, *2*(6), 2104–2109.

Warner, B., & Misra, M. (1996). Understanding Neural Networks as Statistical Tools. *The American Statistician*, *50*, 284–293.

White, H. (1988). Economic Prediction Using Neural Networks: The Case of IBM Daily Stock Returns. In *Proc. of the IEEE International Conference on Neural Networks*. doi:10.1109/ICNN.1988.23959

Xiangwei, L. (2012). Based on BP Neural Network Stock Prediction. *Journal of Curriculum and Teaching*, *1*(1), 45–50.

Yao, , Teng, , Poh, , & Tan, . (1998). Forecasting and Analysis of Marketing Data Using Neural Networks. *J. Inf. Sci. Eng.*, *14*(4), 843–862.

Zhang, C., Pan, H., & Zhou, K. (2015). Comparision of Back Propagation Neural Networks and EMD-Base Neural Networks in Forecasting the Three Asian Stock Markets. *Journal of Applied Sciences*, *15*(1), 90–99. doi:10.3923/jas.2015.90.99

Zuo, Y., & Kita, E. (2012). Stock Price Forecasting Using Bayesian Network. *Expert Systems with Applications*, *39*(8), 6729–6737. doi:10.1016/j.eswa.2011.12.035

KEY TERMS AND DEFINITIONS

Artificial Neural Network (ANN): In machine learning and cognitive science, artificial neural networks (ANNs) are a family of models inspired by biological neural networks (the central nervous systems of animals, in particular the brain) and are used to estimate or approximate functions that can depend on a large number of inputs.

Association Rule Learning (ARL): ARL is one of the most popular data mining techniques. ARL is a method for discovering interesting relations between variables in large databases. It is intended to identify strong rules discovered in databases using some measures of interestingness.

Bombay Stock Exchange (BSE): The Bombay Stock Exchange (BSE) is an Indian stock exchange Established in 1875; the BSE is Asia's first stock exchange and the world's fastest stock exchange with a median trade speed of 6 microseconds. The BSE is the world's 11th largest stock exchange with an overall market capitalization of $1.7 trillion as of January 23rd, 2015. More than 5500 companies are publicly listed on the BSE.

Data Mining: Data Mining is an interdisciplinary subfield of computer science. It is the computational process of discovering patterns in large data involving methods at the intersection of artificial intelligence, machine learning, statistics, and database systems. The overall goal of the data mining process is to extract information from a data set and transform it into an understandable structure for further use.

K-Means Clustering: K-Means clustering is a method of vector quantization, originally from signal processing, that is popular for cluster analysis in data mining. K-means clustering aims to partition n observations into k clusters in which each observation belongs to the cluster with the nearest mean, serving as a prototype of the cluster. This results in a partitioning of the data space into Voronoi cells.

Linear Regression: In statistics, Linear Regression is an approach for modeling the relationship between a scalar dependent variable Y and one or more explanatory variables (or independent variables) denoted X. The case of one explanatory variable is called simple linear regression.

Multiple Regression: Multiple Regression is an extension of simple linear regression. It is used when we want to predict the value of a variable based on the value of two or more other variables. The variable we want to predict is called the dependent variable (or sometimes, the outcome, target or criterion variable).

Prediction: Prediction is also one form of data analysis task, where the model constructed predicts a continuous valued function or ordered value, as opposed to a categorical label. This model is a predictor. Regression analysis is a statistical methodology that is most often used for numeric prediction.

Stock Market: A stock market, equity market or share market is the aggregation of buyers and sellers (a loose network of economic transactions, not a physical facility or discrete entity) of stocks (also called shares); these may include securities listed on a stock exchange as well as those only traded privately.

Chapter 11
Profit Pattern Mining Using Soft Computing for Decision Making:
Pattern Mining Using Vague Set and Genetic Algorithm

Vivek Badhe
MANIT, India

R. S. Thakur
MANIT, India

G. S. Thakur
MANIT, India

ABSTRACT

Problem of decision making is a crucial task in every business. Profit Pattern Mining hit the target by minimizes the gap between statistical based pattern generation and value base decision making. But this job is found very difficult when it depends on the large, imprecise and vague environment, which is frequent in recent years. The concept of soft computing with data mining is novel way to address this difficulty. The general approaches to association rule mining focus on inducting rule by using correlation among data and finding frequent occurring patterns. The major technique uses support and confidence measures for generating rules which is not adequate nowadays as a measure of interest, since the data have become more multifaceted these days, it's a necessary to find solution that deals with such problems and uses some new measures like profit, significance etc. In this chapter, authors apply concept of pattern mining with vague set theory, Genetic algorithm theory and related properties to the commercial management to deal with business decision making problem.

DOI: 10.4018/978-1-5225-0536-5.ch011

INTRODUCTION

In last few decades, information is being generated at rapid pace. If Moore's law be applicable in information generation, then we surely can say it will be a 100 or 1000 times faster than the normal chipset designing rate to new trends. Because of this huge amount of information, database systems have been and are being developed to manage such a pile. To store information is one thing, but to deal with it is another. To recognize and extract the hidden knowledge and potentially interesting patterns from these large databases is accomplished by Data Mining. We know that the association rule mining algorithm is capable to generate the thousands or even millions of rules, but all the rules generate by mining algorithms may not be interesting. As the rules generated by association rule mining algorithms have only statistical significance and alone not capable to give the interesting results. Thus require additional technique like *genetic algorithm* to discover the interesting rules.

Data Mining is a research area where large databases are processed and knowledge discovery is done by application of algorithms that have both statistical and logical significance. As these databases have information from various sources, they are liable to have some magnitude of uncertainty and vagueness in them. To administer with vagueness in databases, *vague rule generation* is a new direction in finding out the correlations and rules that eventually maximize the business profit as well as an inclination towards decision making process.

Data Mining

Data Mining (DM) Techniques (Pujari, 2001) is being highly used for extracting the hidden predictive information from large databases. data mining is also an interesting research area that raises several challenging problems. Profit Pattern Mining is one of them which is a new direction of data mining that deals with prime goal of any business that is to maximize profit.

Data mining (Han et al. 2001) may also be viewed as the process of turning the data into information, the information into action, and action into value or profit. The Figure 1 shows the typical major components of data mining system:

Knowledge Discovery in Databases

Knowledge Discovery in Databases (KDD) (Han et al. 2001) refers to the nontrivial unknown and potentially useful information from data in databases. There is a series of steps/stages involved in KDD shown in Figure 2.

1. **Data Integration:** It is a stage, where multiple data sources often heterogeneous, may be combined in a common source.
2. **Data Selection and Cleaning:** It is a stage, concerned with selecting or segmenting the data that are relevant to some criteria and removes noise, irrelevant and incorrect data from the data collection.
3. **Data Transformation:** This stage is also known as data consolidation, where data are transformed or consolidate into forms appropriate for mining by perfoffiling summary or aggregation operations, for instance.
4. **Data Mining/Pattern Discovery:** An essential process where intelligent methods are applied in order to extract potential useful patterns.

Figure 1. Architecture of a typical data mining system

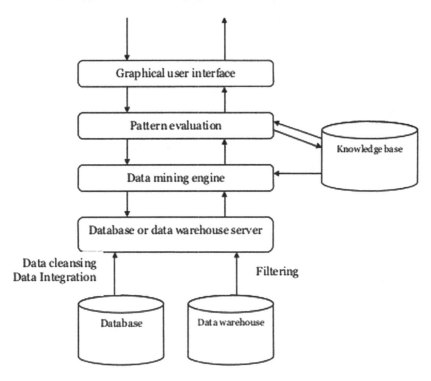

Figure 2. Stages involved in knowledge discovery in database

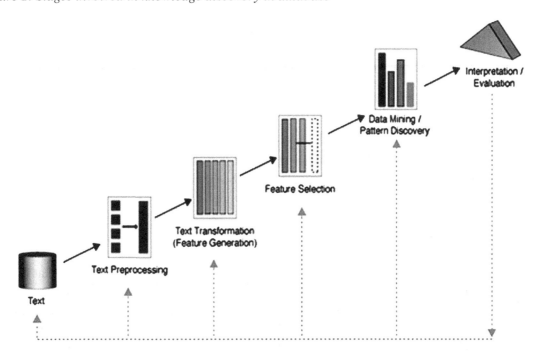

5.   **Interpretation / Pattern Evaluation:** This stage identifies the truly intersecting patterns representing knowledge based on some interestingness measures and uses visualization technique to help, understand and intercept the data mining results to users.

Data Mining Methodology

Mining methodology (Han et al. 2001) has two fundamental goals: *Prediction* and *description*. Prediction allows existing objects in a database to predict unknown or hidden values which has some interesting measure. Description on the other hand focuses on discovering patterns which describe the data and then following it with presentation and visualization techniques for interpretation. Different methodologies are:

- Association Rules Mining
- Classification
- Clustering

Association Rule Mining

Association rules (Han et al. 2001) are, in general, if-then rules that work on some conditional probability. The two main parameters used for such conditions are support and confidence. The support can be concocted of as the percentage that all the items in the rules will satisfy. The confidence on the other hand can be defined as the degree of certainty that an association will hold.

Classification

Classification (Han et al. 2001) is basically done by categorizing data into classes, and then with the help of a model it predicts for an individual data where it may be assigned a label for particular class. It is a categorical classification and supervised learning technique which organize data into its class.

Clustering Techniques

In clustering (Han et.al. 2001) the data is divided into groups of objects having similar characteristics. The data objects in a cluster are similar to other objects of that cluster. Any two or more cluster differs in their physical characteristics. Clustering analysis has been widely used in numerous applications, including pattern recognition, data analysis, image processing and market research.

Data Mining using Soft Computing Techniques

Classical approach to data mining was based on statistical analysis. It was profitable at that time but since then, the database has grown immensely and there is a need to employ and embed some techniques that could enhance the data mining capabilities. As the databases today are pervasive and closer to real world, it has become mandatory to use methods that mines real world data. Reasoning based computing was introduced with the capability to deal with conditions that were unable to process in traditional techniques. Thus, reasoning is employed using soft computing techniques (Kanhaiya et al. 2011). The basic soft computing techniques are neural network, fuzzy logic and genetic algorithms.

Vague Set Theory

The vague set theory (Wen-Lung et al. 1993) was first proposed by W. L. Gau in 1993. This theory gives the viewpoint of vague concepts. It deals with the data having vagueness and can easily apply.

Data Mining Using Genetic Algorithms

The application of the genetic algorithm (Kanhaiya et al. 2011) in the context of data mining is generally for the task of hypothesis testing, refinement and optimization. Data mining can be thought of as a search problem. The problem is to search a large space for interesting information (rules). The absolute size of the search spaces involved in data mining requires that algorithm be explored that can determine interesting rules by examining subsets of this data. The main motivation for using GAs in the discovery of high-level rules by optimization is that they perform a global search and cope better with attribute interaction. GA requires no prior knowledge about the search space and discontinuities preset on the search space have little effect on overall search process.

Profit Pattern Mining

Profit Pattern Mining (Wang et al. 2002) is a new direction of Association Rule Mining it aims to discover those patterns which provides maximum profit (Parvinder et al. 2010). As the major obstacle in the Association Rule Mining application is the gap between the statistical based patterns extraction and valued based decision making, Profit Pattern mining reduces this gap Figure 3 shows the hierarchy of profit pattern mining.

In Profit Pattern Mining a set of past transaction and pre selected target item is given and a model is constructed for recommending target items and promotion strategies to new customers, with the goal of maximizing the net profit.

Figure 3. Hierarchy of profit pattern mining

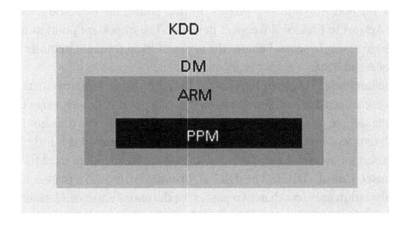

BACKGROUND: A BRIEF REVIEW OF THE WORK ALREADY DONE

The literature review is categorized into *three* sections. In the first section, the mining techniques are introduced that have been developed over the years and how other reasoning based methodology are used which affect the association rule generation. The second section discusses about the related work that have been done so far in association rule mining with vague sets. The Third and last section contains some of the Genetic Algorithms approaches in different aspects.

Classical Association Rule Mining Algorithms

The following section describes some notable literature for Association Rule mining. This can be done on basis of data representation formats for rule mining-horizontal format or vertical format.

Mining Frequent Itemsets Using Horizontal Data Layout

- **AIS:** The foremost method which was developed was the AIS (Agrawal et al. 1993). It was proposed by considering a very large database and mining through it and generating association rules.
- **Apriori Algorithm:** The Apriori (Agrawal et al. 1994) is considered the milestone in data mining. It is a successor to AIS and had the capability of performing better than it in orders of magnitude. The reason why apriori was more effective than AIS is because of the pruning optimization done by following downward and upward closure property. The downward closure property states that if any itemsets are frequent than all of the subsets are frequent. Also, if any itemset is infrequent than all its supersets are infrequent. The issue with the algorithm is that for n length of frequent itemsets it takes n database scans (iterations).
- **Variants/Extensions of Traditional Apriori Algorithm:** AIS and Apriori are the foremost algorithms developed in association rule mining, but as the database became more and larger, so does the mining process also progressed. Many other version of Apriori has been developed since then. Some of those variations or extensions are as follows (Tiwari et al. 2010).
- **Partitioning Technique:** The first improvement over Apriori was the partition technique (Savasere et al. 1995) . Developed by Savasere et. al. The method divides the database in logical disjoints partitions. The method works in two phases. In first phase, the database uses n partitions, each partition uses Apriori to find local frequent itemsets. The important point to notice is that it uses only two database scans. In second phase, the union of local frequent itemsets is obtained to form the global frequent itemset.
- **Sampling:** The sampling (Toivonen 1996) algorithm was another improvement over Apriori. Here the data items are selected at random from the database. If n is the data size then m samples are chosen. Also the sample size should be near to the memory size. The threshold values for samples and the overall datasets are kept different, i.e., the sample threshold is a little less than the actual threshold of the entire dataset. Later the itemsets that are frequent are used for rule generation.
- **Dynamic Itemset Count (DIC):** The DIC algorithm (Brin 1997) is also a modification over Apriori. The algorithm uses less than two passes for the entire database/dataset thus reducing a lot of time but increasing performance. The candidates are generated and as soon as the infrequent itemsets are found they are removed and frequent move forward in the process. It allows the addition of candidate itemsets while performing scanning of database.

- **FP Growth:** One of the most interesting association rule mining algorithm developed (Han et al. 2004) denoted as FP-growth. The FP-growth uses a new data structure FP-tree which works on the divide and conquer principle. The method recursively mines the database without generating candidate itemsets directly to frequent itemsets by creating nodes and traversing through the database while counting the items and sorting them in descending order of support.

Mining Frequent Itemsets Using Vertical Data Layout: Equivalence CLAss Transformation (ECLAT)

The essence of ECLAT (Zaki 2000) is to explore and mine the vertical data format efficiently. The algorithm was proposed by Zaki. He proposed that by using lattice theory, a bigger lattice search space can be decomposed into smaller sublattices which can be processed in main memory. MaxClique (Zaki et al. 1997) is one such algorithm used for fast decomposition along with three (bottom-up, top-down, & hybrid) new search strategies. The ECLAT approach uses few database scans and minimal amount of I/O costs.

Association Rule Mining Using Vague Set Theory

Most of the research work in this area is done by An Lu et al. The following discussion gives a brief overview of the vague set theory applied to association rules.

Managing Merged Data by Vague Functional Dependencies (2004)

In traditional (or classical) approach for mining rule, it is impossible to find vagueness.. This vagueness is to be identified first which forms the basis of vague association rules. The application of vague logic by proposing similarity equality measure (SEQ) in a relational database gives an objective to capture vagueness of data. Furthermore, Vague Functional Dependencies (VFDs) (Lu & Ng, 2004) are presented which validate the inference rules operations performed on different vague relations.

Vague Sets (VS) or Intuitionistic Fuzzy Sets (IFS) for Handling Vague Data: Which One Is Better? (2005)

A lot of work has been done considering how can we find rules that are more natural and adjacent to the real world scenario. The plausible difference found between IFS and VS is the membership intervals (Lu et al. 2005).

Mining Vague Association Rules (2007)

VAR (Lu et al. 2007) first proposed that it is possible to identify vagueness in data and use it to enhance the rule mining process. Vague Association Rules (VARs) is the first of the proposed method that incorporates essential properties of vague set theory. The vague association rules uses the notion of intent, attractiveness, hesitation which are derived from median and imprecision membership values of vague sets. With attractiveness (A) and hesitation (H), an AH-pair database is modeled on which four types of vague support and four types of vague confidence are applied instead of generic support and confidence, thus resulting in vague association rules (VARs). The VARs capture richer information as compared to the generalized association rules. The VARs are generated by refining the classical apriori algorithm by MineVFI that mines vague itemsets not of the main dataset but of the vague AH-pair dataset.

Mining Hesitation Information by Vague Association Rules (2007)

In this paper (Lu e al. 2007) authors give a detailed description of where the VARs can be most effective. The paper discusses a new parameter called hesitation information. For an online shopping scenario, each item that was added to the cart but did not go through the purchase contains some amount of hesitation information. This hesitation information can have many pieces called hesitation statuses (HS). Thus, any data object gives three types of evidences in the interval-based membership, namely; support, against and hesitation. Any item that has hesitation status equal to zero has high percentage of attractiveness. Thus by combining the attractiveness and hesitation information, it is easier to identify the evidence for vagueness of that data object.

Handling Inconsistency of Vague Relations with Functional Dependencies (2007)

The authors (Lu et al. 2007) again discussed and gave some measures to deal with vagueness in databases. Since the data collected from automated systems, sensor networks etc. have grown at rapid rate, it is liable to contain vagueness. Thus to maintain the consistency of vague relation in such databases, the well know integrity constraint to use is Functional Dependencies (FDs). In this paper, the author finds the best approximation of a vague relation with respect to the functional dependency by considering the median (m) and imprecision (i) memberships. Also, the author defines the notion of mi-overlap between vague sets relation which are satisfied by FDs.

A Model for Mining Course Information Using Vague (2012)

Another shows (Pandey et al. 2012) a very different aspect of vague association rules employed to a specific problem. The paper first proposes that the vagueness for every database is different, that is to say that to identify data objects with vagueness one has to have the knowledge of a specific domain. The work is composed of in the field of academia where the vague data objects (courses) are in vague relation to the users (students) of that object. The identification of vagueness whether a student is interested in undertaking classes on particular subject will be helpful in enhancing the course structure for any educational institute.

Association Rule Mining Using Genetic Algorithm

Optimization of Association Rule Mining Using Improved Genetic Algorithms

Authors (Saggar et al, 2004) used Genetic algorithms as post mining technique to optimize the rules generated by Association Rule Mining. Generally the rules generated by Association Rule Mining technique do not consider the negative occurrences of attributes in them, but by using Genetic Algorithms (GAs) over these rules the system can predict the rules which contains negative attributes. The motive for using Gas for rule discovery is that they perform a global search and cope better with attribute interaction.

Optimized Association Rule Mining Using Genetic Algorithm

Authors (Anandhavalli et al. 2009) is to find all the possible optimized rules from given data set using genetic algorithm. The rule generated by association rule mining algorithms like priori, partition, pincer-search, incremental, border algorithm etc, does not consider negation occurrence of the attribute in them and also these rules have only one attribute in the consequent part. By using Genetic Algorithm (GAs) the system can predict the rules which contain negative attributes in the generated rules along with more than one attribute in consequent part.

Genetic Algorithm-Based Strategy for Identifying Association Rules Without Specifying Actual Minimum Support

Authors (Xiaowei et al. 2009) developed strategy for identifying association rules without specifying actual minimum support using genetic algorithm. In their approach, they developed an elaborate encoding method and used relative confidence as the fitness function.

Mining Frequent Itemsets Using Genetic Algorithm

Authors (Soumadip et al. 2010) proposed method for frequent itemset mining using Genetic algorithm. The major advantage of using GA in the discovery of frequent itemsets is that they perform global search and its time complexity is less compared to other algorithms as the genetic algorithm is based on the greedy approach.

Optimization of Association Rule Mining through Genetic Algorithm

Authors (Rupali et al. 2011) designed a new method for generation of strong rule, here they used Genetic algorithm as post mining technique where Apriori algorithm is used to generate the rules after that those rules are optimized using Genetic algorithms. In this direction for the optimization of the rule set the design a new fitness function that uses the concept of supervised learning then the GA will be able to generate the stronger rule set.

Role of Soft Computing as a Tool in Data Mining

Authors (Kanhaiya et al. 2011) discussed that Genetic algorithm is the random optimization method based on the principle of the natural selection and biological evolution, which changes the solution of problems into data individuals of a gene string structure in genetic space by a certain coding scheme, converts objective function into fitness value, evaluates advantages and disadvantages of individuals, and as the basis to the genetic operation.

Genetic Algorithms for the Prioritization of Association Rules

Authors (Ramesh et al. 2011) proposed a genetic algorithm based association rule mining algorithm. Genetic algorithm has been used for prioritization of the rules Fitness function is based on the two measures confidence and the collective strength of the rules, other than the classical support and the confidence of the rules generated. The algorithm is been tested for the four data sets like Adult, Chess, Wine, Zoo.

Extraction of Interesting Association Rules Using Genetic Algorithms

Authors (Peter et al. 2008) presents a genetic algorithms based multi objective evolutionary algorithm rule mining method. They used confidence, comprehensibility, and interestingness as objectives of the association rule mining problem. Specific mechanisms for mutations and crossover operators together with elitism have been designed to extract interesting rules from a transaction database.

Mining Frequent Itemsets for Non Binary Data Set Using Genetic Algorithm

Authors (Vijay et al. 2011) proposed frequent itemset mining using Genetic algorithm. The main aim of this paper is to find all possible frequent itemsets from given dataset using the genetic algorithm.

Performance Analysis of Genetic Algorithm for Mining Association Rules

Authors (Indira 2012) presented method for performance analysis of Genetic algorithm for Mining Association rules. This paper analyzes the performance of GA in Mining ARs effectively based on the variations and modification in GA parameters. The recent works in the past seven years for mining association rules using genetic algorithm is considered for the analysis. Genetic algorithm has proved to generate more accurate results when compared to other formal methods available.

MAIN FOCUS OF THE CHAPTER

Association Rule Mining (ARM)

Association rules are employed to discover relationships among different items in a transactional database.

Basic Concept

An association rule mining could be explained with following concepts. Let in a database D there are a number of transactions T. In each transaction there is number of items belonging to itemset I. If n is the distinct number of items in D then $I = \{i_1, i_2...i_n\}$ is a set of all the items present in database. Also any transaction $t \in T$ may contain variable set of items over I, i.e., $i_1, i_2, i_k \subset I$. Each transaction is associated with a unique identifier T_ID. The association rule is of the form of $A \Rightarrow B$, where $A, B \subset I$ and $A \cap B = \emptyset$, where A is the consequent of the rule.

The association $A \Rightarrow B$ holds for any transaction T in D if its *support S* of any item is satisfied. Support S of an association rule R is the percentage of transaction t that contains $A \cup B$ (both A and B) which is the probability $P(A \cup B)$ of the items in transaction $\text{Supp}(A) = \dfrac{\text{count(A)}}{|D|}$. The association rule R, of the form $A \Rightarrow B$ has confidence C in transaction set T in D if the conditional probability satisfies, i.e., the transaction tn containing X also contains Y. It is taken as $P\left(B|A\right) = A \Rightarrow B = \dfrac{\text{Supp}\left(A \cup B\right)}{\text{Supp}\left(A\right)}$.

Association Rule Mining Algorithms

The usual schemes that are used for discovery of efficient frequent itemsets can be motley given by two categories, namely, candidate generation and pattern-growth.

The candidate generation suffers poor performance since to mine large datasets the database read operation rises to match the support for every itemset. Whereas, the pattern growth shows efficient performance for both long and short frequent itemsets and also accounting for support count.

- Apriori & Its Variants (Partitioned Techniques, Sampling, DIC, etc.)
- Without Candidate generation (FP Tree, FP Growth etc)

Frequent Itemset: To mine any frequent itemset for any transaction is a nontrivial task. The itemsets that occur frequently at least with the minimum user defined support are called frequent itemsets. To describe in mathematically, let $\mathbf{D}$ be the database with $\mathbf{T}$ set of transactions, such that the transaction tϵT and ϵ be the user specified threshold. Let $\mathbf{A} = \{\mathbf{I_1}, \mathbf{I_2}, \mathbf{I_3}...\mathbf{I_m}\}$ be the set of m items then, $\mathbf{X} \subset \mathbf{A}$ is called a frequent itemset with respect to ϵ in $\mathbf{T}$, if $\mathbf{S(X)_T} \geq \epsilon.11$

The frequent itemsets in association rules must satisfy some important properties as follows:

- **Downward Closure Property:** Any subset of frequent set is frequent set.
- **Upward Closure Property:** Any superset of an infrequent set is an infrequent set.
- **Maximal Frequent Set:** A frequent set is a maximal frequent set if it is a frequent set and no superset of this is a frequent set.
- **Border Set:** An itemset is a border set if it is not a frequent set, but all its proper subsets are frequent sets.

Application of Association Rule Mining

The association rule mining could be applied to many areas of research. Its first use is in market-basket analysis. Although it has proved to be preeminent in market strategy, it has extended its capabilities to other domains also like,

- Business
- Banking & Finance
- Insurance
- Science
  - *Medical science & research*
  - *Pharmaceutical and Drug discovery*
  - Astronomical science, etc.
- Government & Legal
  - Frauds and outlier detection.

- Education
- Sports, etc.

Challenges of Association Rule Mining

- **Efficiency and Scalability**
  - During the data cleaning process of pre-mining, "missing and noisy data" have effect on the final rule created.
  - The KDD expert or the data analyst must have some prior knowledge of data or domain.
  - The size (extent) of data affects the result.
  - In real world applications, the transactions are of the order of hundreds of thousands or presumably in millions.
  - The databases have usually thousands of distinct items (attributes).
  - It is difficult to define application specific interestingness measures.
  - It is computationally expensive of huge databases.
- **Application Exploration**
  - Gene Expression, DNA sequence analysis and bio-pattern classification
  - "Invisible" data mining
  - Flexibility and Reusability for Generating Association rule
  - Cost of the finding frequent Itemset.
  - Measures of Interestingness
  - Optimization of Association Rules
  - Memory Management

Vague Sets

Overview

The classical (crisp) set theory define sets as the "collection of objects (either similar or dissimilar) called elements of a set as a whole". These are also referred as crisp in nature because they only tells whether an element is a member or not, i.e., either 0 or 1. It may be also given as an element belongs to or does not belong to particular set. The crisp set theory often times is unable to provide a better understanding of any object/element to be of a certain group. Thus, leading to the fact that value might lie in between 0 and 1.

Basics

A *vague* set is a set of element distributed in a universe that has a grade of membership values in the continuous subinterval of [0, 1]. Hence, such a set can be marked by *true membership* and *false membership* functions. The continuous subinterval states both about the evidence that is in favor of the object and also that is opposing it.

Let V be the vague set. If U is the universe of discourse having X objects with x elements than V in U can be defined using the true membership (V_t) and false membership (V_f) functions. Considering that both V_t and V_f consorted as real numbers in the subinterval of [0, 1]. Also V_t is the lower bound on grade of membership of *x* derived in favor of *x*, and V_f is the lower bound on grade of membership derived against *x*, with each element in X where $V_t + V_f \leq 1$ and $V_t:X \to [0,1]$, $V_f:X \to [0, 1]$. Hence, the grade of membership of *x* is bounded to a subinterval $[V_t(x), 1-V_f(x)]$ of [0, 1].

Genetic Algorithm

Overview

A genetic of algorithm (Mitchell, 1996) is a type of searching algorithm. It searches a solution space for an optimal solution to a problem. The key characteristic of the genetic algorithm is how the searching is done. The algorithm creates a "population" of possible solutions to the problem and lets them "evolve" over multiple generations to find better and better solutions.

Cycle of the Algorithm

The algorithm operates through a simple cycle

- Population creation of strings.
- Evaluation of each string.
- Best string selection.
- Genetic manipulation to create a new population of strings.

Figure 4 shows the interconnection of these four stages. Each cycle produces a new generation of possible solutions (individuals) for a given problem.

The manipulation process enables the genetic operators to produce a new population of individual the offspring, by manipulation the genetic information processed by the pairs chosen to reproduce. The

Figure 4. The reproduction cycle

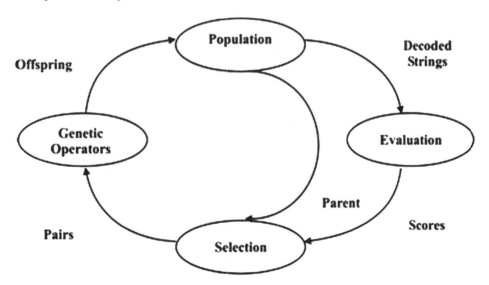

information stored in strings (chromosomes) that describes the individuals. Genetic operators are used. The offspring generated by this process take the place of the older population and the cycle is repeated until a desired level of fitness is attained, or a determined number of cycles are reached.

Biological Terminology

At this point it is useful to formally introduce some biological terminology in brief that will be used in rest of the section of Genetic Algorithm (Mitchell, 1996), the other terminology like Recombination (Crossover) and Mutation are explained in GA operator.

- **Chromosomes:** Strings of DNA that serves as a blueprint for the organism shown in Figure 5 are called chromosomes. A chromosome can be conceptually divided into genes function block of DNA, each of which encodes a particular protein.
- **Genotype:** Many organisms have multiple chromosomes in each cell. The complete collection of genetic material i.e. all chromosomes together is called genome. The term genotype refers to the particular set of genes in a genome.

Genetic Algorithm Terminology

This section explains some basic terminology for the genetic algorithm, including Fitness Functions, Individuals, Populations and Generations Fitness Values and Best Fitness Values Parents and Children.

- **Fitness Functions:** The fitness function is the function we want to optimize. For standard optimization algorithms, this is known as the objective function. Some issues related to fitness function are:
  - Domain specific to goals of problem
  - Single value output: multi-objective must be combined into single function
  - Fast! May need to be executed hundreds or thousands of times

Figure 5. Chromosome structure

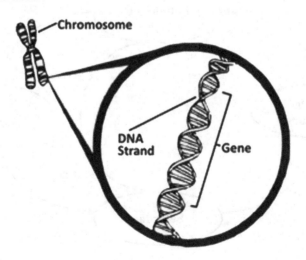

- **Individuals:** An individual is any point to which we can apply the fitness function. The value of the fitness function for an individual is its score.
- **Populations and Generations:** A population is an array of individuals. At each iteration, the genetic algorithm performs a series of computations on the current population to produce a new population. Each successive population is called a new generation.
- **Fitness Values and Best Fitness Values:** The fitness value of an individual is the value of the fitness function for that individual. Because we want to the maximum/minimum of the fitness function, the best fitness value for a population is the largest/smallest fitness value for any individual in the population.
- **Parents and Children:** To create the next generation, the genetic algorithm selects certain individuals in the current population, called parents, and uses them to create individuals in the next generation, called children. Typically, the algorithm is more likely to select parents that have better fitness values.

GAs Operators

Generation of successors is determined by a set of operators that recombine and mutate selected members of the current population; operators correspond to idealized versions of the operations found in biological evolution. The simple form of genetic algorithm involves most common three types of operators: Selection, Crossover and Mutation.

- **Selection:** This operator selects chromosomes in the population for reproduction. The operator filters those chromosomes that are more likely to be selected to reproduce.
- **Crossover:** Crossover is one of the genetic operators used to combine the population's genetic materials. It takes two chromosomes and swaps part of their genetic information to produce new chromosomes.
- **Mutation:** The Mutation operations introduces new genetic structure in the population by randomly changing some of its building blocks since the modifications is totally random and thus not related to any previous structure present in the population. It creates different structure related to other selection of the search space. The mutation is implemented by occasionally altering a random bit from a chromosome (string).

GAs Working Principle

The algorithm (Mitchell, 1996) begins by creating a random initial population. The algorithm then creates a sequence of new population, or generations. At each step, the algorithm uses the individuals in the current generation to create the next generation. For creating the new generation, the algorithm performs the following steps: Scores each member of the current population by computing its fitness value. Scale the raw fitness scores to convert them into a more usable range of values. Selects parents based on their fitness. Produce children from the parents. Children are produced either by making random changes to a single parent – mutation – or by combing the vector entries of a pair of parents – Crossover. Replace the current population with the children to form the next generation. The algorithm stops when one of the five stopping criteria ie generations, time limit, fitness limit, stall generations or stall time limit is met

Decision Making in Uncertainty

Overview

Uncertainty is a natural human concern to deal with. The thesaurus defines uncertainty as doubtfulness and changeableness of a value for a given problem. There are many synonyms of uncertainty and it is possible to allocate each as a "type of uncertainty". As humans correspond with each other in vague and fuzzy manner, the uncertainty is likely to consist. In real world scenario there are very less situation where we find ourselves imparting precise information in context to what we want to communicate and how.

Types of Uncertainty

In mathematics, typology for uncertainty is large. Our discussion limits us to few important types that will help further in our cause for decision making (Terrence et al. 2014). The following types of uncertainty are mostly studied: *vague, fuzzy, confidence, ambiguity, inconsistence, incompleteness, imprecise, general, anomalous, incongruence, ignorant, irrelevant.*

Types of Mathematical Models for Uncertainty

The following section gives a brief overview of the various mathematical tools that deal uncertainty (Wierman, 2010). They are:

1. Set theory
2. Probability theory
3. Fuzzy set theory
4. Rough set theory
5. Vague set theory

Set Theory

The set theory limits *ambiguity*. It is based on the notion of composition or collection. The largest collection is referred as the *universal* set, a universe of discourse, which are to be discussed. A universal set is responsible for the limiting of ambiguity of objects. Sets define whether an object belongs to or does not belong to a set. A collection of objects is called elements. Set theory also uses the concept of intervals (open, closed, or half-open/closed) to limit the values of its objects. Often logics are intertwined with set theory to give conclusions based on some premises. But logical conclusion eliminates uncertainty about the reasoning process.

Probability Theory

The probability theory deals with a different kind of uncertainty: *randomness*. Randomness can be defined as finding the exact outcome of an event is difficult to determine but with long term process will definitely be described. The probability theory follows set theory and logic to portray its functioning. The conditional probability is one of the widely used concepts of the theory. Joint distributions, Bayes theorem, Statistics are some of the extended forms in probability.

Fuzzy Set Theory

There are many other kinds of uncertainties apart from randomness. Things that are not random can still be uncertain. Fuzzy sets (Zadeh, 1965) to a certain extent deal with subjective classification, i.e., classifying objects to a tag or label with the help to a membership function. Fuzzy set can be useful where the source of information is a vague entity. Fuzzy set uses membership values to determine the boundaries of two different regions within a unit interval [0, 1]. Hence, it gives a better understanding of how can an object belong to some set either with full membership, no membership, or mostly partial membership. The theory is applied in mining very easily (Tzung-Pei et al, 2003).

Rough Set Theory

The basis for rough set theory (Pawlak, 1982) is based on the equivalence relations called indiscernibility. The equivalence classes under the indiscernibility relation are called granules. It is defined by partition of a classical set, and then on this partition rough approximations, both upper and lower, are formed on these granules. Pawlak concluded that rough sets are used to deal with vagueness (Pawlak et al. 2006) by defining it as the property of sets described by approximations.

Vague Set Theory

Many set theories are used to deal uncertainty, especially to handle vagueness. The vague se theory, however, was introduced precisely for handling vagueness. It is notion is based on the fuzzy sets but gives a more detailed and defined view for vagueness. Fuzzy uses unit interval to find membership value of the objects. Vague sets also use the unit interval, but classify the membership in two values *true and false membership*. The true membership (V_t) is the evidence of an element of an object present in the universe, and false membership (V_f) is the evidence of negation of element of an object in that universe. Thus vague sets enclose the interval boundary form [0, 1] to [V_t, 1-V_f].

Handling/Dealing Uncertainty in Decision Making

Real world is always certain. It is our understanding of the knowledge of it that makes it uncertain. Hence, uncertainty is filtered by our models of real world, not real world itself. Following is the Categories of Uncertainties in Databases (Motro, 1995).

- Description
- Transaction
- Processing

Description Uncertainty

The information that is stored in the databases is most likely to be percolated with uncertainty. To give a description of these objects as close to real world is the basic aspect of description uncertainty. The three views of the description are:

- **Elements. What are to be described?** The descriptions may take different forms and uncertainty could affect values of each of them depending upon the model used. This could be subcategorized as *Data* level, *Tuple* level, and *Relation* level.
- **Sources. Why uncertain descriptions?** Since reality is not subject to uncertainty but our knowledge of it, *unavailability* of perfect descriptions are the sole sources of uncertain descriptions as perfect descriptions may exist in real world.
- **Degrees. How much uncertainty there is?** The more the relevant information the higher the information is certain. But due to the absence of certain information, uncertainty takes different forms each with a different level. Uncertainty can form a hierarchy where highest degree of uncertainty is due to the doubt of a real world object's *existence*. Moving further in the hierarchy, even the elements existence is assured but some of the information that describes an object is unknown is referred as *incomplete or unavailable*.

Transaction Uncertainty

This category of uncertainty defines the operations that manipulate descriptions. The sole purpose here is to impact the quality of information that is delivered by the system in accordance to a users query. Transaction uncertainty is further defined in terms of transformations and modification made to the system.

- **Transformations:** Transformations are the set of operations which are used to derive more descriptions from stored descriptions. They are usually requests (queries) from the users for the information. There are many reasons why a request may be uncertain, like, *insufficient knowledge* of the database and system to the users. The uncertainty it identifies is *how the information is available* (or the organization of it). This can be considered less for users who have some amount of domain expertise but not all. As mentioned above, not all users have expertise in specific domain. Occasional user access the database system with information that is *vague*. Hence, it defines the uncertainty about *the information needed* (or how to make in acceptable to the system).
- **Modifications:** Modifications are the operations that affect the descriptions stored as information in the database systems. They allow both occasional and expertise users to update and restructure the database. The main sources of uncertainty are similar to transformations. Insufficient knowledge of the system and the specific database. Also the uncertainty about the information embedded in a modification, i.e., vague or imprecise modifications which does not relate to any area of expertise which is not far different from description uncertainty.

Processing Uncertainty

This type of uncertainty arises in the application of transactions to descriptions. The concept of processing uncertainty is to maintain the quality of information too. For that it may allow some of the information systems to process a request with limited computational resources and for other, it may involve random sampling or estimation techniques. And in both processing methods, there would possess uncertainty. Sometimes it is advantageous to be more simple that most accurate.

SOLUTIONS AND RECOMMENDATIONS

Data Mining Using Vague Set Theory

Overview

Data mining can be considered as large problem domain where interesting and valuable information is to be searched. The search depends on the size of dataset of any domain (or the size of a database). Since the database contains real world information it is subject to vagueness. Thus, it requires some efficient mining algorithms that can explore and determine interesting rule hidden within the data.

The approach of vague set theory in data mining is a step towards decision making. To take decision by considering vague parameter into account can be an improvement to a given specific problem domain whilst it was not with classical method. The classical technique limits us to certain extents whereas with vague set a predictive analysis can be done which might govern in the generation of more benefitting rules and patterns.

Vague Sets with Data Mining

Vague set theory is being used in data mining in one of the two different ways:

1. **Vague Sets in Pre-Mining:** Vague sets used in pre-mining results in recognizing the vague item-sets in database. The main functioning of this theory would be to resolve the data cleaning process of knowledge discovery. Data cleaning is an essential process in mining. Usually, in cleaning the databases/datasets in consideration lose some important information. Vague sets however, does not eliminate the cleaning process but enhances it by identifying the vague data available in the database.
2. **Vague Sets in In-Mining:** Vague sets are used formidably for in-mining process (Terrence et al. 2015). The traditional mining approach gives rules that follow support and confidence which considers only Boolean relation between data items, i.e., whether an item belongs with other item or not. But while using vague sets, one can easily identify the degree of vagueness in parameters by incorporating vague sets properties. As opposed to classical technique, the rules incorporated by vague sets results in vague rules (VR).

Performing In-Mining Task on Vague Values Found in Database to Generate VARs

The classical Apriori generates rules by eliminating any parameter related to a vague data object. The VARs, on the other hand, considers the vague aspect of any data object by limiting in within the sub interval [0, 1]. The absence of vagueness in classical rules ensures that the vague set theory is powerful tool to be used when vagueness is taken into account. The vague rules are used for decision making process.

The vague set approach is quite simple. First we need to identify the items that are vague in the database. Once it has been identified, we propose some of the few formulas and later explain what it does. The vague set theory states that the element (or object) of any universe can be limit to the sub interval [0, 1]. Any element belonging to a set is said to have true membership for that set. But element(s) that are variants of the same element that has true membership cannot be considered as false membership, as they also comprise the same item. Those items that are kept aside are termed as vague. Thus, it proves that element having true membership has evidence but those elements that are not present is the evidence against negation of that element termed as false membership. Thus V_t and V_f memberships are denoted as $V_t + V_f \leq 1$, $[V_t, 1-V_f]$ are called vague sets in subinterval [0, 1].

Even though in literature many measures have been describe (Tew et al, 2014). we propose few formulas that are based on vague set theory and satisfy the properties of vague theory. Also, we postulate some new terminologies in context to VARs.

Terminologies Used for Vague Rule Mining

Definitions:

- Variation Matrix/Table
- Vague Percentage
- Actual Support
- True Vague Support
- Actual Confidence
- True Vague Confidence

The following formulas are derived from the vague sets and ARM.

1. **Actual Support (S_{act}):** Actual Support (S_{act}) can also be defined as the classical support used in traditional Apriori algorithm. Here, we find the count of any item, i.e. its true membership (V_t) present in the database D. The vague or non-vague items count is considered in this definition and is denoted by: $S_{act} = V_t / |D|$.

2. **Actual Confidence (C_{act}):** The actual confidence works similarly as the traditional Apriori method. To generate a rule we find the union of any two items A and B (vague or non-vague) divide it with the respective antecedent item's support. It is defined by: $C_{act} = S_{act}(A \cup B) / S_{act}(A)$.

3. **Vague Percentage (V_p):** The vague percentage denotes the amount of vagueness contained in a database for a particular vague item. Since for an item in a database, there exists a true membership (V_t), a false membership (V_f), and a certain amount of vagueness, as in our case vague percentage (V_p). Thus, a database consists of $|D| = V_t + V_f + V_p \leq 1$ all the memberships and percentage values. The vague percentage can be denoted now as $V_p = |D| - (V_t + V_f)$.

The two types of support values are as follows:

1. **True Vague Support (S_{tvg}/S_{vg}):** The True Vague Support (S_{vg}) of a vague item is defined as the sum of true membership (V_t) of that item with the vague percentage (VP) found in the whole database D. it is denoted by: $(V_t + VP) / |D|$ or $(1 - V_f)/ |D|$ Thus we can also state that the lower bound on the negation of the evidence against an item in whole database is called true vague support.

The two confidence values are given as follows:

1. **True Vague Confidence (C_{tvg}/C_{vg}):** The true vague confidence is defined as the union of vague support values of any items A and B to either of its individual vague support. It is denoted by: $C_{vg} = S_{vg}(A \cup B) / S_{vg}(A)$.

Variation Matrix/Table: Once the vague items in the database are identified it is important to make them available during the mining process. For this purpose we design a variation table (or vague table) which consist the number of vague items in its N rows and the variant of that item in its M columns.

Minimum and Maximum Support Boundaries: In a vague set $[V_t, 1 - V_f]$, the true membership tells us about the existence (or occurring) of an item in a database. Hence it is liable to say that it is the minimum support boundary for a particular vague item. Also, the negation of evidence against an item, i.e. $(1-V_f)$ or $(V_t + V_p)$ is the maximum support boundary for that item when vagueness is considered into account.

Data Mining Using Genetic Algorithms

Overview

The application of the genetic algorithm (Mitchell, 1996) in the context of data mining is generally for the task of hypothesis testing, refinement and optimization. Data mining can be thought of as a search problem. The problem is to search a large space for interesting information (rules). The absolute size of the search spaces involved in data mining requires that algorithm be explored that can determine interesting rules by examining subsets of this data. The main motivation for using GAs in the discovery of high-level rules by optimization is that they perform a global search and cope better with attribute interaction. GA requires no prior knowledge about the search space and discontinuities preset on the search space have little effect on overall search process.

Application of Genetic Algorithm in the context of Data Mining is for event prediction. In this generating prediction pattern initializes the population, which contain only a single event. Another crucial component of Genetic Algorithms is the fitness measure. The fitness function must take an individual pattern and return a value indicating how good the pattern is at predicting target events. Conventional quality measures based on accuracy are not appropriate this notion of event prediction.

GA with Data Mining

Genetic Algorithm is used with Data mining in one of the three different ways:

Table 1. Variation matrix

Item(s)/Varients	Var(1)	Var(1)	Var(1)	...	Var(1)
Item(A)	A_1	A_2	A_3	...	A_m
Item(B)	B_1	B_2		...	B_m
...	...	...	...	...	...
Item(N)	N_1	N_2	N_3	...	N_m

1. **GA in Pre-Mining:** Although Genetic Algorithm is rarely applied in pre-mining ie. before mining process, still for some non linear constraints the GA is used in a pure traditional way.
2. **GA in In-Mining**: Genetic Algorithm is applied during mining process in two ways:
    a. **Traditional Genetic Algorithm:** During the mining process Genetic Algorithm is applied between the mining methods ie. association rule mining, clustering or outlier analysis etc. to optimize the results. The traditional GA is rarely used in-mining process.
    b. **Modified Genetic Algorithm:** During the mining process Genetic Algorithm itself is modified ie. the steps of Genetic Algorithm are altered accordingly and this is commonly used approach in in-mining process.
3. **GA in Post Mining:** In post mining, first the traditional mining is done and then Genetic Algorithm is applied to optimize the results. In general Genetic Algorithm is applied in a traditional way but sometimes the encoding method is modified as per the need. The use of Genetic Algorithm in Post mining is most commonly done.

Performing Post-Mining Task on Generated Rules from Conventional Association Rule Mining

The proposed framework and design shown in Figure 6 for mining the profit patterns using Genetic Algorithm covers the following tasks and they are Data Preprocessing, Implementing ARM Algorithm on processed data and optimizing the Rules using GA.

To design the fitness faction for the genetic algorithm we use measure called profit and define the notion of profit because the profit in any business is the key element and the notion of profit may vary depending upon the type of business but in general the notion of profit could be categorized as under:

1. **Value Profit**: Value profit is simply the difference of selling price and the cost price of any product. It is also called the margin of profit.
2. **Percentage of Profit**: It is the percentage of margin of profit with respect to the cost price of any product.
3. **Quantitative Profit**: It is the profit based on the number of items sold, and sometimes it is known as weighted factor.
4. **Interest Measure PROFIT:** It is the profit based on special measure based on the problem domain.

Figure 6. Block diagram of methodology

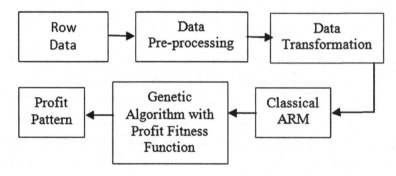

For each rule

Item1 → Item2

The fitness function designed as

$$Fitness(FF) = \frac{C * w1 + I * w2}{w1 + w2}$$

Where w1 and w2 are the user defined weighted factors, and C and I namely Completeness and Interestingness. The value of w1 and w2 are calculated as:

$$w1 = \frac{\text{Percentage profit of Item 1 * Quantity of Item 1}}{\text{Percentage profit of Item 2 * Quantity of Item 2}}$$

$$w2 = \frac{\text{Value profit on Item 1 * Quantity of Item 1}}{\text{Value profit on Item 2 * Quantity of Item 2}}$$

Completeness and Interestingness are defined & calculated as:
Completeness (C): Those rules are considered as complete rules where:

Item1→Item2

Item1 is having lower percentage of profit & Item2 having higher percentage of profit.
Interestingness (I): Those rules are considered as rules of interest where

Item1→Item2

Item1 is having lower value profit & Item2 having higher value profit.

$$C = \frac{TP}{TP + FP} \quad I = \frac{TP}{TP + FP}$$

Where TP, FP, FN are defined as
(For sample rule Item1→ Item2)

- **True Positive (TP):** No. of rules satisfying both Item1 & Item2
- **False Positive (FP):** No. of rules not satisfying Item1 but satisfying Item2.
- **False Negative (FN):** No. of rules satisfying Item1 but not satisfying Item2.

Pseudo-Code of Proposed Methodology

1. Start
2. Preprocess the Row Dataset |RD|

3. Transform the |RD| to Relevant Transaction Dataset |D|
4. Load the Sample Transactions |S| from Dataset |D|
5. Apply Apriori Algorithm to |S| for Rule Generation with defined parameter Support and Confidence.
6. Store the output of Apriori to rule set |R|
7. Apply the GA Cycle on |R|
    a. Selection - Tournament
    b. Crossover – Single Point
    c. Mutation - uniform
    d. Check fitness – Defined Fitness Function FF
    e. Check termination Condition Stall 100
8. Store the outcome of GA as final result to |F|, which contains the optimized (profitable) rules.
9. Mapped the |F| Rule with desire format
10. Stop

CONCLUSION

In this chapter, we formulated a technique for decision making by incorporating vague set theory as a tool in association rule mining. The rules generated by traditional Apriori are compared with the rules generated by our algorithm that finds vague rules. The Apriori algorithm is implemented and the dataset is fed to find rules. Our algorithm uses vague set theory concepts to find rules in the datasets. For that, we give few propositions and definitions regarding the vague terminology of the database, such as, vague percentage, true vague support, and true vague confidence.

We know that the association rule mining algorithm is capable to generate the thousands or even millions of rules, but all the rules generate by mining algorithms may not be interesting. As the rules generated by association rule mining algorithms have only statistical significance and alone not capable to give the interesting results. Thus require additional technique like genetic algorithm to discover the interesting rules. To generate the profit oriented patterns we have designed our fitness function which includes two measures named interestingness and completeness and two user's defined weighted factors that are purely based on profit to discover the profit oriented patterns and fulfill the business needs.

FUTURE RESEARCH DIRECTIONS

Association rule mining has been around for more than two decades as still proving as the most sought out technique for mining hidden knowledge. Association rule mining alone is a powerful method and combination with vague set theory and genetic algorithms improves the accuracy of results and provides interesting rules. Generating interesting rules is not full of reward until it can be utilized to improve the decision making process of business. Some recommender is still required for recommending target items and promotion strategies to new customers, with the goal of business expansion.

REFERENCES

Agrawal, R., Imielinski, T., & Swami, A. (1993). Mining association rules between sets of items in large databases. In *Proceedings of the ACM SIGMOD Int'l Conf. on Management of data*. doi:10.1145/170035.170072

Agrawal, R., & Shrikanth, R. (1994). Fast Algorithm for Mining Association Rules. In *Proceeding of VLBD Conference*.

Anandhavalli, M., Sudhanshu, S.K., Kumar, A., & Ghose, M.K. (2009). Optimized association rule mining using genetic algorithm. *Advances in Information Mining, 1*(2).

Arvind, T.S., & Badhe, V. (2014). Comparative Analysis of Fuzzy, Rough, Vague & Soft set Theories in Association Rule Mining. *International Journal Of Scientific Progress And Research, 2*(1).

Arvind, T.S., & Badhe, V. (2015). The Application of Vague Set Theory in Association Rule Mining: A Survey. *International Journal Advanced Research in Computer Science, 6*(1).

Bhasker, G.V., Shekar, K.C., & Chaitanya, V.L. (2011). Mining Frequent Itemsets for Non Binary Data Set Using Genetic Algorithm. *International Journal of Advanced Engineering Sciences and Technologies, 11*(1), 143-152.

Brin, S., Motwani, R., Ullman, J. D., & Tsurb, S. (1997). Dynamic itemset counting and implication rules for market basket data. *Proc. ACM SIGMOID Int. Conf. Manage. Data*. doi:10.1145/253260.253325

Gau, W.-L., & Buehrer, D. J. (1993). *Vague Sets*. IEEE.

Ghosh, S., Biswas, S., Sarkar, D., & Sarkar, P. P. (2010). Mining Frequent Itemsets Using Genetic Algorithm. *International Journal of Artificial Intelligence & Applications, 1*(4).

Haldulakar & Agrawal. (2011). Optimization of Association Rule Mining through Genetic Algorithm. *International Journal on Computer Science and Engineering, 3*(3), 1252–1259.

Han & Kamber. (2001). *Data Mining: Concepts and techniques*. Morgan Kaufmann Publishers.

Han, J., Pei, I., Yin, Y., & Mao, R. (2004). Mining frequent patterns without candidate generation: A frequent pattern tree approach. *Data Mining and Knowledge Discovery, 8*(1), 53–87. doi:10.1023/B:DAMI.0000005258.31418.83

Indira, K., & Kanmani, S. (2012). Performance Analysis of Genetic Algorithm for Mining Association Rules. *International Journal of Computer Science Issues, 9*(2).

Kanhaiya & Mohanti. (2011). Role of soft computing as a tool in data mining. *International Journal of Computer Science and Information Technologies, 2*(1), 526–537.

Lu, A., Ke, Y., Cheng, J., & Ng, W. (2007). *Mining Vague Association Rules*. Springer. doi:10.1007/978-3-540-71703-4_75

Lu, A., Ke, Y., Cheng, J., & Ng, W. (2007). Mining Hesitation Information by Vague Association Rules. In ER 2007 (LNCS), (vol. 4801, pp. 39–55). Springer-Verlag Berlin Heidelberg.

Lu, A., & Ng, W. (2004). *Managing Merged Data by Vague Functional Dependencies*. Springer. doi:10.1007/978-3-540-30464-7_21

Lu, A., & Ng, W. (2005). *Vague Sets or Intuitionistic Fuzzy Sets for Handling Vague Data- Which One Is Better?* Springer. doi:10.1007/11568322_26

Lu, A., & Ng, W. (2007). *Handling Inconsistency of Vague Relations with Functional Dependencies. In Conceptual Modeling - ER 2007 (LNCS)*, (Vol. 4801, pp. 229–244). Springer.

Mitchell, M. (1996). *An Introduction to Genetic Algorithms*. PHI.

Motro, A. (1995). *Management of Uncertainty in Database Systems*. New York, NY: ACM Press/Addison-Wesley Publishing Co.

Pandey, A., & Pardasani. (2012). A Model for Mining Course Information using Vague Association Rule. *International Journal of Computer Applications, 58*(20).

Pawlak, Z. (1982). *Rough sets*. Elsevier Inc.

Pawlak, Z., & Skowron, A. (2006). Rudiments of rough sets. *Information Sciences*, 177.

Pujari, A. K. (2001). *Data Mining Techniques*. University Press.

Ramesh Kumar & Iyakutti. (2011). Genetic algorithms for the prioritization of Association Rules. *IJCA*, 35-38.

Saggar, M., Agarwal, A. K., & Lad, A. (2004). *Optimization of Association Rule Mining using Improved Genetic Algorithms*. IEEE. doi:10.1109/ICSMC.2004.1400923

Sandhu, Dhaliwal, Panda, & Bisht. (2010). An Improvement in Apriori algorithm Using Profit And Quantity. *Second International Conference on Computer and Network Technology*. IEEE. DOI doi:10.1109/ICCNT.2010.46

Savasere, A., Omieccinski, E., & Navathe, S. (1995). An efficient algorithm for mining association rules in Large databases. *Proceedings of the 21st international Conference on Very Large Databases*.

Tew, C., Giraud-Carrier, C., Tanner, K., & Burton, S. (2014). Behaviour based clustering and analysis of interesting measures for association rule mining: Vol. 28. *Issue 4* (pp. 1004–1045). Springer.

Tiwari, A., Gupta, R. K., & Agrawal, D. P. (2010). A survey on Frequent Pattern Mining: Current Status and Challenging issues. *Information Technology Journal, 9*(7), 1278–1293. doi:10.3923/itj.2010.1278.1293

Toivonen, H. (1996). Sampling large databases for association rules. *Proceedings of 22th International Conference on Very Large Databases*.

Tzung-Pei, H., Kuei-Ying, L., & Shyue-Liang, W. (2003). Fuzzy Data Mining for Interesting Generalized Association Rules. *Fuzzy Sets and Systems, 138*(2), 255–269. doi:10.1016/S0165-0114(02)00272-5

Wakabi-Waiswa & Baryamureeba. (2008). Extraction of Interesting Association Rules Using Genetic Algorithms. *International Journal of Computing and ICT Research, 2*(1).

Wang, K., Zhou, S., & Han, J. (2002). Profit Mining: From Patterns to Actions. In EDBT 2002 (LNCS) (vol. 2287, pp. 70–87). Springer-VerlagBerlin Heidelberg.

Wierman, M. J. (2010). *An Introduction to the Mathematics of Uncertainty*. Center for the Mathematics of Uncerteainty, Creighton University.

Yan, X., Zhang, C., & Zhang, S. (2009). Genetic algorithmbased strategy for identifying association rules without specifying actual minimum support. *Elsevier, Expert Systems with Application, 36*(2), 3066–3077. doi:10.1016/j.eswa.2008.01.028

Zadeh, L. (1965). *Fuzzy Sets*. Elsevier Inc.

Zaki, M. (2000). Scalable algorithms for association mining. *IEEE Transactions on Knowledge and Data Engineering, 12*(3), 372–390. doi:10.1109/69.846291

Zaki, M., Parthasarathy, S., Ogihara, M., & Li, W. (1997). Parallel algorithm for discovery of association rules. *Data Mining and Knowledge Discovery, 1*(4), 343–374. doi:10.1023/A:1009773317876

KEY TERMS AND DEFINITIONS

Association Rule Mining (ARM): One of the important methods of data mining to find hidden correlation from database.

Data Mining: Is the mathematical technique to find hidden pattern from large database.

Genetic Algorithm: It is an unconventional optimization technique based on natural selection.

Knowledge Discovery in Database (KDD): Is the five step process of discovering useful knowledge from a collection of data.

Profit Pattern Mining: Is a new direction of association rule mining aims at finding profitable patterns.

Soft Computing: Is a set of methodologies, which aim to make use of tolerance for imprecision, uncertainty and partial truth to achieve tractability, robustness and low cost solution.

Vague Association Rule Mining: ARM whose measures based on vague set theory.

Vague Set Theory: In mathematics, vague sets are an extension of fuzzy sets.

Chapter 12
Effect of Odia and Tamil Music on the ANS and the Conduction Pathway of Heart of Odia Volunteers

Suraj Kumar Nayak
National Institute of Technology Rourkela, India

Utkarsh Srivastava
National Institute of Technology Rourkela, India

D. N. Tibarewala
Jadavpur University, India

Goutam Thakur
Manipal Institute of Technology, India

Biswajit Mohapatra
Vesaj Patel Hospital, India

Kunal Pal
National Institute of Technology Rourkela, India

ABSTRACT

The current study delineates the effect of Odia and Tamil music on the Autonomic Nervous System (ANS) and cardiac conduction pathway of Odia volunteers. The analysis of the ECG signals using Analysis of Variance (ANOVA) showed that the features obtained from the HRV domain, time-domain and wavelet transform domain were statistically insignificant. But non-linear classifiers like Classification and Regression Tree (CART), Boosted Tree (BT) and Random Forest (RF) indicated the presence of important features. A classification efficiency of more than 85% was achieved when the important features, obtained from the non-linear classifiers, were used. The results suggested that there is an increase in the parasympathetic activity when music is heard in the mother tongue. If a person is made to listen to music in the language with which he is not conversant, an increase in the sympathetic activity is observed. It is also expected that there might be a difference in the cardiac conduction pathway.

DOI: 10.4018/978-1-5225-0536-5.ch012

INTRODUCTION

Studies by various researchers have indicated that the emotional/ mood states of a person may be altered by making them listen to music (Juslin & Sloboda, 2001). Music can also help in reducing the anxiety of the patients in the coronary care units (Haun, Mainous, & Looney, 2001). The change in the state of mind, as mentioned above, affects the functioning of the Autonomic Nervous System (ANS) (Yamashita, Iwai, Akimoto, Sugawara, & Kono, 2006). The ANS comprises of parasympathetic and sympathetic nervous systems (Martini, 2005). The parasympathetic nervous system increases the intensity of contraction of the heart muscles due to the release of acetylcholine (Kiernan & Rajakumar, 2013). This, in turn, results in the decrease in the heart rate. The sympathetic nervous system, on the other hand, releases noradrenaline, which results in the increase in the rate of the heart muscle contraction (Triposkiadis et al., 2009). Hence, there is an increase in the heart rate. The ANS tries to maintain a balance amongst the sympathetic and parasympathetic system (sympathovagal balance) (Goldberger, 1999). A stimulus (either internal or external) may either increase the parasympathetic or the sympathetic activity depending upon the nature of the stimulus. Subsequently, the ANS starts acting to bring both the activities to balance. This results in the cardiac beat-to-beat variation of the cardiac activity (Sztajzel, 2004). Hence, the activity of the ANS can be analyzed by analyzing the ECG signals. The branch of study which allows to understand the ANS by analyzing the ECG signal is known as Heart Rate Variability (HRV) (Sztajzel, 2004). In the present study, we have tried to understand the effect of Odia and Tamil music on the ANS activity of the Odia volunteers. A thorough literature survey suggested that, though researchers have studied the effect of music on the heart rate variability, very few reports were found, which studied the effect of music on the ECG signals (Umemura & Honda, 1998). Hence, the statistical features of the ECG signal and the wavelet processed ECG signal were calculated and analyzed using linear and non-linear statistical processing techniques for classification using Automated Neural Network (ANN).

BACKGROUND

Understanding the effect of music on the physiological parameters of the individuals started more than 125 years ago (Davis, Gfeller, & Thaut, 2008). Music therapy has received much attention in the last decade for treating various physiological disorders (Koelsch, 2009). In music therapy, the patients are subjected to auditory stimulus with music (Watkins, 1997). Various authors have reported the use of music therapy in conjunction with various treatment regimes using allopathic intervention (Metzger, 2004). The auditory stimulation using music has been reported to alter the cardiac autonomic nervous system modulation (Peng, Koo, & Yu, 2009). The music has also been reported to improve the neuro-physiological activity of the persons (Boso, Politi, Barale, & Enzo, 2006). This, in turn, has been reported to not only influence the physiological states of the patients but also drastically alter the hemodynamic parameters. In this regard, positive effects were observed on the cardiovascular system when the patients were stimulated with classical music (Scheufele, 2000). The effect of other types of music, namely, vocals, orchestra and progressive crescendos on the cardiac activity has also been explored (Bernardi, Porta, & Sleight, 2006). In all the studies, an improvement in the cardiovascular regularity was observed when the volunteers were stimulated with the auditory music (Trappe, 2010). Roque AL *et al.* (2013) reported that if the volunteers are subjected to relaxant music, there is every chance of the increased activity of the sympathetic nervous system (Roque et al., 2013). On the contrary, listening to heavy metal music increases the activity of the sympathetic nervous system (Labbé, Schmidt, Babin, & Pharr, 2007). An increase in the activity of the sympathetic nervous system, in individuals who are undergoing stress and anxiety, deteriorates the health condition of the individuals (M. Esler & D. Kaye, 2000). Some of the commonly manifested disorders include disturbed sleep pattern, exhaustion of the individual and a corresponding reduction in the immunologic activity (Solin et al., 2003).

As reported in the previous paragraph, music may alter the cardiac autonomic activity. The autonomic nervous system acts as a bridge between the central nervous system and most of the peripheral organs and organ systems (Paxinos & Mai, 2004). The autonomic nervous system consists of two branches, namely, sympathetic nervous system and parasympathetic nervous system (Appenzeller & Oribe, 1997). These two branches of the autonomic nervous system try to maintain a dynamic flexibility to maintain a balance amongst themselves. This helps in the maintenance of good health. During many diseased conditions, this autonomic balance is lost, which in turn, results in the clinical manifestation of the patho-logical conditions. The set of clinical conditions which affects the health of the individuals are broadly classified as "ANS dysfunction" (Martínez-Lavín & Hermosillo, 2000). The various diseases which occur due to ANS dysfunction include automatic diabetic neuropathy, postural tachycardia syndrome, vasovagal syncope (Stewart, 2000). Additionally, ANS dysfunction manifests itself in conjunction with various neurodegenerative diseases (Alzheimer's and Parkinson's disease) (Zesiewicz, Baker, Wahba, & Hauser, 2003). The alteration in the autonomic nervous system activity can be predicted by measuring the beat-to-beat variation of the heart. The branch of study which analyzes the beat-to-beat variation to understand the autonomic activity of the heart is regarded as heart rate variability (HRV) (Bilchick & Berger, 2006). In general, a lack of variability in the beat-to-beat timing indicates the occurrence of ANS dysfunction (Adeyemi, Desai, Towsey, & Ghista, 1999). Most of the diseases which can provide information about the probability of mortality by analyzing the ANS dysfunction using heart rate vari-ability are related to cardiac system pathologies. Some of the common diseases include hypertension, hypercholesterolemia, multiple sclerosis, ischemic stroke and myocardial infarction (Carney et al., 2001).

Since music can alter the functionality of the autonomic nervous system, researchers were curious to know whether music can be helpful in improving the balance of the ANS in the individuals suffer-ing from the clinical conditions associated with the autonomic dysfunction. This curiosity amongst the researchers and the clinicians promoted them to investigate the effect of music on the health of the individuals suffering from autonomic dysfunction. The investigation results suggested that music can help in bringing back the balance in the autonomic nervous system and hence the auditory stimulus us-ing music may be used for the treatment of the individuals with autonomic dysfunction (Millan et al., 2012). This branch of the study of treating individuals extensively progressed in the last decade and has been named as music therapy (Ruud, 2010). It has benefited individuals suffering from various disorders including depression and autism and also has been useful in pain management (Good, Anderson, Ahn, Cong, & Stanton-Hicks, 2005).

MAIN FOCUS OF THE CHAPTER

The main focus of this study is to understand the effect of music on the functioning of the autonomic nervous system and conduction pathway of the heart of healthy individuals (Odia volunteers). This study was motivated by the keen interest to analyze the physiological alterations, induced by listening to the music of a specific language, which results in the improvement in the performance of the autonomic nervous system and the heart of an individual.

Conduction Pathway of the Heart

The generation of the electrical impulse, which results in the rhythmic contraction of the heart, takes place at the sinoatrial node (S-A node). The S-A node is present close to the superior vena cava on the right atrium (Boyett, Honjo, & Kodama, 2000). The sinoatrial node is composed of specialized cardiac muscles of nearly 1 mm thickness, 3 mm width and 15 mm length. There exists a direct connection between the muscle fibers of the sinoatrial node and the atrial muscle fiber (Monfredi, Dobrzynski, Mondal, Boyett, & Morris, 2010). This connection is responsible for the instantaneous spreading of the electrical impulse generated by the S-A node throughout the atrial wall and finally to the atrioventricular (A-V) node after a time interval of 0.03 msec. The A-V node is present in the backside wall of the right atrium close to the tricuspid valve (Lee, Chen, & Hwang, 2009). The A-V node has a bundle of fibers associated with it, known as A-V bundle (Tawara, Suma, & Shimada, 2000). It is formed of a number of small fascicule, which passes through the fibrous tissue that provides the separation between the atria and the ventricles (Racker & Kadish, 2000). The A-V bundle possesses a special property of restricting the backward conduction of the electrical impulses from the ventricles to the atria. This results in the unidirectional flow of the electrical impulses from the atria to the ventricles (Hall, 2010). The cardiac impulse is subjected to a delay of about 1.3 msec by the A-V node and its associated fiber, in order to facilitate sufficient time to the atria to finish the flow of their blood to the ventricles before the onset of ventricular systole (Burns, 2013). Therefore, the cardiac electrical impulse suffers from a delay of 0.16 msec due to the internodal pathway and the A-V nodal system, before it reaches at the ventricles. A specialized cardiac muscle fiber, known as the Purkinje fiber, extends from the atrioventricular node to the ventricles and passes through the A-V bundle. The characteristics of Purkinje fiber is quite opposite to that of the A-V bundle fiber. It results in the immediate spreading of the cardiac electrical impulse throughout the endocardial surfaces of the ventricles within a short span of 0.03 msec (Rentschler et al., 2001). This is attributed to the fact that it transmits the cardiac excitatory signal with a sufficiently high velocity, about 6 times and 150 times higher than that of the ventricular muscle fiber and atrioventricular bundle fiber respectively. After the Purkinje fiber, spreading of the cardiac electrical impulse throughout the epicardial surfaces of the ventricles is carried out by the ventricular muscle fiber (Torrent-Guasp et al., 2001).

The heart is connected to both the branches of the autonomic nervous system, namely, the parasympathetic and the sympathetic nervous system (Kawashima, 2005). The parasympathetic nerve connection to the heart is also known as the vagi. The parasympathetic nerves are mainly connected to the sinoatrial and the atrioventricular nodes and to a little extent to the atrial and ventricular muscles (Olshansky, Sabbah, Hauptman, & Colucci, 2008). On the other hand, the sympathetic nerves are dispersed throughout the heart with higher connection strength to the ventricular muscle. The activation of the parasympathetic nerves, connected to the heart, results in the release of the hormone acetylcholine at the nerve endings of the vagi. This, in turn, affects the functioning of the heart in two ways. Firstly, it reduces the rate of contraction of the sinoatrial node. Secondly, it reduces the excitability of the atrioventricular junction fibers present between the atrial muscles and the A-V node. Due to this reason, the passage of the cardiac electrical impulse into the ventricle gets slowed down. Therefore the activation of the parasympathetic nervous system can result in a reduction of the heart rate of a person up to half of the normal value (Carney, Freedland, & Veith, 2005). On the other hand, activation of the sympathetic nervous system causes the release of the norepinephrine hormone at the endings of the sympathetic nerves (Triposkiadis et al., 2009). It affects the functioning of the heart in a manner opposite to that of the parasympathetic nervous system. Firstly, it increases the rate of rhythmic contraction of the sinoatrial node. Secondly, the conduction speed of the cardiac electrical impulse increases in every portion of the heart. Thirdly, the contraction strength of the atrial as well as ventricular muscles gets increased (P. D. M. Esler & P. D. D. Kaye, 2000). The stimulation of the sympathetic nervous system can cause an increase in the heart rate of a person up to three times of the normal value and the force of contraction of the cardiac muscles also can increase up to twofold (Floras, 2009).

Electrocardiogram (ECG)

The rhythmic cardiac electrical impulses passing throughout the heart, also, diffuse into the surrounding tissues of the heart. A small amount of the current reaches up to the surface of the body. The placing of electrodes on the skin surface, on either side of the heart, provides information about the electrical potentials generated by the heart (Barr & van Oosterom, 2010). The graphical representation of the same is known as electrocardiogram (ECG) (Harland, Clark, Peters, Everitt, & Stiffell, 2005). A normal ECG signal comprises of various waveforms (the P wave, the QRS complex and the T wave) (Hurst, 1998). The P wave represents the electrical potential generated due to the depolarization of the atria, before the onset of the ventricular systole (Dilaveris & Gialafos, 2001). Similarly, the QRS complex indicates the electrical potential developed during the ventricular depolarization (Wellens, Bär, & Lie, 2000). Therefore, the P wave and the QRS complex are also regarded as depolarization waves. On the other hand, the electrical potential developed during the repolarization of the ventricles is indicated by the T wave (Opthof et al., 2007). As a consequence, the T wave is also known as the repolarization wave. The amplitude of the electrical potentials in different parts of the heart, represented by the various waves of a normal ECG signal, is dependent on the manner of the placement of the electrodes on the body surface and their proximity to the heart (Schijvenaars, Kors, van Herpen, Kornreich, & van Bemmel, 1997). When one of the electrodes is located directly over the ventricles and the other electrode is located anywhere on the body away from the heart, the maximum amplitude of the QRS complex has been observed to be 3 to 4 mV, which is quite low as compared to the electrical potential of 110 mV measured directly on the surface of the heart membrane. When the electrodes are placed either on the arms of the two hands or on one arm and one leg, the amplitude of the QRS complex varies from 1 to 1.5 mV (Bacharova, Selvester, Engblom, & Wagner, 2005). For the afore-mentioned arrangement of the electrodes, the amplitude of the P wave varies from 0.1 to 0.3 mV and that of the T wave varies from 0.2 to 0.3 mV. The time interval between the onset of the P wave and the onset of the Q wave is regarded as P-Q interval. It represents the time elapse between the onsets of the atrial contraction and the ventricular contraction and has a typical value of 0.16 sec. Sometimes, it is also named as P-R interval when the Q wave seems to be absent (Gervais et al., 2009). The contraction of the ventricles lasts for about 0.35 sec and is represented in the normal ECG signal by the time interval between the starting of the Q wave and the end of the T wave, known as Q-T interval (Okin et al., 2000).

Heart Rate Variability

The autonomic nervous system consists of two main branches, namely, the sympathetic nervous system and parasympathetic nervous system (Appenzeller & Oribe, 1997). These systems help in controlling the activity of the most of the peripheral organs and organ systems. The monitoring of the functioning of these organs and/or organ systems are difficult to analyze, except the cardiological function (Ravits, 1997). The cardiological function can be estimated by careful understanding of the ECG signals. Though the normal ECG signal doesn't provide information about the activity of the autonomic nervous system, the analysis of the beat-to-beat timing variations, obtained by analyzing QRS complexes of any two consecutive cycles of the ECG signal might provide information about the function of the autonomic nervous system. This field of study has evolved since last three decades and might provide information about the autonomic stability of an individual (Martínez-Lavín, Hermosillo, Rosas, & Soto, 1998).

An in-depth analysis of the timing of the beat-to-beat variations is regarded as heart rate variability (Stauss, 2003). Heart rate variability has shown promises in understanding not only the autonomic balance but also in the alteration of the cardiac health (Friedman & Thayer, 1998). In the year 1996, a task force was established by the Board of the European Society of Cardiology. The task force was also co-sponsored by the North American Society of Pacing and Electrophysiology. The main task of this task force was to propose guidelines for the measurement, physiological interpretation and clinical use of the information obtained from the heart rate variability analysis (Cardiology & Cardiology, 1996). As per the recommendations of the task force, the measurement of the heart rate variability can be done either in the time domain or in the frequency domain (Hejjel & Gal, 2001). The parameters which are obtained from the time domain methods may be categorized as either statistical or geometric measures (parameters). The detection of the time domain measures is quite simple. The time domain measures are usually associated with the measurement of the heart rate in any specific time period or measurement of the timing variation amongst two consecutive QRS complexes (Umetani, Singer, McCraty, & Atkinson, 1998). The time interval between the two consecutive QRS complexes is regarded as NN interval. The various statistical and the geometric parameters (obtained from different histograms) are basically obtained from the analysis of the NN intervals (Kleiger, Stein, & Bigger, 2005). As per the task force, the analysis of at least 5-minute recording of the ECG signal should be done. The standard deviation of the total number of NN intervals is regarded as SDNN (Sztajzel, 2004). The feature RMSSD is obtained by calculating the mean of the squared differences of successive NN intervals, followed by calculating a square root value of the same (Thayer, Yamamoto, & Brosschot, 2010). NN50 is determined by calculating the differences in the consecutive NN intervals whose differences are more than 50 msec. The pNN50 parameter is calculated by dividing the NN50 value by the total number of NN intervals (Appelhans & Luecken, 2006). The geometric measures are obtained from the histogram plotted amongst the duration of RR-intervals versus the number of RR-intervals (Acharya, Joseph, Kannathal, Lim, & Suri, 2006). Usually, the histograms are made having bin width of approximately 8 msec. The histogram plot appears as triangular in shape. The width of the base of the triangle is regarded as TINN (triangular interpolation of NN interval) (Salahuddin, Cho, Jeong, & Kim, 2007).

During the analysis of the heart rate variability features in the frequency domain, the analysis of very low frequency (VLF) components, low frequency components (LF) and high frequency (HF) components have been proposed for the HRV analysis using short-term ECG signal recording (Parati, Saul, Di Rienzo, & Mancia, 1995). While analyzing HRV using long-term ECG recording (24 hours), the additional analysis of ultra-low frequency components is recommended (Kleiger et al., 2005). In the HRV analysis, the various features obtained from the time domain and frequency domain methods can be subjected to various linear (analysis of variance) as well as non-linear (classification and regression tree, boosted tree, random forest) statistical methods for obtaining the important predictors. Thereafter, the important predictors may be used in various combinations as input for the probable classification using artificial neural network.

It has been reported by various researchers that, in order to understand the effect of music on the conduction pathway of the heart, the time domain analysis and the joint time-frequency analysis of the ECG signals should be carried out. In the time domain analysis, the various statistical features are extracted from the recorded ECG signals. Similar to the HRV analysis, the extracted time domain features are then subjected to various linear (analysis of variance) as well as non-linear (classification and regression tree, boosted tree, random forest) statistical methods for obtaining the statistically significant and important features respectively. The statistically significant and important features may be used in various combinations as input for probable classification using an artificial neural network. The joint time-frequency analysis of the recorded ECG signals can be performed by decomposing the ECG signals using wavelet and reconstructing the decomposed signals. The features of the reconstructed signals can be obtained using the similar procedure as that of the time domain analysis. Finally, the important predictors can be found out and used for classification using an artificial neural network.

Analysis of Variance (ANOVA)

The analysis of variance (ANOVA) is one of the various linear statistical methods used for determining the statistically significant features of more than two groups of data or observations (Bolton, 1997). Although the name of the method is analysis of variance, it actually tests the available groups of data to find out whether a significant difference between the means of the groups exist or not (Larson, 2008). The reason behind its naming lies in the fact that it analyzes the variances in order to test the occurrence of significant differences between the means. In this method, the total variance is divided into the variance because of the variability among the groups (known as mean square effect) and that due to the variability within the groups (known as mean square error). The mean square effect component of variance, which is due to the differences between the means, is then used for estimating the statistical significance. The analysis of variance is based on the assumptions that the expected values of the errors are zero, all the errors possess equal variances, all the errors are independent of each other and are normally distributed.

Classification and Regression Tree (CART)

The classification and regression tree is a supervised learning method, which is used to develop prediction models from data (Lewis, 2000). The data set is subdivided recursively and a prediction model is fitted for every partition, in order to obtain the models. The classification tree is useful for those dependent variables which can take a finite number of disordered values, whereas, the regression tree is suitable for those target variables which either take continuous values or systematic discrete values. In a classification tree, the prediction error is obtained in the form of misclassification cost (Lemon, Roy, Clark, Friedmann, & Rakowski, 2003). However, in a regression tree, the prediction error is obtained in terms of the square of the variation amongst the measured and predicted values (Harrell, 2013).

Boosted Tree (BT)

Boosted trees are regarded as one of the most powerful tools, useful for predictive data mining. They can be utilized for regression problems along with classification problems having continuous or categorically dependent variables (Windeatt & Ardeshir, 2002). The concept of boosted trees has emerged from the effort of applying boosting methods to the regression trees (Elith, Leathwick, & Hastie, 2008). In this method, a sequence of binary trees is produced in which every successive tree is developed for the prediction residuals of the anteceding one. In this method, the binary tree refers to the fact that, at every splitting node, the total data is segregated into two samples.

Random Forest (RF)

The random forest method is another supervised learning method that was introduced by Breiman (Svetnik et al., 2003). The random forest is a collection of the simple tree predictors that are useful for classification and regression problems (Strobl, Malley, & Tutz, 2009). In this method, each tree predictor results in an outcome, whenever provided with a group of predictor values. The outcome of every tree predictor is dependent on a group of values of the predictor, which are chosen independently.

Artificial Neural Network (ANN)

The artificial neural network (ANN) is a non-linear computational method motivated by the functionalities of the biological neural networks (Jain, Mao, & Mohiuddin, 1996). An artificial neural network consists of the interconnection of nodes (neurons), which tries to imitate some functionalities of the biological neurons. Basically, an artificial neural network comprises of several inputs having weights associated with them, a threshold function and an activation function, which finds out the output. The weights are determined during training and classification efficiency of the developed model is tested during testing (Agatonovic-Kustrin & Beresford, 2000).

Wavelet Transform and Multiresolution Analysis

Though the Fourier transform still remains the most powerful tool for frequency domain analysis because of its intuitiveness, its mathematical easefulness and its effective implementation using the FFT algorithm, the major disadvantage of Fourier transform is the analysis of the global behavior of the signals (Cristi, 2004). It is not useful if the goal is to find out the local behavior of a signal (Sneddon, 1995). Wavelet Transform is one of the few methods available for characterizing the local behavior of a signal. It provides the time-frequency analysis of the signal (Polikar, 1996).

According to the uncertainty principle in signal processing, a signal can't be represented in both the time and the frequency domain at the same time with absolute accuracy. Multiresolution analysis is a method for analyzing signals, with the provision of different resolutions at different frequencies (Tsatsanis & Giannakis, 1995). It provides an excellent resolution in time and a poor resolution in frequency at high frequencies. However, at low frequencies, it results in a good resolution in frequency and poor resolution in time. Therefore, it is suitable for analyzing signals having high-frequency components for a short interval of time and low-frequency components for a long interval of time.

MATERIALS AND METHODS

Volunteers

Fifteen male volunteers were chosen for the study. All the volunteers were Odia speaking. The volunteers were in the age group of 21.2 ± 2.242 years. The selection was done such that chosen volunteers neither smoke cigarettes nor were involved in any athletic/swimming activities. This was done to make sure that the above-mentioned activities did not stimulate the autonomic nervous system. The ECG signal of the volunteers was recorded one week after mid-semester examination and at least two weeks before the end-semester examination so as to eliminate any anxiety due to the examination. The volunteers were informed verbally about the study in detail. If they agreed to participate in the study, they were asked to sign an informed consent form. Required ethical clearance was obtained from the Institute ethical committee for the acquisition of the ECG signals for human volunteers vide office order# NITRKL/IEC/ FORM/2/25/4/11/001, dated 13/12/2013.

Recording of the ECG Signal

The volunteers were asked to sit on a wooden chair in a relaxed position. After they had made themselves comfortable, the ECG signals were recorded using a portable ECG sensor (EKG sensor, Vernier Software and Technology, USA). The volunteers were called consecutively for three days. On the first day, the ECG signal of the volunteers was recorded without any stimulus. On the second and the third days, the volunteers were made to listen to Odia and Tamil music, respectively and the ECG signals were recorded. The recording of the ECG signal was done for 7 min.

Analysis of the ECG Signal

5 minutes of the ECG signal was extracted from the recorded ECG signal and was used for calculating the HRV parameters. The HRV parameters were calculated using Biomedical Workbench software (National Instruments, USA). The HRV parameters were tabulated in an Excel sheet. The important features were determined using linear (ANOVA) and non-linear (CART, BT and RF) statistical methods. The important parameters, so obtained, were used for classification using Automated Neural Networks (ANN).

The ECG signals were further processed in the time and the joint time-frequency domains. Five seconds of ECG signal was used for processing. The statistical features of the ECG signal were calculated using the statistical palette of LabVIEW 2013. Further, the ECG signals were decomposed using db06 wavelet and reconstructed using D7 and D8 sub-bands. The statistical features of the reconstituted ECG signal were also calculated. These predictors were used as inputs for probable classification using ANN.

RESULT AND DISCUSSION

HRV Analysis

The results of the HRV analysis indicated that there was a decrease in the heart rate during the post-stimulus condition. The differences in the heart rate were insignificant. This indicated that there was an increase in the parasympathetic activity of the volunteers during the post-stimulus condition. Similar observations have also been made by many researchers. Like the heart rate, the differences in the remaining HRV features were also found to be statistically insignificant.

The HRV parameters were subsequently analyzed using CART, BT and RF methods. All these methods are categorized under decision tree classifiers. CART is the primitive decision tree method. BT classifier is reported to be better than CART due to the increased number of nodes in the decision tree. RF is by far the best amongst the three classifiers. This is due to the fact that RF uses a series of the decision tree for making the decision. Using the above classifiers, some of the HRV features were found to be statistically significant (Table 1). It suggested that, even though the linear classifier (ANOVA) was not able to classify the signals, the non-linear classifiers can predict some of the features that can be used for probable classification using ANN. CART and BT indicated that LF n.u. (FFT) was the important predictor. The average of the LF n.u. (FFT) parameter was nearly equal during no stimulus condition and Odia music stimulus condition and was much lower than the Tamil music stimulus condition. This suggested that either the sympathetic or mixed sympathetic-vagal activity was higher in the volunteers during post-Tamil music stimulus. The RF classifier indicated that the average value of high-frequency HRV spectral components (HF % (FFT)) was higher during the Odia music stimulus as compared to the no- stimuli. On the contrary, the average HF % (FFT) value was lowest after Tamil music stimulus. An increase in the HF % (FFT) value is an indicator of the parasympathetic activity. This indicated that Tamil music increased the sympathetic activity in the Odia volunteers, whereas, Odia music stimulated the parasympathetic activity of the volunteers as compared to the no stimulus condition. The LF n.u. (FFT) and HF % (FFT) were used for probable classification using ANN. The results indicated that when LF n.u. (FFT) was used as the predictor, a classification efficiency of greater than 90% was achieved using RBF algorithm (RBF 1-33-3). The network utilized Gaussian function as the hidden activation function for the hidden layer. The Softmax function was chosen as the output activation function and the network used Entropy as the error function. The classification efficiency was found to be 90.66%. The details of the classifying network and confusion matrix have been tabulated in Table 2 and Table 3. Similarly when HF % (FFT) was used, a classification efficiency of greater than 85% was achieved

Table 1. Important predictors obtained from HRV features

Classifiers	HRV Features	Mean±SD			Predictor Importance
		Control Group	Odia Music	Tamil Music	
CART	L.F (n.u.) FFT	27.9200 ± 8.5335	27.7266 ± 7.1151	30.4933 ± 5.1520	1.0000
BT	LF n.u. FFT	27.9200 ± 8.5335	27.7266 ± 7.1151	30.4933 ± 5.1520	1.0000
RF	HF FFT	53.2666 ± 10.4640	54.8666 ± 8.9031	50.8000 ± 6.6138	1.0000

Table 2. Parameters of 1-33-3 RBF network

Networks	Features Used	Classification efficiency	Algorithm	Error function	Hidden Act.	Output Act.
RBF 1-33-3	LF norm (n.u.)	90.66%	RBFT	Entropy	Gaussian	Softmax

Table 3. Confusion matrix of 1-33-3 RBF network

	Catagory-WM	Catagory-OM	Catagory-TM	Result
Total	15.00	15.00	15.00	45.00
Correct	13.00	15.00	13.00	41.00
Incorrect	2.00	0.00	2.00	4.00
Correct (%)	86.00	100.00	86.00	90.66
Incorrect (%)	13.00	0.00	13.00	9.34

(result not shown). Any classification efficiency of greater than 80% is considered as acceptable for classification. These results suggest that there is a non-linear mathematical relationship amongst the LF n.u. (FFT) and HF % (FFT) features with that of the stimuli and no-stimuli conditions. Hence, LF n.u. (FFT) and HF % (FFT) can be used as the features for classifying the stimuli and non-stimuli conditions.

ECG Signal Analysis in Time Domain

The statistical features of the ECG signal were calculated. ANOVA analysis indicated that, the statistical differences among the features were insignificant and no important predictors were identified. Hence, the non-linear classifiers were used for determining the important predictors. A summary of the important predictors obtained from the analysis has been tabulated in Table 4. These important predictors were used in various combinations as input for ANN classifiers to determine the best classification efficiency. The result indicated that, when the arithmetic mean (AM) and the Kurtosis of the signal were used as the input for the ANN classifier, a classification efficiency of more than 90% was achieved using the RBF network (RBF 2-30-3). The network used the Gaussian function as the hidden activation function for the hidden layer. The output activation function of the network was softmax and the network used entropy as the error function. The classification efficiency was observed to be 90.66%. The details of the classifier and the confusion matrix for the best classification efficiency are tabulated in Table 5 and Table 6.

ECG Signal Analysis in Joint Time-Frequency Domain

The ECG signals were further analyzed in the joint time- frequency domain. The processing in the joint time- frequency domain was performed using Discrete Wavelet Transform (DWT). The db06 wavelet

Table 4. Important predictors from time-domain features

Classifiers	Time-Domain Features	Mean±SD			Predictor Importance
		Control Group	Odia Music	Tamil Music	
CART	Mode	0.0047±0.0271	0.0090±0.0180	0.0116±0.0126	1.0000
BT	AM	0.0009±0.0043	0.0008±0.0044	-0.0005±0.0046	1.0000
	Kurtosis	14.3003±4.5384	14.8617±4.0589	14.8474±4.3499	0.9665
	Summation	4.9892±21.6202	4.0493±22.2041	-2.8514±23.4587	1.0000
RF	AM	0.0009±0.0043	0.0008±0.0044	-0.0005±0.0046	1.0000

Table 5. Parameters of 2-30-3 RBF network

Networks	Features Used	Classification Efficiency	Algorithm	Error Function	Hidden Act.	Output Act.
RBF 2-30-3	AM, Kurtosis	90.66%	RBFT	Entropy	Gaussian	Softmax

Table 6. Confusion matrix of 2-30-3 RBF network

	Catagory-WM	Catagory-OM	Catagory-TM	Result
Total	15.00	15.00	15.00	45.00
Correct	13.00	14.00	14.00	41.00
Incorrect	2.00	1.00	1.00	4.00
Correct (%)	86.00	93.00	93.00	90.66
Incorrect (%)	13.00	6.00	6.00	8.33

was used for processing of the signals. The signal was decomposed into eight levels and subsequently reconstituted using D7 and D8 sub-bands (Figure 1). The analysis of the features using ANOVA didn't divulge any information about the important parameters. The non-linear classifiers indicated that some of the features (as tabulated in Table 7) were important predictors. The features were used in various combinations as input for the ANN classifier. The results indicated that when the AM and the standard deviation (SD) of the wavelet processed signals were used as the predictors, a classification efficiency of 86.66% was achieved for the RBF network (RBF 2-33-3). Gaussian function was used as the hidden activation function for the hidden layer. The Softmax function was used as the output activation function of the network. The network used Entropy as the error function. The details of the classifier and the confusion matrix for the best classification efficiency are tabulated in Table 8 and Table 9.

FUTURE RESEARCH DIRECTIONS

The authors propose potential directions for the future research. Though the results and inferences obtained from the current study are encouraging, the involvement of more number of volunteers in the future studies is recommended. In this study, the effect of music of two different languages on the auto-

Table 7. Important predictors from time-domain wavelet features

Classifiers	Wavelet Features	Mean±SD			Predictor Importance
		Control Group	Odia Music	Tamil Music	
CART	Kurtosis	13.5210±4.2349	14.2664±3.3059	13.8271±3.4893	1.0000
BT	Kurtosis	13.5210±4.2349	14.2664±3.3059	13.8271±3.4893	1.0000
RF	AM	0.00007±0.0010	0.0001±0.0007	0.0002±0.0012	0.9679
	SD	0.1754±0.0426	0.1677±0.0403	0.1683±0.0436	1.0000

Figure 1. Wavelet decomposition and reconstruction of ECG signal

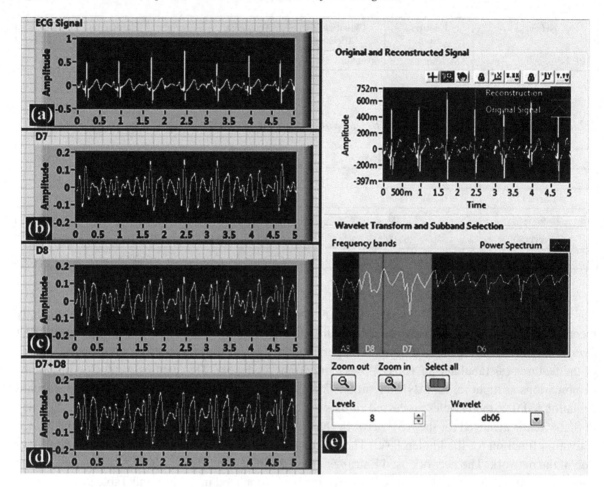

Table 8. Parameters of 2-33-3 RBF network

Networks	Features Used	Classification Efficiency	Algorithm	Error Function	Hidden Act.	Output Act.
RBF 2-33-3	AM, SD	86.33%	RBFT	Entropy	Gaussian	Softmax

Table 9. Confusion matrix of 2-33-3 RBF network

	Catagory-WM	Catagory-OM	Catagory-TM	Result
Total	15.00	15.00	15.00	45.00
Correct	12.00	14.00	13.00	39.00
Incorrect	3.00	1.00	2.00	6.00
Correct (%)	80.00	93.00	86.00	86.33
Incorrect (%)	20.00	6.00	13.00	13.00

nomic nervous system and conduction pathway of the heart of a specific language speaking volunteers has been analyzed. Future research can be done using different types of music to discover their effects on an individual so that a particular type of music with best positive effects on the health can be recommended for patients practicing music therapy. Also, an in-depth study can be performed to divulge more information regarding the effect of music on the functioning of the heart, other organs and organ systems.

CONCLUSION

The current study describes the effect of Odia and Tamil music on the ANS of the Odia volunteers. It was observed that none of the features, which were calculated using HRV analysis, time-domain analysis and joint time-frequency analysis, were able to predict the different conditions using ANOVA. But, when non-linear classifiers were used, many of the predictors showed a predictor importance of 100%. This indicated that the features obtained from the above-mentioned analysis can be effectively classified using the non-linear domain. The HF% (FFT) was found to be an important predictor from the HRV analysis. The results suggested that if a person is made to listen to music in his mother tongue, there is a slight increase in the parasympathetic activity. This can be explained by the fact that, listening to the music in the mother tongue soothes the volunteers and helps the volunteers to relief from anxiety. On the other hand, if a volunteer is made to listen to music which he can't completely understand, an increase in the sympathetic activity was seen. This can be attributed to the fact that when the volunteer is not accustomed to the language, listening to the music may create emotional irritation to the volunteers which, in turn, might increase the anxiety of the volunteers.

To have an understanding whether the exposure of the music in mother tongue and a completely unknown language have any effect on the conduction pathway of the heart, the ECG signal was analyzed in the time-domain and joint time-frequency domain. The analysis of the results suggests that, though no statistically different parameters were observed using ANOVA analysis, some of the features could be classified using non-linear classifiers with an efficiency of more than 95%. The results suggested that, there might be physiological changes in the conduction pathway of the heart. An in-depth analysis has to be conducted to have an idea about the exact changes. The important features, which were obtained from the HRV analysis, time-domain analysis and joint time-frequency analysis, were used as the categorical inputs for the ANN classifiers. The classification efficiencies using specific networks were found to be more than 85%. The highest classification efficiencies were achieved using RBF algorithm as compared to the MLP algorithm (results not shown).

REFERENCES

Acharya, U. R., Joseph, K. P., Kannathal, N., Lim, C. M., & Suri, J. S. (2006). Heart rate variability: A review. *Medical & Biological Engineering & Computing*, *44*(12), 1031–1051. doi:10.1007/s11517-006-0119-0 PMID:17111118

Adeyemi, E. O., Desai, K., Towsey, M., & Ghista, D. (1999). Characterization of autonomic dysfunction in patients with irritable bowel syndrome by means of heart rate variability studies. *The American Journal of Gastroenterology*, *94*(3), 816–823. doi:10.1111/j.1572-0241.1999.00861.x PMID:10086672

Agatonovic-Kustrin, S., & Beresford, R. (2000). Basic concepts of artificial neural network (ANN) modeling and its application in pharmaceutical research. *Journal of Pharmaceutical and Biomedical Analysis*, *22*(5), 717–727. doi:10.1016/S0731-7085(99)00272-1 PMID:10815714

Appelhans, B. M., & Luecken, L. J. (2006). Heart rate variability as an index of regulated emotional responding. *Review of General Psychology*, *10*(3), 229–240. doi:10.1037/1089-2680.10.3.229

Appenzeller, O., & Oribe, E. (1997). *The autonomic nervous system: an introduction to basic and clinical concepts*. Elsevier Health Sciences.

Bacharova, L., Selvester, R. H., Engblom, H., & Wagner, G. S. (2005). Where is the central terminal located?: In search of understanding the use of the Wilson central terminal for production of 9 of the standard 12 electrocardiogram leads. *Journal of Electrocardiology*, *38*(2), 119–127. doi:10.1016/j.jelectrocard.2005.01.002 PMID:15892021

Barr, R. C., & van Oosterom, A. (2010). *Genesis of the electrocardiogram. In Comprehensive electrocardiology* (pp. 167–190). Springer. doi:10.1007/978-1-84882-046-3_5

Bernardi, L., Porta, C., & Sleight, P. (2006). Cardiovascular, cerebrovascular, and respiratory changes induced by different types of music in musicians and non-musicians: The importance of silence. *Heart (British Cardiac Society)*, *92*(4), 445–452. doi:10.1136/hrt.2005.064600 PMID:16199412

Bilchick, K. C., & Berger, R. D. (2006). Heart rate variability. *Journal of Cardiovascular Electrophysiology*, *17*(6), 691–694. doi:10.1111/j.1540-8167.2006.00501.x PMID:16836727

Bolton, S. (1997). Analysis of variance. In *Pharmaceutical statistics: Practical and clinical applications*. Basel: Marcel Dekker.

Boso, M., Politi, P., Barale, F., & Enzo, E. (2006). Neurophysiology and neurobiology of the musical experience. *Functional Neurology*, *21*(4), 187–191. PMID:17367577

Boyett, M. R., Honjo, H., & Kodama, I. (2000). The sinoatrial node, a heterogeneous pacemaker structure. *Cardiovascular Research*, *47*(4), 658–687. doi:10.1016/S0008-6363(00)00135-8 PMID:10974216

Burns, N. (2013). *Cardiovascular physiology*. Retrieved from School of Medicine, Trinity College, Dublin: http://www.medicine.tcd.ie/physiology/assets/docs12_13/lecturenotes/NBurns/Trinity%20CVS%20lecture

Cardiology, T. F. E. S., & Cardiology, T. F. E. S. (1996). the North American Society of Pacing and Electrophysiology. Heart rate variability: Standards of measurement, physiological interpretation and clinical use. *Circulation*, *93*(5), 1043–1065. doi:10.1161/01.CIR.93.5.1043 PMID:8598068

Carney, R. M., Blumenthal, J. A., Stein, P. K., Watkins, L., Catellier, D., Berkman, L. F., & Freedland, K. E. et al. (2001). Depression, heart rate variability, and acute myocardial infarction. *Circulation*, *104*(17), 2024–2028. doi:10.1161/hc4201.097834 PMID:11673340

Carney, R. M., Freedland, K. E., & Veith, R. C. (2005). Depression, the autonomic nervous system, and coronary heart disease. *Psychosomatic Medicine*, *67*, S29–S33. doi:10.1097/01.psy.0000162254.61556.d5 PMID:15953797

Cristi, R. (2004). *Modern digital signal processing*. Cl-Engineering.

Davis, W. B., Gfeller, K. E., & Thaut, M. H. (2008). *An introduction to music therapy: Theory and practice*. ERIC.

Dilaveris, P. E., & Gialafos, J. E. (2001). P-wave dispersion: A novel predictor of paroxysmal atrial fibrillation. *Annals of Noninvasive Electrocardiology*, *6*(2), 159–165. doi:10.1111/j.1542-474X.2001. tb00101.x PMID:11333174

Elith, J., Leathwick, J. R., & Hastie, T. (2008). A working guide to boosted regression trees. *Journal of Animal Ecology*, *77*(4), 802–813. doi:10.1111/j.1365-2656.2008.01390.x PMID:18397250

Esler, M., & Kaye, D. (2000). Sympathetic nervous system activation in essential hypertension, cardiac failure and psychosomatic heart disease. *Journal of Cardiovascular Pharmacology*, *35*, S1–S7. doi:10.1097/00005344-200000004-00001 PMID:11346214

Esler, P. D. M., & Kaye, P. D. D. (2000). Measurement of sympathetic nervous system activity in heart failure: The role of norepinephrine kinetics. *Heart Failure Reviews*, *5*(1), 17–25. doi:10.1023/A:1009889922985 PMID:16228913

Floras, J. S. (2009). Sympathetic nervous system activation in human heart failure: Clinical implications of an updated model. *Journal of the American College of Cardiology*, *54*(5), 375–385. doi:10.1016/j. jacc.2009.03.061 PMID:19628111

Friedman, B. H., & Thayer, J. F. (1998). Autonomic balance revisited: Panic anxiety and heart rate variability. *Journal of Psychosomatic Research*, *44*(1), 133–151. doi:10.1016/S0022-3999(97)00202-X PMID:9483470

Gervais, R., Leclercq, C., Shankar, A., Jacobs, S., Eiskjaer, H., Johannessen, A., & Daubert, C. et al. (2009). Surface electrocardiogram to predict outcome in candidates for cardiac resynchronization therapy: A sub-analysis of the CARE-HF trial. *European Journal of Heart Failure*, *11*(7), 699–705. doi:10.1093/ eurjhf/hfp074 PMID:19505883

Goldberger, J. J. (1999). Sympathovagal balance: How should we measure it? *American Journal of Physiology. Heart and Circulatory Physiology*, *276*(4), H1273–H1280. PMID:10199852

Good, M., Anderson, G. C., Ahn, S., Cong, X., & Stanton-Hicks, M. (2005). Relaxation and music reduce pain following intestinal surgery. *Research in Nursing & Health*, *28*(3), 240–251. doi:10.1002/ nur.20076 PMID:15884029

Hall, J. E. (2010). *Guyton and Hall textbook of medical physiology*. Elsevier Health Sciences.

Harland, C., Clark, T., Peters, N., Everitt, M. J., & Stiffell, P. (2005). A compact electric potential sensor array for the acquisition and reconstruction of the 7-lead electrocardiogram without electrical charge contact with the skin. *Physiological Measurement*, *26*(6), 939–950. doi:10.1088/0967-3334/26/6/005 PMID:16311443

Harrell, F. E. (2013). *Regression modeling strategies: with applications to linear models, logistic regression, and survival analysis*. Springer Science & Business Media.

Haun, M., Mainous, R. O., & Looney, S. W. (2001). Effect of music on anxiety of women awaiting breast biopsy. *Behavioral Medicine (Washington, D.C.)*, 27(3), 127–132. doi:10.1080/08964280109595779 PMID:11985186

Hejjel, L., & Gal, I. (2001). Heart rate variability analysis. *Acta Physiologica Hungarica*, 88(3-4), 219–230. doi:10.1556/APhysiol.88.2001.3-4.4 PMID:12162580

Hurst, J. W. (1998). Naming of the waves in the ECG, with a brief account of their genesis. *Circulation*, 98(18), 1937–1942. doi:10.1161/01.CIR.98.18.1937 PMID:9799216

Jain, A. K., Mao, J., & Mohiuddin, K. (1996). Artificial neural networks: A tutorial. *Computer*, 29(3), 31–44. doi:10.1109/2.485891

Juslin, P. N., & Sloboda, J. A. (2001). *Music and emotion: Theory and research*. Oxford University Press.

Kawashima, T. (2005). The autonomic nervous system of the human heart with special reference to its origin, course, and peripheral distribution. *Anatomy and Embryology*, 209(6), 425–438. doi:10.1007/s00429-005-0462-1 PMID:15887046

Kiernan, J., & Rajakumar, R. (2013). *Barr's the human nervous system: an anatomical viewpoint*. Lippincott Williams & Wilkins.

Kleiger, R. E., Stein, P. K., & Bigger, J. T. (2005). Heart rate variability: Measurement and clinical utility. *Annals of Noninvasive Electrocardiology*, 10(1), 88–101. doi:10.1111/j.1542-474X.2005.10101.x PMID:15649244

Koelsch, S. (2009). A neuroscientific perspective on music therapy. *Annals of the New York Academy of Sciences*, 1169(1), 374–384. doi:10.1111/j.1749-6632.2009.04592.x PMID:19673812

Labbé, E., Schmidt, N., Babin, J., & Pharr, M. (2007). Coping with stress: The effectiveness of different types of music. *Applied Psychophysiology and Biofeedback*, 32(3-4), 163–168. doi:10.1007/s10484-007-9043-9 PMID:17965934

Larson, M. G. (2008). Analysis of variance. *Circulation*, 117(1), 115–121. doi:10.1161/CIRCULATIONAHA.107.654335 PMID:18172051

Lee, P.-C., Chen, S.-A., & Hwang, B. (2009). Atrioventricular node anatomy and physiology: Implications for ablation of atrioventricular nodal reentrant tachycardia. *Current Opinion in Cardiology*, 24(2), 105–112. doi:10.1097/HCO.0b013e328323d83f PMID:19225293

Lemon, S. C., Roy, J., Clark, M. A., Friedmann, P. D., & Rakowski, W. (2003). Classification and regression tree analysis in public health: Methodological review and comparison with logistic regression. *Annals of Behavioral Medicine*, 26(3), 172–181. doi:10.1207/S15324796ABM2603_02 PMID:14644693

Lewis, R. J. (2000). *An introduction to classification and regression tree (CART) analysis*. Paper presented at the Annual Meeting of the Society for Academic Emergency Medicine, San Francisco, CA.

Martínez-Lavín, M., & Hermosillo, A. G. (2000). *Autonomic nervous system dysfunction may explain the multisystem features of fibromyalgia*. Paper presented at the Seminars in arthritis and rheumatism. doi:10.1016/S0049-0172(00)80008-6

Martínez-Lavín, M., Hermosillo, A. G., Rosas, M., & Soto, M. E. (1998). Circadian studies of autonomic nervous balance in patients with fibromyalgia: A heart rate variability analysis. *Arthritis and Rheumatism*, *41*(11), 1966–1971. doi:10.1002/1529-0131(199811)41:11<1966::AID-ART11>3.3.CO;2-F PMID:9811051

Martini, F. (2005). *Human anatomy.* San Francisco, CA: Pearson/Benjamin Cummings.

Metzger, L. K. (2004). Assessment of use of music by patients participating in cardiac rehabilitation. *Journal of Music Therapy*, *41*(1), 55–69. doi:10.1093/jmt/41.1.55 PMID:15157124

Millan, M. J., Agid, Y., Brüne, M., Bullmore, E. T., Carter, C. S., Clayton, N. S., & Young, L. J. et al. (2012). Cognitive dysfunction in psychiatric disorders: Characteristics, causes and the quest for improved therapy. *Nature Reviews. Drug Discovery*, *11*(2), 141–168. doi:10.1038/nrd3628 PMID:22293568

Monfredi, O., Dobrzynski, H., Mondal, T., Boyett, M. R., & Morris, G. M. (2010). The anatomy and physiology of the sinoatrial node—a contemporary review. *Pacing and Clinical Electrophysiology*, *33*(11), 1392–1406. doi:10.1111/j.1540-8159.2010.02838.x PMID:20946278

Okin, P. M., Devereux, R. B., Howard, B. V., Fabsitz, R. R., Lee, E. T., & Welty, T. K. (2000). Assessment of QT interval and QT dispersion for prediction of all-cause and cardiovascular mortality in American Indians the Strong Heart Study. *Circulation*, *101*(1), 61–66. doi:10.1161/01.CIR.101.1.61 PMID:10618305

Olshansky, B., Sabbah, H. N., Hauptman, P. J., & Colucci, W. S. (2008). Parasympathetic nervous system and heart failure pathophysiology and potential implications for therapy. *Circulation*, *118*(8), 863–871. doi:10.1161/CIRCULATIONAHA.107.760405 PMID:18711023

Opthof, T., Coronel, R., Wilms-Schopman, F. J., Plotnikov, A. N., Shlapakova, I. N., Danilo, P. Jr, & Janse, M. J. et al. (2007). Dispersion of repolarization in canine ventricle and the electrocardiographic T wave: T pe interval does not reflect transmural dispersion. *Heart Rhythm*, *4*(3), 341–348. doi:10.1016/j.hrthm.2006.11.022 PMID:17341400

Parati, G., Saul, J. P., Di Rienzo, M., & Mancia, G. (1995). Spectral analysis of blood pressure and heart rate variability in evaluating cardiovascular regulation a critical appraisal. *Hypertension*, *25*(6), 1276–1286. doi:10.1161/01.HYP.25.6.1276 PMID:7768574

Paxinos, G., & Mai, J. K. (2004). *The human nervous system.* Academic Press.

Peng, S.-M., Koo, M., & Yu, Z.-R. (2009). Effects of music and essential oil inhalation on cardiac autonomic balance in healthy individuals. *Journal of Alternative and Complementary Medicine (New York, N.Y.)*, *15*(1), 53–57. doi:10.1089/acm.2008.0243 PMID:19769477

Polikar, R. (1996). *The Wavelet Transform* (2nd ed.). Part I, Fundamental Concepts and An Overview of the Wavelet Theory.

Racker, D. K., & Kadish, A. H. (2000). Proximal atrioventricular bundle, atrioventricular node, and distal atrioventricular bundle are distinct anatomic structures with unique histological characteristics and innervation. *Circulation*, *101*(9), 1049–1059. doi:10.1161/01.CIR.101.9.1049 PMID:10704174

Ravits, J. M. (1997). AAEM minimonograph# 48: Autonomic nervous system testing. *Muscle & Nerve*, *20*(8), 919–937. doi:10.1002/(SICI)1097-4598(199708)20:8<919::AID-MUS1>3.0.CO;2-9 PMID:9236782

Rentschler, S., Vaidya, D. M., Tamaddon, H., Degenhardt, K., Sassoon, D., & Morley, G. E. (2001). Visualization and functional characterization of the developing murine cardiac conduction system. *Development*, *128*(10), 1785–1792. PMID:11311159

Roque, A. L., Valenti, V. E., Guida, H. L., Campos, M. F., Knap, A., Vanderlei, L. C. M., & Abreu, L. C. et al. (2013). The effects of auditory stimulation with music on heart rate variability in healthy women. *Clinics (Sao Paulo)*, *68*(7), 960–967. doi:10.6061/clinics/2013(07)12 PMID:23917660

Ruud, E. (2010). *Music therapy: A perspective from the humanities*. Barcelona Publishers.

Salahuddin, L., Cho, J., Jeong, M. G., & Kim, D. (2007). *Ultra short term analysis of heart rate variability for monitoring mental stress in mobile settings*. Paper presented at the Engineering in Medicine and Biology Society, 2007. EMBS 2007. 29th Annual International Conference of the IEEE. doi:10.1109/IEMBS.2007.4353378

Scheufele, P. M. (2000). Effects of progressive relaxation and classical music on measurements of attention, relaxation, and stress responses. *Journal of Behavioral Medicine*, *23*(2), 207–228. doi:10.1023/A:1005542121935 PMID:10833680

Schijvenaars, B. J., Kors, J. A., van Herpen, G., Kornreich, F., & van Bemmel, J. H. (1997). Effect of electrode positioning on ECG interpretation by computer. *Journal of Electrocardiology*, *30*(3), 247–256. doi:10.1016/S0022-0736(97)80010-6 PMID:9261733

Sneddon, I. N. (1995). *Fourier transforms*. Courier Corporation.

Solin, P., Kaye, D. M., Little, P. J., Bergin, P., Richardson, M., & Naughton, M. T. (2003). Impact of sleep apnea on sympathetic nervous system activity in heart failure. *CHEST Journal*, *123*(4), 1119–1126. doi:10.1378/chest.123.4.1119 PMID:12684302

Stauss, H. M. (2003). Heart rate variability. *American Journal of Physiology. Regulatory, Integrative and Comparative Physiology*, *285*(5), R927–R931. doi:10.1152/ajpregu.00452.2003 PMID:14557228

Stewart, J. M. (2000). Autonomic nervous system dysfunction in adolescents with postural orthostatic tachycardia syndrome and chronic fatigue syndrome is characterized by attenuated vagal baroreflex and potentiated sympathetic vasomotion. *Pediatric Research*, *48*(2), 218–226. doi:10.1203/00006450-200008000-00016 PMID:10926298

Strobl, C., Malley, J., & Tutz, G. (2009). An introduction to recursive partitioning: Rationale, application, and characteristics of classification and regression trees, bagging, and random forests. *Psychological Methods*, *14*(4), 323–348. doi:10.1037/a0016973 PMID:19968396

Svetnik, V., Liaw, A., Tong, C., Culberson, J. C., Sheridan, R. P., & Feuston, B. P. (2003). Random forest: A classification and regression tool for compound classification and QSAR modeling. *Journal of Chemical Information and Computer Sciences*, *43*(6), 1947–1958. doi:10.1021/ci034160g PMID:14632445

Sztajzel, J. (2004). Heart rate variability: A noninvasive electrocardiographic method to measure the autonomic nervous system. *Swiss Medical Weekly, 134*, 514–522. PMID:15517504

Tawara, S., Suma, K., & Shimada, M. (2000). *The conduction system of the mammalian heart: an anatomico-histological study of the atrioventricular bundle and the Purkinje fibers*. Imperial College Press.

Thayer, J. F., Yamamoto, S. S., & Brosschot, J. F. (2010). The relationship of autonomic imbalance, heart rate variability and cardiovascular disease risk factors. *International Journal of Cardiology, 141*(2), 122–131. doi:10.1016/j.ijcard.2009.09.543 PMID:19910061

Torrent-Guasp, F., Ballester, M., Buckberg, G. D., Carreras, F., Flotats, A., Carrió, I., & Narula, J. et al. (2001). Spatial orientation of the ventricular muscle band: Physiologic contribution and surgical implications. *The Journal of Thoracic and Cardiovascular Surgery, 122*(2), 389–392. doi:10.1067/mtc.2001.113745 PMID:11479518

Trappe, H.-J. (2010). The effects of music on the cardiovascular system and cardiovascular health. *Heart (British Cardiac Society), 96*(23), 1868–1871. doi:10.1136/hrt.2010.209858 PMID:21062776

Triposkiadis, F., Karayannis, G., Giamouzis, G., Skoularigis, J., Louridas, G., & Butler, J. (2009). The sympathetic nervous system in heart failure: Physiology, pathophysiology, and clinical implications. *Journal of the American College of Cardiology, 54*(19), 1747–1762. doi:10.1016/j.jacc.2009.05.015 PMID:19874988

Tsatsanis, M. K., & Giannakis, G. B. (1995). Principal component filter banks for optimal multiresolution analysis. *Signal Processing. IEEE Transactions on, 43*(8), 1766–1777. doi:10.1109/78.403336

Umemura, M., & Honda, K. (1998). Influence of Music on Heart Rate Variability and Comfort. A Consideration Through Comparison of Music and Noise. *Journal of Human Ergology, 27*(1/2), 30–38. PMID:11579697

Umetani, K., Singer, D. H., McCraty, R., & Atkinson, M. (1998). Twenty-four hour time domain heart rate variability and heart rate: Relations to age and gender over nine decades. *Journal of the American College of Cardiology, 31*(3), 593–601. doi:10.1016/S0735-1097(97)00554-8 PMID:9502641

Watkins, G. R. (1997). Music therapy: Proposed physiological mechanisms and clinical implications. *Clinical Nurse Specialist CNS, 11*(2), 43–50. doi:10.1097/00002800-199703000-00003 PMID:9233140

Wellens, H. J., Bär, F. W., & Lie, K. (2000). *The value of the electrocardiogram in the differential diagnosis of a tachycardia with a widened QRS complex*. Springer.

Windeatt, T., & Ardeshir, G. (2002). *Boosted tree ensembles for solving multiclass problems. In Multiple Classifier Systems* (pp. 42–51). Springer.

Yamashita, S., Iwai, K., Akimoto, T., Sugawara, J., & Kono, I. (2006). Effects of music during exercise on RPE, heart rate and the autonomic nervous system. *The Journal of Sports Medicine and Physical Fitness, 46*(3), 425. PMID:16998447

Zesiewicz, T. A., Baker, M. J., Wahba, M., & Hauser, R. A. (2003). Autonomic nervous system dysfunction in Parkinson's disease. *Current Treatment Options in Neurology, 5*(2), 149–160. doi:10.1007/s11940-003-0005-0 PMID:12628063

ADDITIONAL READING

Addison, P. S. (2002). *The illustrated wavelet transform handbook: introductory theory and applications in science, engineering, medicine and finance*. CRC press. doi:10.1887/0750306920

Akay, M. (1998). *Time Frequency andWavelets in Biomedical Signal Processing*: IEEE press series in Biomedical Engineering.

Baharav, A., Kotagal, S., Gibbons, V., Rubin, B., Pratt, G., Karin, J., & Akselrod, S. (1995). Fluctuations in autonomic nervous activity during sleep displayed by power spectrum analysis of heart rate variability. *Neurology*, *45*(6), 1183–1187. doi:10.1212/WNL.45.6.1183 PMID:7783886

Bannister, R. (1983). *Autonomic failure: a textbook of clinical disorders of the autonomic nervous system*. USA: Oxford University Press.

Baxt, W. G. (1991). Use of an artificial neural network for the diagnosis of myocardial infarction. *Annals of Internal Medicine*, *115*(11), 843–848. doi:10.7326/0003-4819-115-11-843 PMID:1952470

Baxt, W. G. (1995). Application of artificial neural networks to clinical medicine. *Lancet*, *346*(8983), 1135–1138. doi:10.1016/S0140-6736(95)91804-3 PMID:7475607

Benedetto, J. J., & Li, S. (1998). The theory of multiresolution analysis frames and applications to filter banks. *Applied and Computational Harmonic Analysis*, *5*(4), 389–427. doi:10.1006/acha.1997.0237

Chon, T.-S., Park, Y. S., Moon, K. H., & Cha, E. Y. (1996). Patternizing communities by using an artificial neural network. *Ecological Modelling*, *90*(1), 69–78. doi:10.1016/0304-3800(95)00148-4

Chui, C. K. (1992). Wavelets: a tutorial in theory and applications. Wavelet Analysis and its Applications, San Diego, CA: Academic Press,| c1992, edited by Chui, Charles K., 1.

De'Ath, G. (2007). Boosted trees for ecological modeling and prediction. *Ecology*, *88*(1), 243–251. doi:10.1890/0012-9658(2007)88[243:BTFEMA]2.0.CO;2 PMID:17489472

Demirkir, C., & Sankur, B. (2004). *Face detection using boosted tree classifier stages*. Paper presented at the Signal Processing and Communications Applications Conference, 2004. Proceedings of the IEEE 12th. doi:10.1109/SIU.2004.1338594

Dreiseitl, S., & Ohno-Machado, L. (2002). Logistic regression and artificial neural network classification models: A methodology review. *Journal of Biomedical Informatics*, *35*(5), 352–359. doi:10.1016/S1532-0464(03)00034-0 PMID:12968784

Fonarow, G. C., Adams, K. F., Abraham, W. T., Yancy, C. W., Boscardin, W. J., & Committee, A. S. A. (2005). Risk stratification for in-hospital mortality in acutely decompensated heart failure: Classification and regression tree analysis. *Journal of the American Medical Association*, *293*(5), 572–580. doi:10.1001/jama.293.5.572 PMID:15687312

Gabella, G. (2001). Autonomic nervous system. *eLS*.

Gil, E., Mendez, M., Vergara, J. M., Cerutti, S., Bianchi, A. M., & Laguna, P. (2009). Discrimination of sleep-apnea-related decreases in the amplitude fluctuations of PPG signal in children by HRV analysis. *Biomedical Engineering. IEEE Transactions on, 56*(4), 1005–1014.

Goto, M., Nagashima, M., Baba, R., Nagano, Y., Yokota, M., Nishibata, K., & Tsuji, A. (1997). Analysis of heart rate variability demonstrates effects of development on vagal modulation of heart rate in healthy children. *The Journal of Pediatrics, 130*(5), 725–729. doi:10.1016/S0022-3476(97)80013-3 PMID:9152280

Gupta, R., Mitra, M., & Bera, J. (2014). *ECG Signal Analysis ECG Acquisition and Automated Remote Processing* (pp. 15–49). Springer. doi:10.1007/978-81-322-1557-8_2

Ham, J., Chen, Y., Crawford, M. M., & Ghosh, J. (2005). Investigation of the random forest framework for classification of hyperspectral data. *Geoscience and Remote Sensing. IEEE Transactions on, 43*(3), 492–501.

Haykin, S., & Network, N. (2004). A comprehensive foundation. *Neural Networks, 2*.

Iacobucci, D., Tybout, A., Sternthal, B., Kepper, G., Verducci, J., & Meyers-Levy, J. (2001). Analysis of variance. *Journal of Consumer Psychology, 10*(1/2), 5–35.

Kim, J., & André, E. (2008). Emotion recognition based on physiological changes in music listening. *Pattern Analysis and Machine Intelligence. IEEE Transactions on, 30*(12), 2067–2083.

Kingsbury, N. (2001). Complex wavelets for shift invariant analysis and filtering of signals. *Applied and Computational Harmonic Analysis, 10*(3), 234–253. doi:10.1006/acha.2000.0343

Kuo, R. J., Chen, C., & Hwang, Y. (2001). An intelligent stock trading decision support system through integration of genetic algorithm based fuzzy neural network and artificial neural network. *Fuzzy Sets and Systems, 118*(1), 21–45. doi:10.1016/S0165-0114(98)00399-6

Lang, M., Guo, H., Odegard, J. E., Burrus, C. S., & Wells, R. Jr. (1996). Noise reduction using an undecimated discrete wavelet transform. *Signal Processing Letters, IEEE, 3*(1), 10–12. doi:10.1109/97.475823

Lundqvist, L.-O., Carlsson, F., Hilmersson, P., & Juslin, P. (2008). Emotional responses to music: Experience, expression, and physiology. *Psychology of Music, 37*(1), 61–90. doi:10.1177/0305735607086048

Niskanen, J.-P., Tarvainen, M. P., Ranta-Aho, P. O., & Karjalainen, P. A. (2004). Software for advanced HRV analysis. *Computer Methods and Programs in Biomedicine, 76*(1), 73–81. doi:10.1016/j.cmpb.2004.03.004 PMID:15313543

Rangayyan, R. M. (2015). *Biomedical signal analysis* (Vol. 33). John Wiley & Sons. doi:10.1002/9781119068129

Samanta, B., & Al-Balushi, K. (2003). Artificial neural network based fault diagnostics of rolling element bearings using time-domain features. *Mechanical Systems and Signal Processing, 17*(2), 317–328. doi:10.1006/mssp.2001.1462

Saper, C. B. (2002). The central autonomic nervous system: Conscious visceral perception and autonomic pattern generation. *Annual Review of Neuroscience, 25*(1), 433–469. doi:10.1146/annurev.neuro.25.032502.111311 PMID:12052916

Saritha, C., Sukanya, V., & Murthy, Y. N. (2008). ECG signal analysis using wavelet transforms. *Bulg. J. Phys*, *35*(1), 68–77.

Scherer, K. R., & Zentner, M. R. (2001). Emotional effects of music: Production rules. *Music and emotion: Theory and research*, 361-392.

Selesnick, I. W., Baraniuk, R. G., & Kingsbury, N. G. (2005). The dual-tree complex wavelet transform. *Signal Processing Magazine, IEEE*, *22*(6), 123–151. doi:10.1109/MSP.2005.1550194

Tarvainen, M. P., Niskanen, J.-P., Lipponen, J., Ranta-Aho, P., & Karjalainen, P. (2009). *Kubios HRV—a software for advanced heart rate variability analysis*. Paper presented at the 4th European Conference of the International Federation for Medical and Biological Engineering. doi:10.1007/978-3-540-89208-3_243

Tarvainen, M. P., Ranta-Aho, P. O., & Karjalainen, P. A. (2002). An advanced detrending method with application to HRV analysis. *IEEE Transactions on Bio-Medical Engineering*, *49*(2), 172–175. doi:10.1109/10.979357 PMID:12066885

Tu, J. V. (1996). Advantages and disadvantages of using artificial neural networks versus logistic regression for predicting medical outcomes. *Journal of Clinical Epidemiology*, *49*(11), 1225–1231. doi:10.1016/S0895-4356(96)00002-9 PMID:8892489

Wang, S.-C. (2003). *Artificial neural network Interdisciplinary Computing in Java Programming* (pp. 81–100). Springer. doi:10.1007/978-1-4615-0377-4_5

Wu, S.-D., & Lo, P.-C. (2008). Inward-attention meditation increases parasympathetic activity: A study based on heart rate variability. *Biomedical Research*, *29*(5), 245–250. doi:10.2220/biomedres.29.245 PMID:18997439

KEY TERMS AND DEFINITIONS

Analysis of Variance (ANOVA): It is a linear statistical method, useful to determine the statistically significant features of three or more groups of data. It analyzes the variance to find out the differences between the means.

Artificial Neural Network: It is a non-linear computational method which tries to imitate some functioning of the biological neurons. An interconnection of the nodes (neurons) exists in it, either in the feed-forward or in the feedback manner.

Autonomic Nervous System: It is that part of the nervous system which is responsible for the control of most of the visceral and unconscious functions of the human body.

Classification and Regression Tree (CART): The classification and regression tree is a supervised learning method that is used to develop prediction models from data.

Electrocardiogram (ECG): Electrocardiogram is the graphical representation of the electrical activities occurring within the heart. It comprises of various waves, namely, P-wave, QRS-complex and T-wave.

Heart Rate Variability: Heart Rate Variability can be defined as the variation in the time duration between the successive cardiac cycles.

Parasympathetic Nervous System: The parasympathetic nervous system is that branch of the autonomic nervous system which acts to slow down the heart rate, increase the activity of the intestine and glands.

Sympathetic Nervous System: The sympathetic nervous system is one of two branches of the autonomic nervous system that acts to increase the heart rate and blood pressure and contract the blood vessels.

Chapter 13
Document Clustering:
A Summarized Survey

Harsha Patil
Maulana Azad National Institute of Technology, India

R. S. Thakur
Maulana Azad National Institute of Technology, India

ABSTRACT

As we know use of Internet flourishes with its full velocity and in all dimensions. Enormous availability of Text documents in digital form (email, web pages, blog post, news articles, ebooks and other text files) on internet challenges technology to appropriate retrieval of document as a response for any search query. As a result there has been an eruption of interest in people to mine these vast resources and classify them properly. It invigorates researchers and developers to work on numerous approaches of document clustering. Researchers got keen interest in this problem of text mining. The aim of this chapter is to summarised different document clustering algorithms used by researchers.

INTRODUCTION

Clustering is the process of subseting data objects. Subsets are based on characteristics of the objects. Objects with similar characteristics are come together and make a set.So, objects from one set have high similarity while objects from other set.(C. C. Aggarwalet al, 2012). Example: Suppose we have collection of 10 objects. Here we consider shape characteristic of objects .So objects of same shape are come together in one set.This set is known as cluster and process of dividing similar objects in setwise is known as clustering.After partitioning we get three clusters of objects.

In clustering problem, defining concepts of Optimization criteria is very important. In above example partitioning objects on the basis of their shapes is very easy task, but this is not the always case. In reality, finding the properties of object by which we can make cluster is very difficult, basically it's very important that objects which belongs to different cluster somehow must be more dissimilar to each other. Suppose, we have collection of n objects lets o1,o2,o3..........on. Lets s= {o1,o2,o3......on} and

DOI: 10.4018/978-1-5225-0536-5.ch013

Figure 1. Clustering based on OBJECTS shape

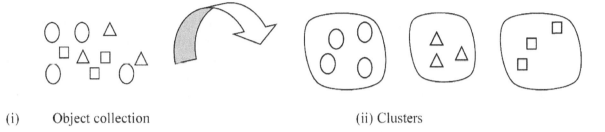

(i)   Object collection   (ii) Clusters

suppose number of clusters are k.so we need to partition n objects into k clusters. That means we need to make k partitions. So suppose those partitions are: P1,P2,P3......Pk. So properties that are shared by these parttions are:

(i) Pi≠ Φ ∀i=1,2,3...k
(ii) Pi∩Pj= Φ ∀i≠j
k
(iii) ∪Pi=S
i=1

We need to find some similarity or some disimilarity among objects by which we can partition objects into different sets. Some of widely used similarity and dissimilarity measures are Euclidean distance, Cosine similarity and so on.

Euclidean Distance

The purpose of a measure of similarity is to compare two lists of numbers (i.e. vectors), and compute a single number which evaluates their similarity. The basis of many measures of similarity and dissimilarity is euclidean distance. The distance between vectors X and Y is defined as follows:

$$d(x, y) = \sqrt{\sum_{i}^{n} (x_i - y_i)^2}$$

In other words, euclidean distance is the square root of the sum of squared differences between corresponding elements of the two vectors. Note that the formula treats the values of X and Y seriously: no adjustment is made for differences in scale. Euclidean distance is only appropriate for data measured on the same scale. As you will see in the section on correlation, the correlation coefficient is (inversely) related to the euclidean distance between standardized versions of the data.

Euclidean distance is most often used to compare profiles of respondents across variables. For example, suppose our data consist of demographic information on a sample of individuals, arranged as a respondent-by-variable matrix. Each row of the matrix is a vector of m numbers, where m is the number of variables. We can evaluate the similarity (or, in this case, the distance) between any pair of rows. Notice that for this kind of data, the variables are the columns. A variable records the results of a measurement. For our purposes, in fact, it is useful to think of the variable as the measuring device itself. This means that it has its own scale, which determines the size and type of numbers it can have. For instance, the income measurer might yield numbers between 0 and 79 million, while another variable, the education measurer, might yield numbers from 0 to 30. The fact that the income numbers are larger in general than the education numbers is not meaningful because the variables are measured on different scales. In order to compare columns we must adjust for or take account of differences in scale. But the row vectors are different. If one case has larger numbers in general then another case, this is because that case has more income, more education, etc., than the other case; it is not an artifact of differences in scale, because rows do not have scales: they are not even variables. In order to compute similarities or dissimilarities among rows, we do not need to (in fact, must not) try to adjust for differences in scale. Hence, Euclidean distance is usually the right measure for comparing cases.

Cosine Similarity

Cosine similarity is a measure of similarity between two vectors of an inner product space that measures the cosine of the angle between them. The cosine of $0°$ is 1, and it is less than 1 for any other angle. It is thus a judgment of orientation and not magnitude: two vectors with the same orientation have a cosine similarity of 1, two vectors at $90°$ have a similarity of 0, and two vectors diametrically opposed have a similarity of -1, independent of their magnitude. Cosine similarity is particularly used in positive space, where the outcome is neatly bounded in [0,1] (G. Saltonet al, 1983).

Note that these bounds apply for any number of dimensions, and cosine similarity is most commonly used in high-dimensional positive spaces. For example, in information retrieval and text mining, each term is notionally assigned a different dimension and a document is characterised by a vector where the value of each dimension corresponds to the number of times that term appears in the document (Y. Yang, 1995). Cosine similarity then gives a useful measure of how similar two documents are likely to be in terms of their subject matter.

BACKGROUND

Document clustering had been widely studied in computer science literature. Document clustering has been an interesting topic of study since a long time. There are many method (C. C. Aggarwalet al, 2006). which are discussed earlier are used by researcher for clustering as per their requirements. Many algorithms are developed my researchers in this era. For agglomerative clustering UPAGMA (Unweighted Pair Group Method with Arithmetic Mean) work very well. Bisecting K-means has best results as compare to K-means for partition clustering. Many researcher work with frequent item sets for document clustering (F Beil et al, 2002).Hierarchical Frequent Term based Clustering (HFTC) has been great contribution in this regards. In which author (R. Agrawal et al., 1994) used Apriori calculate frequent. But HFTC result depends on the order of selected item sets, which in turn depends on the greedy heuristic used also HFTC was not scalable. Fung, et al,2003 came up with Hierarchical Document Clustering using Frequent item sets (FIHC) which provides light on limitation of HFTC. According to researchers FIHC is "cluster centered" .It means FIHC measures cohesiveness of cluster directly using frequent item sets. Some of the drawbacks of FIHC include (i) using all the frequent item sets to get the clustering (number of frequent item sets may be very large and redundant) (ii) Not comparable with previous methods like UPGMA and Bisecting K-means in terms of clustering quality (C. C. Aggarwal et al, 2000). (iii) Use hard clustering (each document can belong to at most one cluster), etc. Then Yu, et al came up with a much more efficient algorithm using closed frequent item sets for clustering (TDC). They also provide a method for estimating the support correctly. But they use closed item sets which also may be redundant. Hasan H Malik et al, 2006 proposed Hierarchical Clustering using Closed Interesting Item sets, (which we refer to as HCCI) which is the current state of the art in clustering using frequent item sets.

Research is also being done about improving the clustering quality by using an ontology to enhance the document representation. Some of the most commonly available ontologies include WordNet, MESH, Wikipedia etc. Several works have been done to include these ontologies to enhance document representation by replacing the words with their synonyms or the concepts related to them. But all these methods have a very limited coverage. It can also happen that addition of new words could bring in noise into the document or while replacing the original content, there might be some information loss. Existing knowledge repositories like Wikipedia and ODP (open directory project) can be used as background knowledge. Gabrilovich and Markovitch propose a method to improve text classification performance by enriching document representation with Wikipedia concepts. Wang P. Et al.,2009 has great contribution in semantic analysis of text. They proposed method in which they automatically construct a thesaurus of concepts from Wikipedia. They also introduce framework to expand the BOW representation with semantic relation (synonymy, hyponymy and associative relations). Xiaoke Su et al.,2009suggested a fast incremental hierarchical clustering algorithm which was feasible and effective. Theoretical analysis and experiments results shows that it not only overcome the inadequate impact of memory while clustering large data set but also reflect the accurate features of the data set. Over the past decades, many researchers have been proposed several approaches of document clustering some of them are briefly summarized here:

Table 1. Literature review summary

Authors	Problem Address	Clustering Concept
(Lin and Kondadadi,2001)	Clustering efficiency	Soft document clustering
(Beil et al.,2002)	Clustering accuracy	Frequent item set based
(Hortho et al., 2003)	Semantic analysis for text	Partitioning
(Fung et al., 2003)	Quality of cluster in large document set	Frequent item set based
(Sedding and Kazakov, 2004)	Semantic analysis for text	Partitioning
(Yu et al., 2004)	Topic directory and clustering accuracy	Frequent item set based
(Xiaohui Cui et al.,2005)	Clustering large datasets	hybrid Particle Swarm Optimization (PSO)+K-means
(Wang et al., 2006)	Semantic analysis for text	Partitioning
(Chen et al., 2009)	Semantic analysis for text	Frequent item set based
(Cai et al., 2010)	Document labeling	Partitioning
(Daniel R.M. et al., 2014)	Text reduction and Feature extraction	Partitioning

MAIN FOCUS OF THE CHAPTER

Text data is ubiquitous in nature. In age of Internet generation of digital documents are very fast. As the volume of text data increases, management and analysis of text data becomes unprecedentedly important. Text mining is an emerging technology for handling the increasing text data. Document clustering is one of the widely used application of text mining. Text clustering is to divide a collection of text documents into different category groups so that documents in the same category group describe the same topic, such as movie description or sports details. Document clustering technique needs to handle large and high dimensional data and should be able to handle sparsity and semantics. Due to the sparsity nature of documents it's become impossible to finalized general technique of document clustering which is suitable for all kinds of text data. The main objective of document clustering technique is to minimize intra cluster distance between documents. Document Clustering can be categorised in two broad category on the basis of their assignment pattern (Chun-Ling Chen et al., 2010):

1. Hard document clustering: Each document is exactly belong to only one cluster.
2. Soft document clustering: Each document has probabilistic membership to each cluster.

Challenges in Document Clustering

Document clustering is being studied from many decades but still it is far from a trivial and solved problem (Pankaj Jajoo, 2008). The challenges are:

1. Selecting appropriate features of the documents that should be used for clustering.
2. Selecting an appropriate similarity measure between documents.
3. Selecting an appropriate clustering method utilising the above similarity measure.
4. Implementing the clustering algorithm in an efficient way that makes it feasible in terms of required.
5. Memory and CPU resources.
6. Finding ways of assessing the quality of the performed clustering.

Furthermore, with medium to large document collections (10,000+ documents), the number of term-document relations is fairly high (millions+), and the computational complexity of the algorithm applied is thus a central factor in whether it is feasible for real-life applications. If a dense matrix is constructed to represent term-document relations, this matrix could easily become too large to keep in memory - e.g. $100,000 documents \times 100,000 terms = 1010$ entries ~ 40 GB using 32-bit floating point values. If the vector model is applied, the dimensionality of the resulting vector space will likewise be quite high (10,000+). This means that simple operations, like finding the Euclidean distance between two documents in the vector space, become time consuming tasks.

Document Clustering Process

Document clustering is a step by step process. It consist first document retrieval, preprocessing, clustering and then evaluation.

The first step of document clustering is locating interesting documents. An IR system accepts a query from a user and responds with a set of documents. This document collection may have some non-

Figure 2. Clustering process

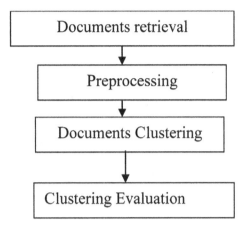

relevant documents. Document collection process may include crawling, indexing, filtering etc. After retrieving documents the next step is document preprocessing, which are used to, indexing documents to store and retrieve them in a better way, and filter them to remove the extra data, for example, stop words. Preprocessing also includes representing the documents in a way that can be used for clustering. There are many ways of representing the documents like, Vector-Model, graphical model, etc. Many measures are also used for weighing the documents and their similarities. Document Clustering, which is the main focus of this chapter is used to group the documents in a way that one group contain the similar documents. Clustering evaluation step includes evaluate the performance of the clustering technique for given document collection.

SOLUTIONS AND RECOMMENDATIONS

Document Clustering Techniques

- **Distance Based:** Distance-based clustering algorithms are based on finding similarity between the text objects. As defined earlier cosine similarity function is used commonly in the text domain. Computation of text similarity is a fundamental problem in information retrieval. Although most of the work in information retrieval has focused on how to assess the similarity of a keyword query and a text document, rather than the similarity between two documents, many weighting heuristics and similarity functions can also be applied to optimize the similarity function for clustering. Effective information retrieval models generally capture three heuristics, i.e., TF weighting, IDF weighting, and document length normalization (Brown et al.,1992)
- **Partitioning Based:** Partitioning algorithms are widely used techniques for document clustering. The two most widely used distance-based partitioning algorithms (Chakrabarti et al.,2000) are as follows:
- **k-Medoid Clustering Algorithms**: In k-medoid clustering algorithms, we use a set of points from the original data as the anchors(or medoids) around which the clusters are built. The key aim of the algorithm is to determine an optimal set of representative documents from the original

Figure 3. Clustering techniques

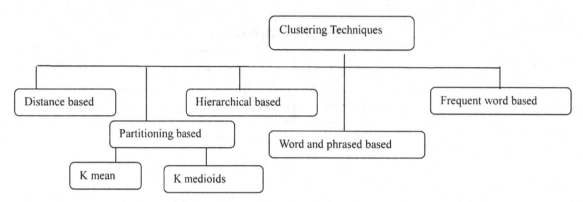

corpus around which the clusters are built. Each document is assigned to its closest representative from the collection. This creates a running set of clusters from the corpus which are successively improved by a randomized process. The algorithm works with an iterative approach in which the set of k representatives are successively improved with the use of randomized inter-changes. Specifically, we use the average similarity of each document in the corpus to its closest representative as the objective function which needs to be improved during this interchange process. In each iteration, we replace a randomly picked representative in the current set of medoids with a randomly picked representative from the collection, if it improves the clustering objective function. This approach is applied until convergence is achieved. There are two main disadvantages of the use of k-medoids based clustering algorithms, one of which is specific to the case of text data. One general disadvantage of k-medoids clustering algorithms is that they require a large number of iterations in order to achieve convergence and are therefore quite slow. This is because each iteration requires the computation of an objective function whose time requirement is proportional to the size of the underlying corpus (A. Jain et al., 1998) The second key disadvantage is that k-medoid algorithms do notwork very well for sparse data such as text (Charu C. Agrawal et al., 2003). This is because a large fraction of document pairs do not have many words in common, and the similarities between such document pairs are small (and noisy) values. Therefore, a single document medoid often does not contain all the concepts required in order to effectively build a cluster around it. This characteristic is specific to the case of the information retrieval domain, because of the sparse nature of the underlying text data.

- **k-Means Clustering Algorithms**: The k-means clustering algorithm also uses a set of k representatives around which the clusters are built. However, these representatives are not necessarily obtained from the original data and are refined somewhat differently than a k-medoids approach. The simplest form of the k-means approach is to start off with a set of k seeds from the original corpus, and assign documents to these seeds on the basis of closest similarity (L. Kaufman et al., 1990). In the next iteration, the centroid of the assigned points to each seed is used to replace the seed in the last iteration. In other words, the new seed is defined, so that it is a better central point for this cluster. This approach is continued until convergence.

- **Hierarchical Based**: Partitioning methods organized a set of objects into number of exclusive groups but hierarchical algorithm partition objects into groups at different levels (A. Jain et al.,1998). Hierarchical algorithms can be agglomerative or divisive (L. Kaufman et al.,1990).

Agglomerative algorithms, also called the bottom -up algorithms, initially treat each object as a separate cluster and successively merge the couple of clusters that are close to one another to create new clusters until all of the clusters are merged into one (M. Dash et al.,1997).

Inter cluster distance is calculated by following methods:

Singly Linkage Distance

Single link algorithm is an example of agglomerative hierarchical clustering method. We recall that is a bottom-up strategy: compare each point with each point. Each object is placed in a separate cluster, and at each step we merge the closest pair of clusters, until certain termination conditions are satisfied. This requires defining a notion of cluster proximity (E. M. Voorghees et al.,1986).

For the single link, the proximity of two clusters is defined as the minimum of the distance between any two points in the two clusters.

Using graph terminology, if we start with all points, each one a separate cluster on its own (called a singleton cluster), and then add links between all points one at a time – shortest links first, then these single links combine the points into clusters. (i.e. the points with the shortest distance between each other are combined into a cluster first, then the next shortest distance are combined, and so on)

Dendogram shows the same information as in the graph above, however distance threshold is vertical, and points are at the bottom (horizontal). The height at which two clusters are merged in the dendogram reflects the distance of the two clusters.

Complete Linkage Distance Omplete

Linkage clustering is one of several methods of agglomerative hierarchical clustering. At the beginning of the process, each element is in a cluster of its own. The clusters are then sequentially combined into larger clusters until all elements end up being in the same cluster. At each step, the two clusters separated by the shortest distance are combined. The definition of 'shortest distance' is what differentiates between the different agglomerative clustering methods. In complete-linkage clustering, the link between two clusters contains all element pairs, and the distance between clusters equals the distance between those two elements (one in each cluster) that are farthest away from each other. The shortest of these links that remains at any step causes the fusion of the two clusters whose elements are involved. The

Figure 4. Dendogram diagram

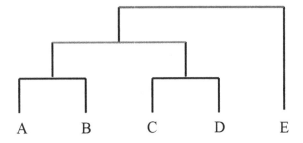

method is also known as farthest neighbour clustering. The result of the clustering can be visualized as a dendrogram, which shows the sequence of cluster fusion and the distance at which each fusion took place*(T. Sorensen, 1948; Ligendre, 1998)*.

Mathematically the complete linkage function, the distance $D(X, Y)$ between clusters X and Y, is described by the following expression:

$$D(X,Y) = \max_{x \in X, y \in Y} d(x, y)$$

where, $d(x, y)$ is the distance between elements $x \in X$ and $y \in Y$; X and Y are two sets of elements.

The worst case time complexity of complete-link clustering is at most O(n^2 log n) (A. Jain et al.,1998). One O(n^2 log n) algorithm is to compute the n^2 distance metric and then sort the distances for each data point (overall time: O(n^2 log n)). After each merge iteration, the distance metric can be updated in O(n). We pick the next pair to merge by finding the smallest distance that is still eligible for merging. If we do this by traversing the n sorted lists of distances, then, by the end of clustering, we will have done n^2 traversal steps. Adding all this up gives you O(n^2 log n).

Average Linkage Distance

In group-average linkage clustering, the similarity between two clusters is the average similarity between the pairs of documents in the two clusters. Clearly, the average linkage clustering process is somewhat slower than single-linkage clustering, because we need to determine the average similarity between a large number of pairs in order to determine group-wise similarity. On the other hand, it is much more robust in terms of clustering quality, because it does not exhibit the chaining behavior of single linkage clustering. It is possible to speed up the average linkage clustering algorithm by approximating the average linkage similarity between two clusters C1 and C2 by computing the similarity between the mean document of C1 and the mean document of C2. While this approach does not work equally well for all data domains, it works particularly well for the case of text data. In this case, the running time can be reduced to O(n2) (Charu C. Agrawal et al., 2000), where n is the total number of nodes. The method can be implemented quite efficiently in the case of document data, because the centroid of a cluster is simply the concatenation of the documents in that cluster. Divisive algorithms, also called the top - down algorithms, proceed with all of the objects in the same cluster and in each successive iteration a cluster is split up using a flat clustering algorithm recursively until each object is in its own singleton cluster. The Hierarchical Frequent Term-based Clustering (HFTC) method proposed by (Beil et al., 2002) introduced document clustering using frequent item sets. HFTC method select item set one by one which are frequent, on the basis of which new clusters are created. So the clustering result depends on the order of selected item sets, but HFTC is not scalable (Fung et al., 2003). The Frequent Item set Hierarchical Cluster (FIHC) proposed by (Fung et al., 2003) is very scalable method. First step of the method is to find all global frequent item sets from document set. Then assign each global frequent item set in separate cluster. FIHC assigns documents to the best cluster from among all available clusters. Initial clusters are overlapping because one document may contain multiple global frequent item sets. For removing this overlapping the next step of the algorithm finds the best cluster for the document. In which for each document, the "best" initial cluster is identified and the document is assigned only to the best matching initial cluster. Any cluster Ci is best cluster for docj if it achieve the minimum score for cluster membership. The minimum score can be measured with the help of score function based on cluster frequent item.

Incremental Hierarchical Document Clustering

Most of the document clustering algorithms are executed in static mode, it means that for the execution of algorithm its required that document should be store one place and then cluster them by making multiple iterations over them. But, in the current scenario when digital media is continuously growing and the number of documents being generated everyday has increased considerably. This rapid growth of online documents is become the reason of inception for Incremental hierarchical document clustering. N. Sahoo et al., 2006 applied Cobweb algorithm for text document clustering by using Negative Binomial distribution and Katz's distributions.

Word and Phrased Based

Since text documents are drawn from an inherently high-dimensional domain, it can be useful to view the problem in a dual way, in which important clusters of words may be found and utilized for finding clusters of documents. In a corpus containing d terms and n documents, one may view a term-document matrix as an n × d matrix, in which the (i, j)th entry is the frequency of the jth term in the ith document. We note that this matrix is extremely sparse since a given document contains an extremely small fraction of the universe of words. We note that the problem of clustering rows in this matrix is that of clustering documents, whereas that of clustering columns in this matrix is that of clustering words. In reality, the two problems are closely related, as good clusters of words may be leveraged in order to find good clusters of documents and vice-versa. For example, the work in determines frequent item sets of words in the document collection, and uses them to determine compact clusters of documents. This is somewhat analogous to the use of clusters of words for determining clusters of documents. The most general technique for simultaneous word and document clustering is referred to as co-clustering . This approach simultaneous clusters the rows and columns of the term-document matrix, in order to create such clusters. This can also be considered to be equivalent to the problem of re-ordering the rows and columns of the term-document matrix so as to create dense rectangular blocks of non-zero entries in this matrix. In some cases, the ordering information among words may be used in order to determine good clusters. The work in determines the frequent phrases in the collection and leverages them in order to determine document clusters. It is important to understand that the problem of word clusters and document clusters are essentially dual problems which are closely related to one another. The former is related to dimensionality reduction, whereas the latter is related to traditional clustering. The boundary between the two problems is quite fluid, because good word clusters provide hints for finding good document clusters and vice-versa. For example, a more general probabilistic framework which determines word clusters and document clusters simultaneously is referred to as topic modeling (Croft,1997). Topic modeling is a more general framework than either clustering or dimensionality reduction.

Frequent Word Based

Frequent pattern mining is a technique which has been widely used in the data mining literature in order to determine the most relevant patterns in transactional data. The clustering approach in is designed on the basis of such frequent pattern mining algorithms. A frequent item set in the context of text data is also referred to as a frequent term set, because we are dealing with documents rather than transactions. The main idea of the approach is to not cluster the high dimensional document data set, but consider the low dimensional frequent term sets as cluster candidates. This essentially means that a frequent terms set is a description of a cluster which corresponds to all the documents containing that frequent term set. Since a frequent term set can be considered a description of a cluster, a set of carefully chosen frequent terms sets can be considered a clustering. The appropriate choice of this set of frequent term sets is defined on the basis of the overlaps between the supporting documents of the different frequent term sets.

FUTURE RESEARCH DIRECTION

However many researcher have lots of findings as output of their research work, but still many gates are remain unopened. According to survey locality of documents in corpus have great contribution in output of clustering algorithms. In case of semantic based document clustering result effected by expert knowledge repositories. Another open problem is the choice of initialization strategy for most kmeans or em based algorithms. The choice of cluster labels is another issue that remains largely unaddressed in the literature. An interesting direction for future research would be to investigate other measures of similarity not captured by the vector model, such as matches in mathematical formula. For improving quality of clustering, fusion of different document clustering algorithms with ontology based database will help.

CONCLUSION

The main objective of this chapter is to provide a brief overview of the document clustering algorithms which are often used in the area. The chapter is very useful for the researcher who are doing research on document clustering and it can be a good direction for them. Research are going on various algorithm of document clustering. Main focus are on increasing algorithm effectiveness and reducing the complexity. However various techniques are available, but distance based methods are widely used techniques because of its simplicity. Documents are created in large amount from social networks or online chat applications. These types of document text needs application of streaming. Because text received from online resources are not pure text. Other types of documents are increasingly arise in heterogeneous applications in which the text is available in the context of links, and other heterogeneous multimedia data.it is critical to effectively adapt text-based algorithms to heterogeneous multimedia scenarios. Area of Document clustering is very vast area of research.

REFERENCES

Aggarwal, C. C., Gates, S. C., & Yu, P. S. (2004). On Using Partial Supervision for Text Categorization. *IEEE Transactions on Knowledge and Data Engineering, 16*(2), 245–255. doi:10.1109/TKDE.2004.1269601

Aggarwal, C. C., Procopiuc, C., Wolf, J., Yu, P. S., & Park, J.-S. (1999). Fast Algorithms for Projected Clustering. *ACM SIGMOD Conference*. doi:10.1145/304181.304188

Aggarwal, C. C., & Yu, P. S. (2000). Finding Generalized Projected Clusters in High Dimensional Spaces. *ACM SIGMOD Conference.*

Aggarwal, C. C., & Yu, P. S. (2001). On Effective Conceptual Indexing and Similarity Search in Text. In *ICDM, Proceedings IEEE International Conference*. doi:10.1109/ICDM.2001.989494

Aggarwal, C. C., & Yu, P. S. (2006). A Framework for Clustering Massive Text and Categorical Data Streams. In *SIAM Proceedings, Conference on Data Mining.*

Aggarwal, C. C., Zhao, Y., & Yu, P. S. (2012). Text Clustering with Side Information. In *ICDE Conference*, (pp 894-904).

Agrawal, R., Gehrke, J., Raghavan, P., & Gunopulos, D. (1999). Automatic Subspace Clustering of High Dimensional Data for Data Mining Applications. *ACM SIGMOD Conference.*

Agrawal, R., & Srikant, R. (1994). Fast algorithms for mining association rules. In *Proc. 20th Int. Conf. Very Large Data Bases.*

Allan, J., Papka, R., & Lavrenko, V. (1998). Online new event detection and tracking. In *ACM SIGIR Proc 21st Int.Conf. On Research and development in information retrieval.*

Andritsos, P., Tsaparas, P., Miller, R., & Sevcik, K. (2004). LIMBO: Scalable Clustering of Categorical Data. In *Proc. 9th international conference EDBT.*

Angelova, R., & Siersdorfer, S. (2006) A neighborhood-based approach for clustering of linked document collections. In *CIKM Proc. Of 15th Int.Conf. On Information and knowledge management.*

Anick, P., & Vaithyanathan, S. (1997). Exploiting Clustering and Phrases for Context-Based Information Retrieval. In *Proc. 20th Int. Conf. ACM SIGIR.*

Baeza-Yates, R. A., & Ribeiro-Neto, B. A. (2011). *Modern Information Retrieval- the concepts and technology behind search* (2nd ed.). Harlow, UK: Pearson Education Ltd.

Baker, L., & McCallum, A. (1998). Distributional Clustering of Words for Text Classification. In *SIGIR Proc. Of 21st Int.ACM Conf. On Research and development in information retrieval.*

Basu, S., Banerjee, A., & Mooney, R. J. (2002). Semi-supervised Clustering by Seeding. In *ICML Proc. Of 19th Int.Conf. On Machine Learning.*

Basu, S., Bilenko, M., & Mooney, R. J. (2004). A probabilistic framework for semi-supervised clustering. In *KDD Proc. Of 10th ACM SIGKDD Int.Conf. On knowledge discovery and data mining.*

Beil, F., Ester, M., & Xu, X. (2002). Frequent term-based text clustering. In *Proc. of International conf. ACMKDD*. doi:10.1145/775047.775110

Bekkerman, R., El-Yaniv, R., Winter, Y., & Tishby, N. (2001) On Feature Distributional Clustering for Text Categorization. In *SIGIR Proc. Of 24th Int.ACM Conf. On development in information retrieval*.

Blei, D., & Lafferty, J. (2006) Dynamic topic models. In *ICML Proc. Of 23rd Int.Conf. On Machine Learning*.

Blei, D., Ng, A., & Jordan, M. (2003). Latent Dirichlet allocation, *In Journal of Machine Learning Research. Vole, 3*, 993–1022.

Brown, P. F., deSouza, P. V., Mercer, R. L., & Della Pietra, V. J. (1992). Class-based n-gram models of natural language. Journal of Computational Linguistics, 18(4).

Chakrabarti, K., & Mehrotra, S. (2000). Local Dimension reduction: A new Approach to Indexing High Dimensional Spaces. In *VLDB Proc. Of 26th Int. conf. on Very Large Databases*.

Chang, J., & Blei, D. (2009). Topic Models for Document Networks. In *Proc. Of 12th Int.Conf. Artificial Intelligence and Statistics*.

Chen, C. L., Tseng, F. S. C., & Liang, T. (2010). Mining fuzzy frequent item sets for hierarchical document clustering. Process Manag, 46(2), 193–211.

Chen, C.-L., Tseng, F. S. C., & Liang, T. (2010, November). An integration of WordNet and Fuzzy association rule mining for multi-label document clustering. *Data & Knowledge Engineering, 69*(11), 1208–1226. doi:10.1016/j.datak.2010.08.003

Croft, W. B. (1977). Clustering large files of documents using the single-link method. *Journal of the American Society for Information Science, 28*(6), 341–344. doi:10.1002/asi.4630280606

Cui & Potok. (2005). Document Clustering Analysis Based on Hybrid PSO+K-means Algorithm. *Journal of Computer Sciences*, 27-33.

Cutting, D., Karger, D., Pedersen, J., & Tukey, J. (1992). A Cluster-based Approach to Browsing Large Document Collections. In *SIGIR Proc. Of 15th Int.ACM SIGIR Conf. on Research and Development in information retrieval*.

Cutting, D., Karger, D., & Pederson, J. (n.d.). Constant Interaction-time Scatter/Gather Browsing of Large Document Collections. In *SIGIR Proc. Of 16th Int.ACM SIGIR Conf. on Research and Development in information retrieval*.

Daniel, R. M., & Shukla, A. K. (2014). Improving Text Search Process using Text Document Clustering Approach. *International Journal of Science and Research, 3*(5), 14-24.

Dash, M., & Liu, H. (1997). Feature Selection for Clustering. In *Proc. of Int. Conf. PAKDD*. doi:10.1007/3-540-45571-X_13

Deerwester, S., Dumais, S., Landauer, T., Furnas, G., & Harshman, R. (1990). Indexing by Latent Semantic Analysis. *JASIS, 41*(6), 391–407. doi:10.1002/(SICI)1097-4571(199009)41:6<391::AID-ASI1>3.0.CO;2-9

Dhillon, I. (2001). Co-clustering Documents and Words using bipartitespectral graph partitioning. In *KDD Proc. Of 7th Int.ACM SIGKDD Conf. on Knowledge discovery and data mining.*

Dhillon, I., & Modha, D. (2001). Concept Decompositions for Large Sparse Data using Clustering. Springer.

Ding, C., He, X., Zha, H., & Simon, H. D. (2002). Adaptive Dimension Reduction for Clustering High Dimensional Data. In *ICDM Proc. Of 24th Int Conf. on Machine Learning.*

Dorow, B., & Widdows, D. (2003). Discovering corpus-specific word senses. In *Proceedings of the tenth conference on European chapter of the Association for Computational Linguistics.*

Everitt, B. S., Landau, S., & Leese, M. (2001). *Cluster Analysis* (4th ed.). London: Arnold.

Fang, H., Tao, T., & Zhai, C. (2004). A formal study of information retrieval heuristics. *Proceedings of ACM SIGIR Int. conf. On research and development in Information retrieval.* doi:10.1145/1008992.1009004

Fisher, D. (1979). Knowledge Acquisition via incremental conceptual clustering.Machine Learning, 2, 139–172.

Franz, M., Ward, T., McCarley, J., & Zhu, W.-J. (2001). Unsupervised and supervised clustering for topic tracking.*Proceedings of ACM SIGIR 24th Int. conf. On research and development in Information retrieval.* doi:10.1145/383952.384013

Fung, B., Wang, K., & Ester, M. (2003). Hierarchical Document Clustering using Frequent Itemsets. In *Proc. of SIAM Intl. Conf. on Data Mining.*

Fung, G. P. C., Yu, J. X., Yu, P., & Lu, H. (2005). Parameter Free Bursty Events Detection in Text Streams. In *Proceeding of 31st int. conf. VLDB.*

Gennari, J. H., Langley, P., & Fisher, D. (1989). Models of incremental concept formation. Journal of Artificial Intelligence, 40, 11–61.

Gibson, D., Kleinberg, J., & Raghavan, P. (1998). Clustering Categorical Data. An Approach Based on Dynamical Systems. In *Proc. of 24th Int. conf.VLDB Conference.*

Girolami, M., & Kaban, A. (2003). On the Equivalence between PLSI and LDA. *SIGIR Conference.* doi:10.1145/860435.860537

Guha, S., Rastogi, R., & Shim, K. (1998). CURE: An Efficient Clustering Algorithm for Large Databases. *ACM SIGMOD Conference.* doi:10.1145/276304.276312

Guha, S., Rastogi, R., & Shim, K. (1999). ROCK a robust clustering algorithm for categorical attributes. In *15th International Conference on Data Engineering.* doi:10.1109/ICDE.1999.754967

He, Q., Chang, K., Lim, E.-P., & Zhang, J. (2007). Bursty feature representation for clustering text streams.*SDM Conference.* doi:10.1137/1.9781611972771.50

Hofmann, T. (1999). Probabilistic Latent Semantic Indexing. In *Proc. of 22nd Int. conf. On Research development in information retrieval ACM SIGIR Conference.*

Hotho, A., Staab, S., & Stumme, G. (2003). Wordnet improves text document clustering. In SIGIR international conference on Semantic Web Workshop.

Jajoo, P. (2008). *Document Clustering*. (Masters' Thesis). IIT Kharagpur.

Jardine, N., & van Rijsbergen, C. J. (1971). The use of hierarchical clustering in information retrieval. *Information Storage and Retrieval, 7*(5), 217–240. doi:10.1016/0020-0271(71)90051-9

Ji, X., & Xu, W. (2006). Document clustering with prior knowledge. In *Proc. of ACM SIGIR 29th int. conf. On research development on information retrieval.*

Kaufman, L., & Rousseeuw, P. J. (1990). *Finding Groups in Data: An Introduction to Cluster Analysis.* Wiley Interscience. doi:10.1002/9780470316801

Ke, W., Sugimoto, C., & Mostafa, J. (2009) Dynamicity vs. effectiveness: studying online clustering for scatter/gather.*ACM SIGIR Conference, 2009.A Survey of Text Clustering Algorithms 125.* doi:10.1145/1571941.1571947

Kim, H., & Lee, S. (2000). A Semi-supervised document clustering technique for information organization. *CIKM Conference.* doi:10.1145/354756.354777

Kleinberg, J. (2002).Bursty and hierarchical structure in streams. In *Proc. of Int conf.ACMKDD Conference.*

Lee, D. D., & Seung, H. S. (1999). Learning the parts of objects by non negative matrix factorization. *Nature, 401*(6755), 788–791. doi:10.1038/44565 PMID:10548103

Legendre, P., & Legendre, L. (1998). *Numerical Ecology* (2nd ed.). Academic Press.

Li, T., Ding, C., & Zhang, Y. (2008). Knowledge transformation from word space to document space. *ACM SIGIR Conference.*

Li, T., Ma, S., & Ogihara, M. (2004). Document Clustering via Adaptive Subspace Iteration. In *Proc. Of 27th Int. conf.ACM SIGIR Conference.*

Liu, T., Lin, S., Chen, Z., & Ma, W.-Y. (2003). An Evaluation on Feature Selection for Text Clustering. *ICML Conference.*

Liu, Y.-B., Cai, J.-R., Yin, J., & Fu, A. W.-C. (2008). Clustering Text Data Streams. *Journal of Computer Science and Technology, 23*(1), 112–128. doi:10.1007/s11390-008-9115-1

Lu, Y., Mei, Q., & Zhai, C. (2011). Investigating task performance of probabilistic topic models: An empirical study of PLSA and LDA.*Information Retrieval, 14*(2), 178–203. doi:10.1007/s10791-010-9141-9

Malik, H. H., & Kender, J. R. (2006).High Quality, Efficient Hierarchical Document Clustering Using Closed Interesting Itemsets. In *Proc. of IEEE Intl. Conf. on Data Mining.*

Mei, Q., Cai, D., Zhang, D., & Zhai, C.-X. (2008). Topic Modeling with Network Regularization. In *Proc. of 17th international conf.On WWW Conference.*

Metzler, D., Dumais, S. T., & Meek, C. (2007). Similarity Measures for Short Segments of Text. *Proceedings of ECIR.* doi:10.1007/978-3-540-71496-5_5

Ming, Z., Wang, K., & Chua, T.-S. (2010). Prototype hierarchy-based clustering for the categorization and navigation of web collections.*ACMSIGIR Conference*. doi:10.1145/1835449.1835453

Mitchell, T. M. (1999). The role of unlabeled data in supervised learning.*Proceedings of the Sixth International Colloquium on Cognitive Science*.

Murtagh, F. (1983). A Survey of Recent Advances in Hierarchical Clustering Algorithms. *The Computer Journal*, *26*(4), 354–359. doi:10.1093/comjnl/26.4.354

Murtagh, F. (1984). Complexities of Hierarchical Clustering Algorithms: State of the Art. *Computational Statistics Quarterly*, *1*(2), 101–113.

Pantel, P., & Lin, D. (2002). Document Clustering with Committees. In *Proc. of 25th int. conf.ACMSIGIR Conference*.

Qi, G., Aggarwal, C., & Huang, T. (2012). Community Detection with Edge Content in Social Media works. *ICDE Conference*.

Rege, M., Dong, M., & Fotouhi, F. (2006). Co-clustering Documents and Words Using Bipartite Isoperimetric Graph Partitioning.*ICDM Conference*. doi:10.1109/ICDM.2006.36

Robertson, S. E., & Walker, S. (1994). Some simple effective approximations to the 2-poisson model for probabilistic weighted retrieval. In SIGIR.

Sahami, M., & Heilman, T. D. (2006). A web-based kernel function for measuring the similarity of short text snippets. *Proceedings of WWW2006*, 377–386.

Sahoo, N., Callan, J., Krishnan, R., Duncan, G., & Padman, R. (2006). Incremental Hierarchical Clustering of Text Documents. In *Proc. of Int. conf.ACM CIKM Conference*.

Salton, G. (1983). *An Introduction to Modern Information Retrieval*. McGraw Hill.

Salton, G., & Buckley, C. (1988). Term Weighting Approaches in Automatic Text Retrieval. *Information Processing & Management*, *24*(5), 513–523. doi:10.1016/0306-4573(88)90021-0

Schutze, H., & Silverstein, C. (1997). Projections for Efficient Document Clustering. In *Proc. of 20th Int. conf.ACM SIGIR Conference*.

Sedding, J., & Kazakov, D. (2004). WordNet-based text document clustering. In COLING-2004 workshop on robust methods in analysis of natural language data. doi:10.3115/1621445.1621458

Shi, J., & Malik, J. (2000). Normalized cuts and image segmentation. *IEEE Transactions on Pattern Analysis and Machine Intelligence*, 888–905.

Silverstein, C., & Pedersen, J. (1997). Almost-constant time clustering of arbitrary corpus subsets.*ACM SIGIR Conference*.

Singhal, A., Buckley, C., & Mitra, M. (1996). Pivoted Document Length Normalization. *ACM SIGIR Conference*.

Slonim, N., Friedman, N., & Tishby, N. (2002). Unsupervised document classification using sequential information maximization.*ACM SIGIR Conference*. doi:10.1145/564376.564401

Slonim, N., & Tishby, N. (2000). Document Clustering using word clusters via the information bottleneck method. *ACM SIGIR Conference*. doi:10.1145/345508.345578

Sorensen, T. (1948). A method of establishing groups of equal amplitude in plant sociology based on similarity of species and its application to analyses of the vegetation on Danish commons. *Biologiske Skrifter, 5*, 1–34.

Steinbach, M., Karypis, G., & Kumar, V. (2000). A Comparison of Document Clustering Techniques. *KDD Workshop on text mining.*

Su, X., Lan, Y., Wan, R., & Qin, Y. (2009). A Fast Incremental Clustering Algorithm. *Proceedings of the 2009 International Symposium on Information Processing (ISIP'09).*

Sun, Y., Han, J., Gao, J., & Yu, Y. (2009). iTopicModel: Information Network Integrated Topic Modeling. *ICDM Conference.*

van Rijsbergen, C. J., & Croft. Document Clustering, W. B. (1975). An Evaluation of some experiments with the Cranfield 1400 collection. *Information Processing & Management, 11*(5-7), 171–182. doi:10.1016/0306-4573(75)90006-0

Voorhees, E. M. (1986). *Implementing Agglomerative Hierarchical Clustering for use in Information Retrieval.* Technical Report TR86–765. Cornell University.

Wang, F., & Zhang, C. (2007) T. Li. Regularized clustering for documents.*ACM SIGIR Conference.*

Wang, P., Hu, J., Zeng, H.-J., & Chen, Z. (2009). Wikipedia knowledge to improve text classification. *Knowledge and Information Systems, 19*(3), 265–281. doi:10.1007/s10115-008-0152-4

Wilbur, J., & Sirotkin, K. (1992). The automatic identification of stop words. *Information Sciences, 18*, 45–55.

Willett, P. (1980). Document Clustering using an inverted file approach. *Journal of Information Science, 2*(5), 223–231. doi:10.1177/016555158000200503

Willett, P. (1988). Recent Trends in Hierarchical Document Clustering: *A Critical Review. Information Processing & Management, 24*(5), 577–597. doi:10.1016/0306-4573(88)90027-1

Xu, W., Liu, X., & Gong, Y. (2003). Document Clustering based on negative matrix factorization. In *Proc. of ACM SIGIR 26th International Conference.*

Yang, T., Jin, R., Chi, Y., & Zhu, S. (2009). Combining link and content for community detection: a discriminative approach. In *Proc. of Int. conf.ACM KDD Conference.*

Yang, Y. (1995). Noise Reduction in a Statistical Approach to Text Categorization. In *Proc. Of 18th Int. conf. ACM SIGIR.*

Yang, Y., & Pederson, J. O. (1995). A comparative study on feature selection in text categorization. In *Proc. of Int. conf.ACM SIGIR Conference.*

Yao, L., & Mimno, D. (2009). Efficient methods for topic model inference on streaming document collections. In *Proc. of 15th Int. conf.ACM KDD Conference.*

Zamir, O., & Etzioni, O. (1998). Web Document Clustering: A Feasibility Demonstration. *ACM SIGIR Conference*.

Zamir, O., Etzioni, O., Madani, O., & Karp, R. M. (1997). Fast and Intuitive Clustering of Web Documents. *ACM KDD Conference*.

Zhang, D., Wang, J., & Si, L. (2011). Document clustering with universum. In *Proc. of Int. conf. On ACM SIGIR Conference*.

Zhang, J., Ghahramani, Z., & Yang, Y. (2005). A probabilistic model for online document clustering with application to novelty detection. Advances in Neural Information Processing Letters, 17.

Zhang, T., Ramakrishnan, R., & Livny, M. (1996). BIRCH: An Efficient Data Clustering Method for Very Large Databases. In *Proc. Of International conference on Management of Data ACM SIGMOD*. doi:10.1145/233269.233324

Zhang, X., Hu, X., & Zhou, X. (2008). A comparative evaluation of different link types on enhancing document clustering. In *Proc. Of 31st international ACM SIGIR Conference*. doi:10.1145/1390334.1390429

Zhao, Y., & Karypis, G. (2002). Evaluation of hierarchical clustering algorithms for document data set. *CIKM Conference*.

Zhao, Y., & Karypis, G. (2004). Empirical and Theoretical comparisons of selected criterion functions for document clustering. *Machine Learning*, *55*(3), 311–331. doi:10.1023/B:MACH.0000027785.44527.d6

Zhong, S. (2005). Efficient Streaming Text Clustering. *Neural Networks*, *18*(5–6), 2005. PMID:16085385

Zhou, Y., Cheng, H., & Yu, J. X. (2009). Graph Clustering based on Structural/Attribute Similarities. In *Proceeding of VLDB Conference*.

KEY TERMS AND DEFINITIONS

Centroid: Centroid is an arithmetic mean of all data points of the cluster. It is rarely one of the original data points.

Corpus: Collection of text documents.

Digital Document: Documents in electronic form.

Frequent Itemset: Itemsets that meet minimum support threshold are called frequent itemset.

Inverse Document Frequency: Inverse document frequency is a factor which give weightage to the term, that occurs rarely in documents of corpus.

Medoid: A medoid is most centrally located object of cluster whose average dissimilarity to all the objects in the cluster is minimal.

Term Frequency: The number of times a term occurs in document.

Text Mining: It is a process of finding high quality information from text.

Chapter 14
Cluster Analysis with Various Algorithms for Mixed Data

Abha Sharma
Maulana Azad National Institute of Technology, India

R. S. Thakur
Maulana Azad National Institute of Technology, India

ABSTRACT

Analyzing clustering of mixed data set is a complex problem. Very useful clustering algorithms like k-means, fuzzy c-means, hierarchical methods etc. developed to extract hidden groups from numeric data. In this paper, the mixed data is converted into pure numeric with a conversion method, the various algorithm of numeric data has been applied on various well known mixed datasets, to exploit the inherent structure of the mixed data. Experimental results shows how smoothly the mixed data is giving better results on universally applicable clustering algorithms for numeric data.

INTRODUCTION

The fast growth in real world data has generated need for new techniques that can convert huge datasets into useful information and data mining is one which has a power to do this transformation. Information retrieval, medical diagnosis, financial fraud, image processing, bioinformatics are various applications of data mining. According to Han et al. (2001) proposes clustering is one of the important unsupervised learning which is the process of grouping a set of objects such that the objects in the same groups are similar but are very dissimilar with objects in other clusters.

Many clustering algorithms have been developed for numeric, categorical and mixed data, special attention has been paid to mixed data analysis, where data objects are neither pure categorical, nor pure numeric and very useful for real world datasets from statistics to psychology. According to MacQueen (1967)k-means clustering is a very fast and simple method for clustering high-dimensional numerical data.

Sharma et al. (2014) discuss in their paper that the absence of inherent ordering of data the clustering of mixed data has became a challenge along with the high dimensionality of mixed data. So it is not a simple and straight forward to develop clustering technique of high quality as well as the functions, models, algorithms, methods which applied on the numeric datasets are not applicable to the mixed datasets.

DOI: 10.4018/978-1-5225-0536-5.ch014

Hsu et al. (2008) discusses that usually real world datasets are mixed contain both numeric and categorical attributes. However, most existing clustering algorithms assume all attributes are either numeric or categorical, examples of which includes the k-means, Huang (1997) proposed k-modes, again Huang et al. (1999) discovered fuzzy k-modes, He et al. (2012) proposed the TGCA algorithm, Barbara et al. (2002) proposed COOLCAT, and Deng etal. (2010) proposed G-ANMI algorithms. When mixed data are encountered, most of them usually exploit transformation approaches to convert one type of the attributes to the other and then apply traditional single-type clustering algorithms. However, in most cases, transformation scheme may result in loss of information, leading to undesired clustering outcomes.

Uptill now there has been some research carried out for directly dealing with mixed data. Cheessman and Stutz (1996) proposed the approach AutoClass for mixed data, which exploited mixture model and Bayesian method to deal with mixed data. Li etal. (2002) presented the Similarity-Based Agglomerative Clustering (SBAC), which is a hierarchical agglomerative algorithm. The SBAC algorithm adopts the similarity measure defined by Goodall et al. (1966) to evaluate similarities among data objects. Hsu et al. (2006) Clustering Algorithm based on the Variance and Entropy (CAVE) for clustering mixed data. The CAVE algorithm needs to build a distance hierarchy for every categorical attribute, and the determination of the distance hierarchy requires domain expertise. Hsu et al. (2011) extended self-organizing map to analysis mixed data. In their method, the distance hierarchy can be automatically constructed by using the values of class attributes. Chatzis (2011) proposed the KL-FCM-GM algorithm, which is based on the assumption that data deriving from clusters are in the Gaussian form and designed for the Gauss Multinomial distributed data. David et al. (2012) presented SpectralCAT to deal with mixed data SpectralCAT system, the numeric values were transformed to the categorical ones. Huang (1997) presented a k-prototypes algorithm, which integrated the k-means with k-modes methods to partition mixed data. Jinchao et al. (2012) proposed the fuzzy k-prototypes which took into account the fuzzy nature of data objects.

The sections of this chapter are as follows: Background, Experimental analysis, Conclusion, Future work, and References.

BACKGROUND

The k-means algorithm which is the base of all the clustering algorithms and implemented in various areas. But the algorithm has major drawback of not handling the type of data other than numeric. Huang (1997) proposed k-prototype algorithm which combines the k-modes and the k-means algorithm using two types of distance measures Euclidian distance and match mismatch measure respectively, therefore it can handle mixed numeric and categorical datasets.

One more big challenge for clustering pure categorical data Sharma et al. (2012, 2016) or mixed data is to preprocess the mixed data or categorical data into pure numeric such as in binary or any other formats. In this work the transformation of mixed data into pure numeric data has been done using first step of TMCM algorithm Ming-Yi et al. (2010) to use the power of existing pure numeric algorithm such as k-means, single linkage, fuzzy c means, Stephen (1994) proposed subtractive with fuzzy *C*-means all algorithms is made for numeric data. According to Yinghua et al. (2013) to convert mixed data into binary formats is simple and fast to process but lack of resemblance a similarity information of categorical values, therefore slightly not relevant.

K-prototype mixed data clustering algorithm directly cluster the whole data. According to Maulik et al. (2000) many integrated similarity measures had been developed during some decades for mixed data clustering, still computationally fast and relevant similarity measure remains challenging. So it is advantageous to resolve this difficulty by finding the resemblance or similarity between numeric and categorical values of a particular data object.

Subsequently in this paper all the real world mixed data can be cluster with a general clustering algorithm applicable to mixed data with more accuracy. Compare to either binary conversion of data then cluster or directly cluster the mixed data.

Jain et al. (1999) discussed about many significant and popular clustering algorithms developed with same issue of finding out the value of k i.e. number of clusters present in the datasets.

K-modes algorithm for categorical data clustering, k-prototype for mixed data clustering, k-means for numeric data clustering needs the user to specify number of clusters in advance which leads a direct influence on the construction of final cluster formation.

Fisher et al. (1987) revel that it is still the significant work for cluster analysis when the external knowledge of number of classes are not present in the whole scene and to design an algorithm which perform clustering with no knowledge of number of clusters. This paper address the above issue of not handling the combined FCM and subtractive algorithm for mixed datasets and has done an analysis where no need to assign number of clusters in advance. To the best of our knowledge there is no analysis has been done in the direction of pure numeric algorithms like k-means, FCM etc on mixed datasets. So to select the number of clusters automatically is a unsolved area of research.

This paper hybridized the conversion technique to cluster the more accurately which is more capable to find number of clusters automatically for mixed datasets.

This paper prepared a concurrence metric after partition the data into pure numeric and pure categorical attributes. Then among the pure categorical attribute the base attribute is chosen based on the higher categories. Base numeric attributes has been chosen based on lowest variance.

Some Pure Numeric Algorithms Which Applied on Mixed Datasets Are Explained as Follows

A very basic approaches to manage the dimensionality of data is to decrease the number of attributes via either feature extraction or feature selection. The feature selection discards the attributes based on the class requirement for example the student performance needs only the most relevant attributes i.e. grades attribute and rest can skip such as behaviour, attendance etc. But the feature extraction extract the features by either making the combinations of attributes to make it most relevant attributes or derive any new attribute using any function or model, in feature extraction the derived attributes are most relevant and gives good results to discover clusters.

- **Silhouette:** According to Kaufman et al. (2009) to get an idea of how well-separated the resulting clusters are, you can make a silhouette plot using the cluster indices output from k-means. The silhouette plot displays a measure of how close each point in one cluster is to points in the neighbouring clusters. This measure ranges from +1, indicating points that are very distant from neighbouring clusters, through 0, indicating points that are not distinctly in one cluster or another, to -1, indicating points that are probably assigned to the wrong cluster. silhouette returns these values in its first output.

- **k-Means:** Rokach et al. (2005) discussed that The *k*-means method is used only when the mean of a cluster is available and users need to specify the number of clusters k in advance, which is the only disadvantage of this most popular and simple . The *k*- means method is not suitable for discovering clusters sphere shaped clusters only.

- **Hierarchical Clustering:** Hierarchical clustering is a widely used method for detecting clusters in genomic data. Clusters are defined by cutting branches off the dendrogram. A common but inflexible method uses a constant height cut-off value; this method exhibits suboptimal performance on complicated dendrogram. According to Manning et al. (2009) hierarchical clustering groups data over a variety of scales by creating a cluster tree or dendrogram. The tree is not a single set of clusters, but rather a multilevel hierarchy, where clusters at one level are joined as clusters at the next level. This allows you to decide the level or scale of clustering that is most appropriate for your application.

- **Fuzzy *C*-means Clustering:** According to Yinghua et al. (2013) Fuzzy *C*-means clustering (FCM) shows the fuzziness of the belongingness of each object and can retain more information of the dataset than the hard k-means clustering's. Although FCM has many advantages compared to k-means having one main disadvantage that it is sensitive to noise. By minimising the cost i.e. sum of all the membership degree of each data object correspond to all clusters and the sum should be equal to one. therefore this paper used the Principal Component Analysis (PCA) to eliminate the drawback of membership to the noise also. Since in reality noise should not assign very low or even zero membership .

- **Principal Component Analysis (PCA):** Han et al. (2001) in their book showed approximately all the algorithms into one platform and according to that principal components analysis (PCA) projected the original data onto a much smaller space as it searches for *k n*-dimensional orthogonal vectors which represent the whole data in a best way, where $k \leq n$., resulting in dimensionality reduction. Unlike attribute subset selection, which reduces the attribute set size by retaining a subset of the initial set of attributes, PCA "combines" the essence of attributes by creating an alternative, smaller set of variables. The initial data can then be projected onto this smaller set. PCA often reveals relationships that were not previously suspected and thereby allows interpretations that would not ordinarily result.

- **Subtractive Method:** Dutta et al. (2010) shows the major drawback of k-means and FCM is to assign cluster number initially in a prior. In this paper subtractive method is used to estimate the number of clusters in FCM. Subtractive method is modified form of mountain method where each data point is considered as a cluster centre of equal importance. This method is based on finding out the potential value of each data point or say cluster centres. the data point with highest potential value is chosen as a first cluster centre. Therefore the main idea behind this is once the cluster is found the potential of all the data points are reduced according to their distance from the cluster centre.

Fuzzy *C*-means (FCM) is a method of clustering for numeric datasets. Subtractive method is a method used to define number of cluster where no need to give number of clusters in advance. So in literature the implementation and results of both the FCM and subtractive methods are not available.

The major steps of analysis of pure numeric clustering algorithms on mixed data has two steps:

1.   To convert the mixed data into pure numeric datasets using the first step of TMCM clustering algorithm.
2.   Apply the k-means, FCM, FCM with subtractive, Hierarchical clustering, Silhouette clustering etc.

Then the evaluation of cluster numbers k has been done based on cost.

This analysis has been done on various mixed datasets such as abalone, Credit Approval, Servo, Zoo etc. Major i.e. broad partitions has been calculated in case of higher number of classes.

ANALYSIS AND REPRESENTATION OF DATA

The main aim of this section is to evaluate the clustering and scalability of the mixed data on pure numeric clustering algorithm. The motivation for this paper is to cluster high-dimensional mixed data using existing best numeric data clustering algorithm. To better understand the properties of this work, real world data were used to investigate the structure of the data using different parameter to enhance the performance of the algorithms.

Several real data sets downloaded from the UCI Machine Learning Repository by Catherine et al. (1998) These data sets are shown in Table 1. The transformed mixed data is shown in Tables 2, 3, 4, and 5.

Table 1. The four datasets from UCI repository

Dataset	Objects	Attributes	Actual classes
Servo	167	4	.2-5.7
Abalone	4177	8	29
Zoo	101	17	7
Credit Approval	690	15	2

Table 2. Abalone dataset

0.015138	0.0455	0.0365	0.0095	0.0514	0.02245	0.0101	0.015
0.015138	0.035	0.0265	0.009	0.02255	0.00995	0.00485	0.007
0.015801	0.053	0.042	0.0135	0.0677	0.02565	0.01415	0.021
0.015138	0.044	0.0365	0.0125	0.0516	0.02155	0.0114	0.0155

Table 3. Credit approval dataset

0.00107357	0.001067896	0.00065906	0.000643	0.000722945	0.00054038	0.00054038	0.000565569
0.00093129	0.001067896	0.00065906	0.000674	0.000805525	0.00054038	0.00054038	0.000565569
0.00093129	0.001067896	0.00065906	0.000674	0.000805525	0.00054038	0.00057949	0.000565569
0.00107357	0.001067896	0.00065906	0.000643	0.000722945	0.00054038	0.00054038	0.000540378

Table 4. Zoo dataset

0.4	0.024851	0.02932	0.0145	0.022393	0.024687	0.0252945	0.020817	0.0242918
0.4	0.024851	0.02932	0.0145	0.022393	0.024687	0.0252945	0.016749	0.0242918
0	0.016646	0.02932	0.01585	0.0199014	0.024687	0.008219	0.020817	0.0242918
0.4	0.024851	0.02932	0.0145	0.022393	0.024687	0.0252945	0.020817	0.0242918

Table 5. Servo dataset

0.415151515	0.55965224	0.5	0.4
0.416666667	0.528611117	0.6	0.5
0.381818182	0.528611117	0.4	0.3
0.416666667	0.582612022	0.3	0.2

And the analysis of the above converted data is shown in this section. Where Figure 1 shows Silhouette clustering of abalone data When k=2, Figure 2 shows Silhouette clustering of abalone data When k=3, Figure 3 shows Silhouette clustering of abalone data When k=4, Figure 4 shows Silhouette clustering of CA data When k=2, Figure 2 shows Silhouette clustering of abalone data When k=3, Figure 3 shows Silhouette clustering of abalone data When k=4, Figure 4 shows Silhouette clustering of CA data When k=2, Figure 5 shows Silhouette clustering of CA data When k=3, Figure 6 shows Silhouette clustering of CA data When k=4, Figure 7 shows Silhouette clustering of Servo data When k=2, Figure 8 shows

Figure 1. Silhouette clustering of abalone data when k=2

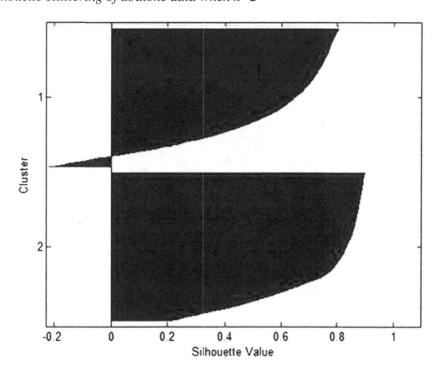

Figure 2. Silhouette clustering of abalone data when k=3

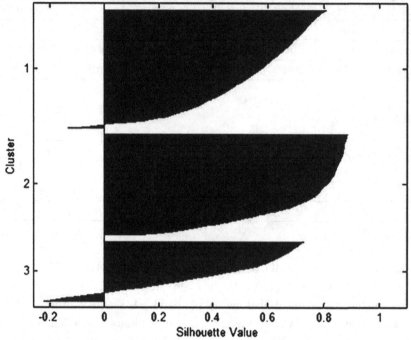

Figure 3. Silhouette clustering of abalone data when k=4

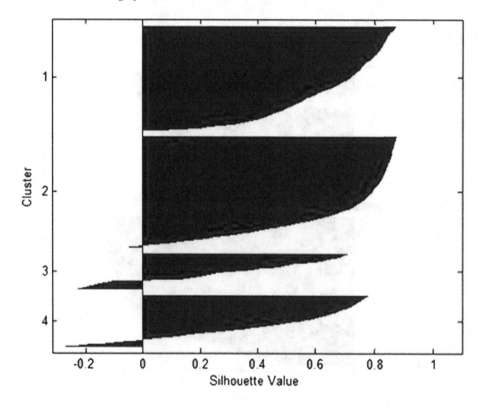

Figure 4. Silhouette clustering of CA data when k=2

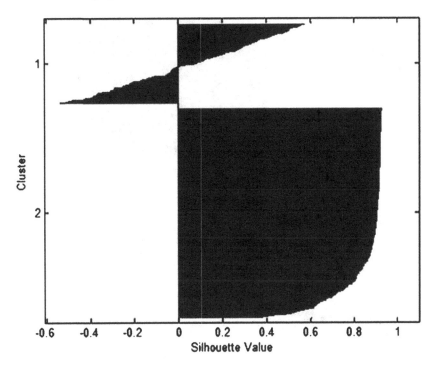

Figure 5. Silhouette clustering of CA data when k=3

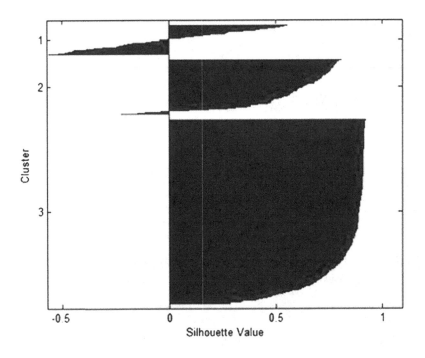

Figure 6. Silhouette clustering of CA data when k=4

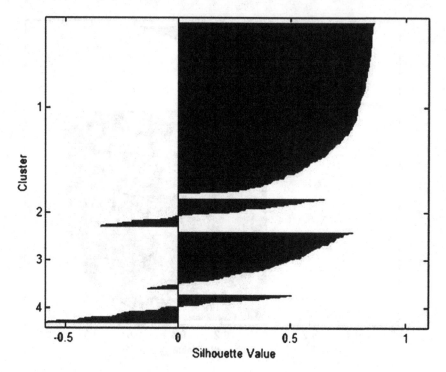

Figure 7. Silhouette clustering of Servo data when k=2

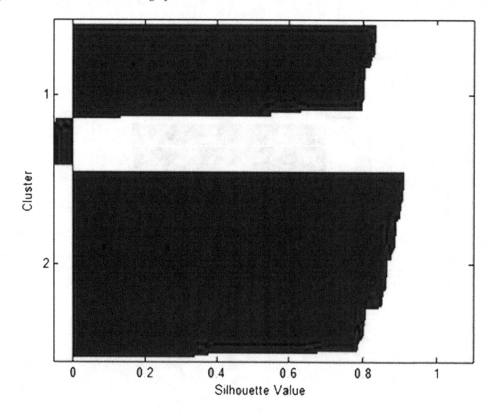

Figure 8. Silhouette clustering of Servo data when k=3

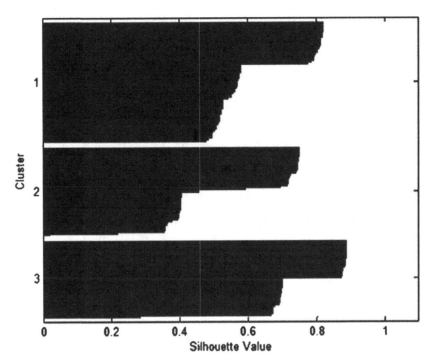

Figure 9. Silhouette clustering of Servo data when k=4

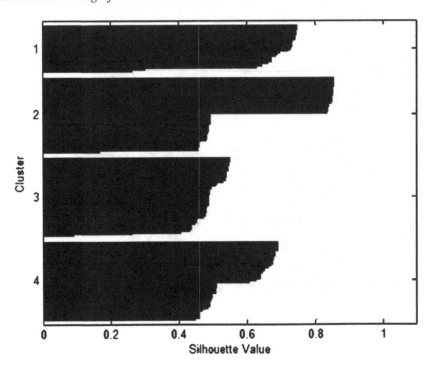

Silhouette clustering of Servo data When k=3, Figure 9 showsSilhouette clustering of Servo data When k=4, Figure 10 shows Silhouette clustering of Zoo data When k=2, Figure 11 shows Silhouette clustering of Zoo data When k=3, Figure 12 shows Silhouette clustering of Zoo data When k=4, Figure 13 shows K-means clustering of abalone data using PCA on k=2, Figure 14 shows K-means clustering of abalone data using PCA on k=3, Figure 15 shows K-means clustering of Servo data using PCA on k=2, Figure 16 shows K-means clustering of Servo data using PCA on k=3, Figure 17 shows K-means clustering of Credit Approval using PCA on k=2, Figure 18 shows K-means clustering of Credit Approval data using PCA on k=3, Figure 19 shows K-means clustering of Zoo data using PCA on k=2, Figure20 shows K-means clustering of Zoo data using PCA on k=3, Figure 21 shows Hierarchical cluster tree of Abalone data using a 3-dimensional scatter plot, Figure 22 shows Hierarchical cluster tree of CA data using a 3-dimensional scatter plot, Figure 23 shows Hierarchical linkage clustering tree of Servo data, Figure 24 shows Hierarchical cluster tree of Zoo data using a 3-dimensional scatter plot, Figure 25 shows Hierarchical linkage clustering tree abalone data, Figure 26 shows Hierarchical linkage clustering tree CA data, Figure 27 shows Hierarchical linkage clustering tree Servo data, Figure 28 shows K-means clustering of Zoo data using PCA on k=3, Figure 29 shows Cluster Evaluation of Zoo data with PCA using k-means, Figure 30 shows Cluster Evaluation of Abalone data with PCA using k-means, Figure 31 shows Cluster

Figure 10. Silhouette clustering of Zoo data when k=2

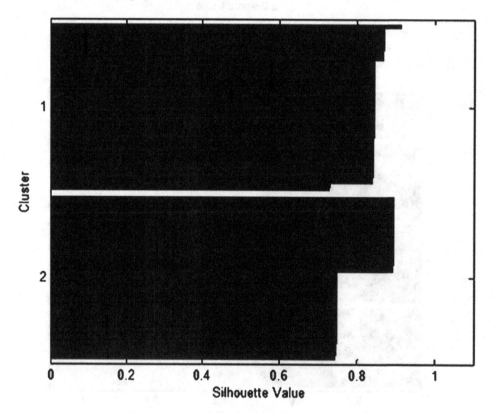

Figure 11. Silhouette clustering of Zoo data when k=3

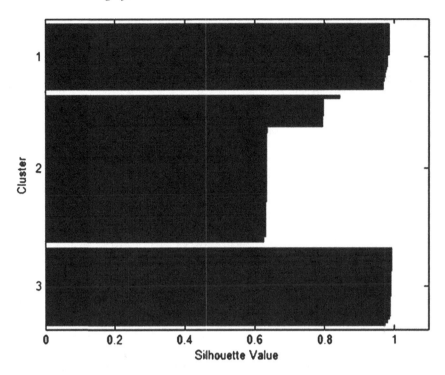

Figure 12. Silhouette clustering of Zoo data when k=4

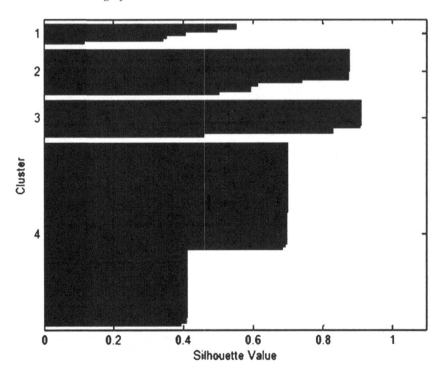

Figure 13. K-means clustering of abalone data using PCA on k=2

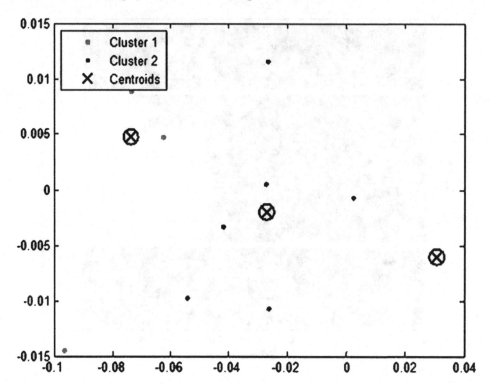

Figure 14. K-means clustering of Abalone data using PCA on k=3

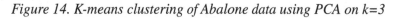
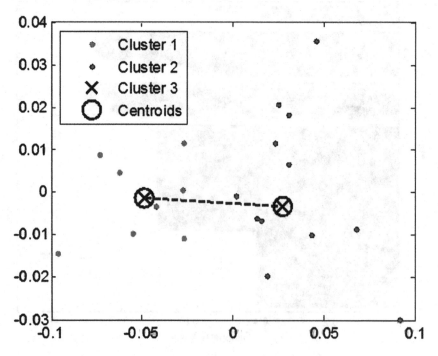

Figure 15. K-means clustering of credit approval data using PCA on k=2

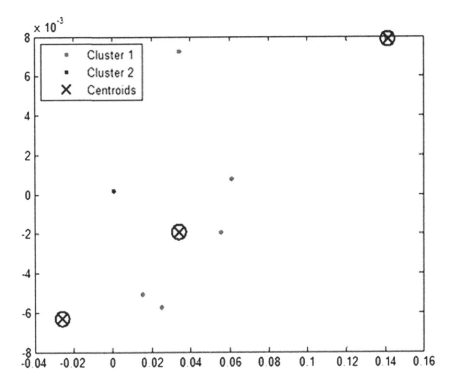

Figure 16. K-means clustering of credit approval data using PCA on k=3

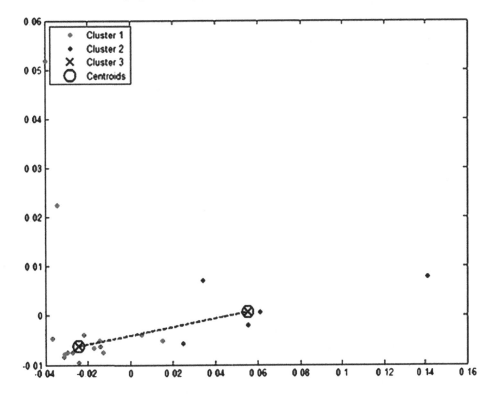

Figure 17. K-means clustering of Servo data using PCA on k=2

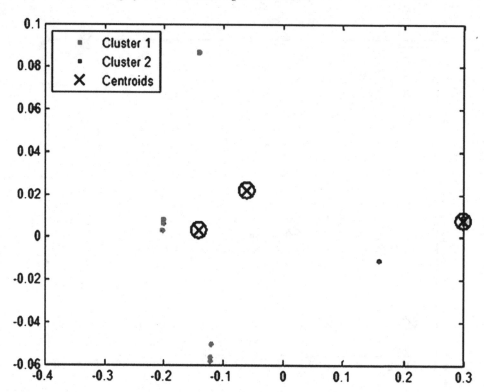

Figure 18. K-means clustering of Servo data using PCA on k=3

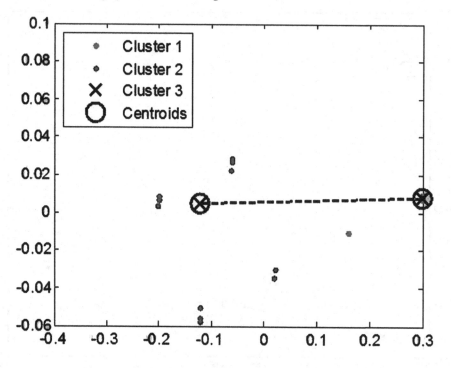

Figure 19. K-means clustering of Zoo data using PCA on k=2

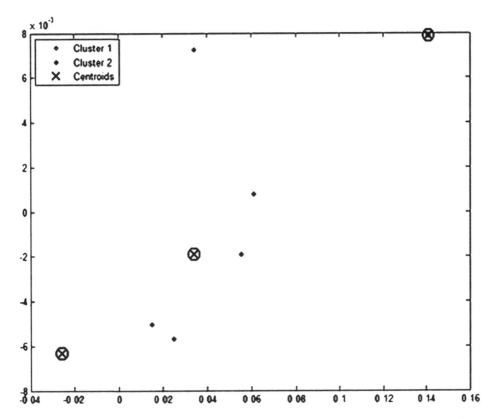

Figure 20. K-means clustering of Zoo data using PCA on k=3

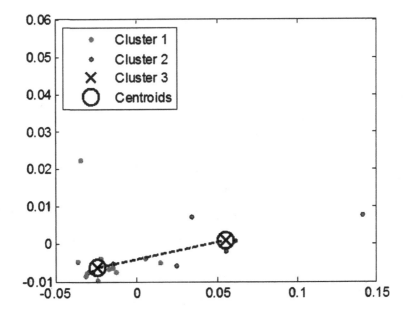

Figure 21. Hierarchical cluster tree of Abalone data using a 3-dimensional scatter plot

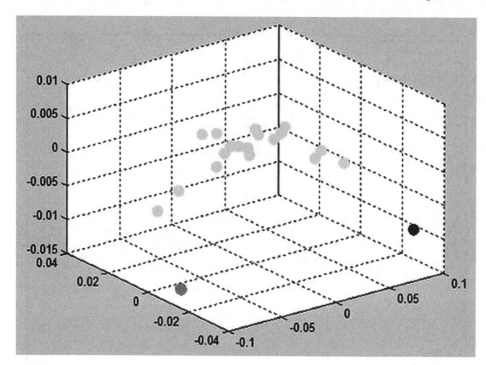

Figure 22. Hierarchical cluster tree of CA data using a 3-dimensional scatter plot

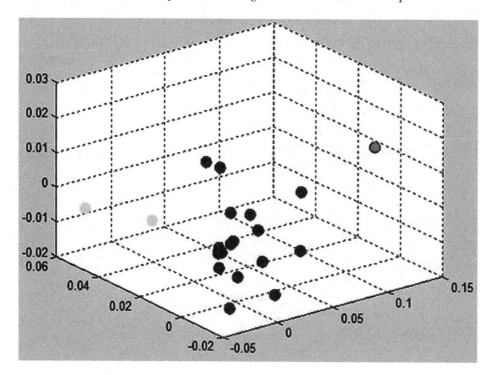

Figure 23. Hierarchical cluster tree of Servo data using a 3-dimensional scatter plot

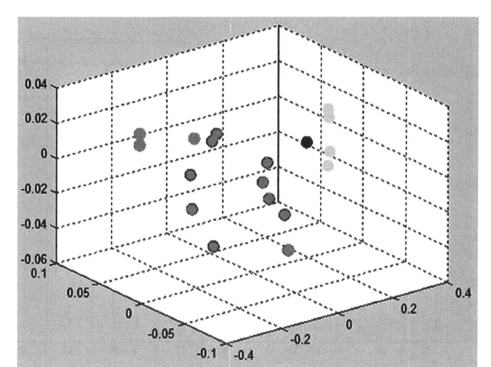

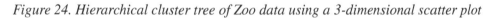

Figure 24. Hierarchical cluster tree of Zoo data using a 3-dimensional scatter plot

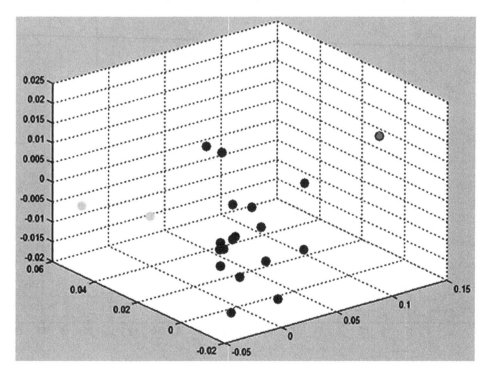

Figure 25. Hierarchical linkage clustering tree of Abalone data

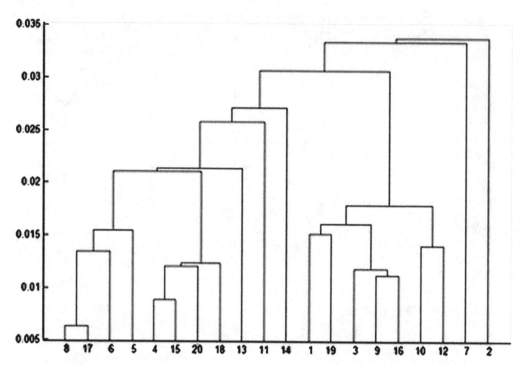

Figure 26. Hierarchical linkage clustering tree CA data

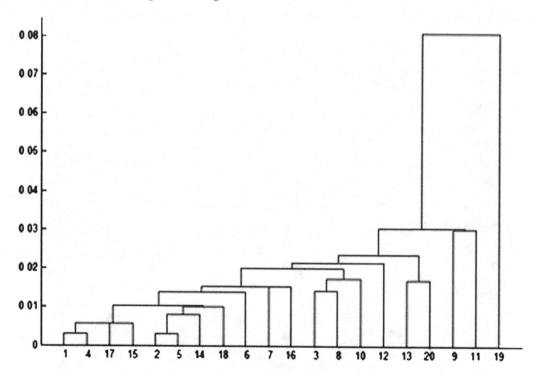

Figure 27. Hierarchical linkage clustering tree Servo data

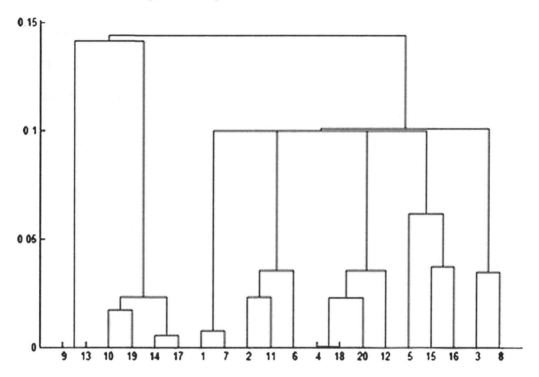

Figure 28. Hierarchical linkage clustering tree Zoo data

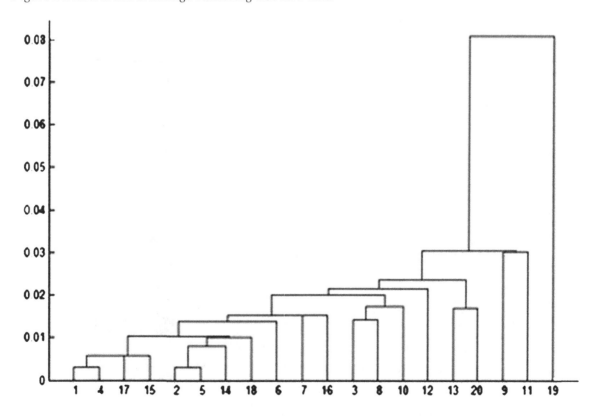

Figure 29. FCM clustering of Abalone data when user assign k=2

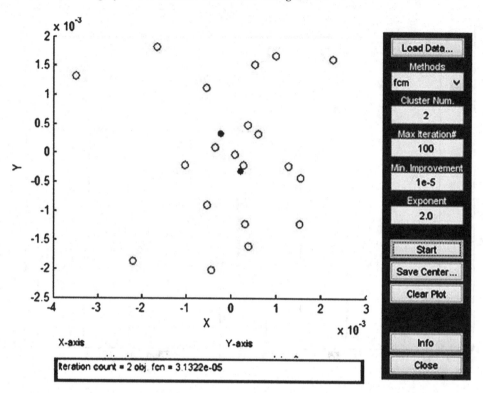

Figure 30. FCM clustering of Abalone data when user assign k=3

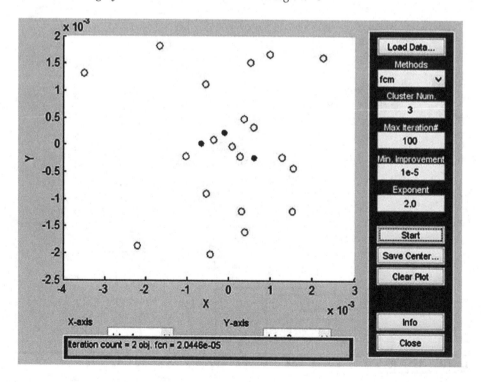

Figure 31. FCM clustering of Abalone data when user assign k=4

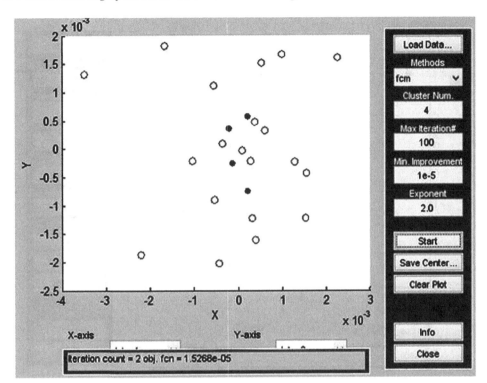

Figure 32. FCM clustering of abalone data when user assign k=5

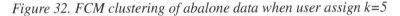

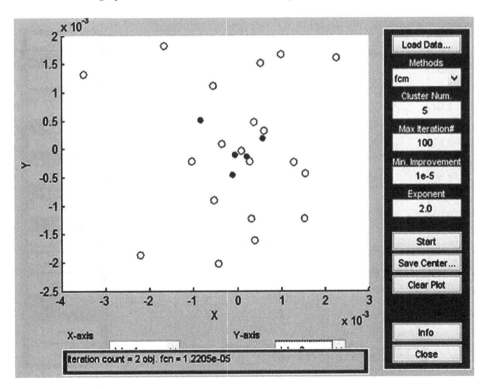

Figure 33. FCM with subtractive clustering of abalone data which automatically assign k

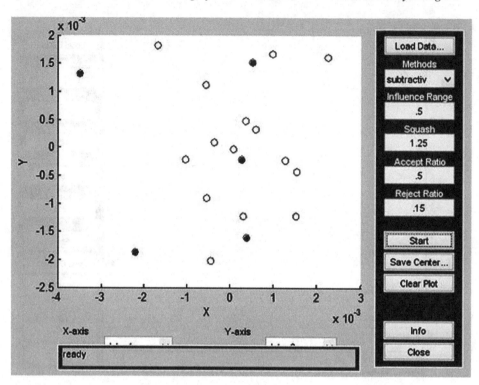

Figure 34. FCM clustering of CA data when user assign k=2

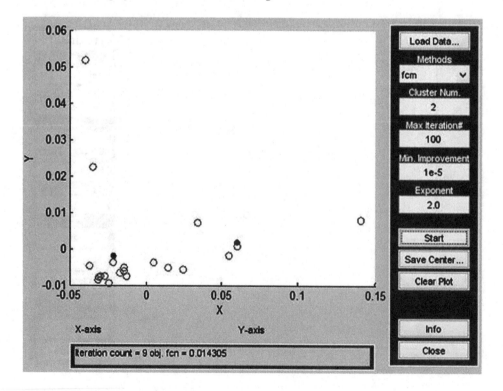

Evaluation of Servo data with PCA using k-means, Figure 32 shows Cluster Evaluation of CA data with PCA using k-means, Figure 29 shows FCM clustering of Abalone data when user assign k=2, Figure 30 shows FCM clustering of Abalone data when user assign k=3, Figure31 shows FCM clustering of Abalone data when user assign k=4, Figure 32 shows FCM clustering when user assign k=5, Figure 33 shows FCM with subtractive clustering which automatically assign k, Figure34 shows FCM clustering of CA data when user assign k=2, Figure35 shows FCM clustering of CA data when user assign k=3,

Figure 35. FCM clustering of CA data when user assign k=3

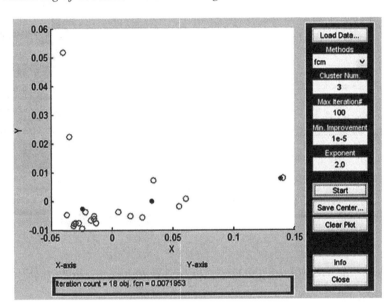

Figure 36. FCM clustering of CA data when user assign k=4

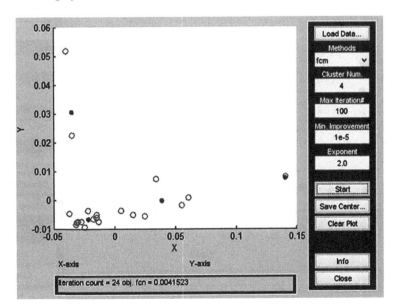

Figure 37. FCM clustering of CA data when user assign k=5

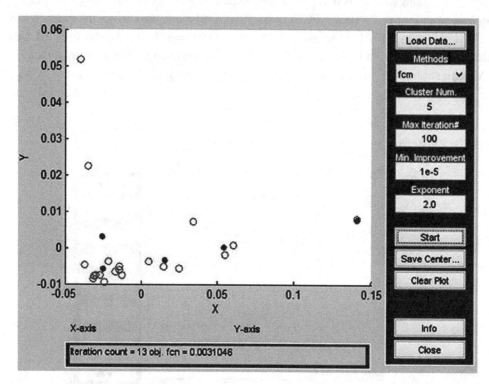

Figure 38. FCM clustering with subtractive method of CA data which automatically assigns k

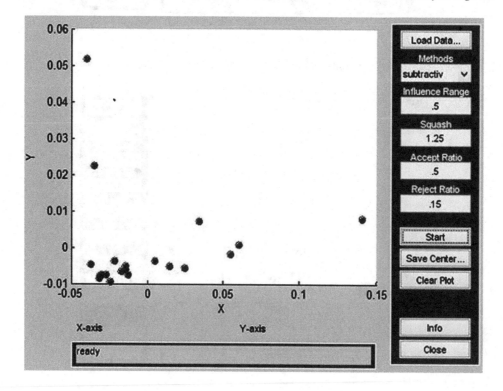

Figure 39. FCM clustering of Servo data when user assign k=2

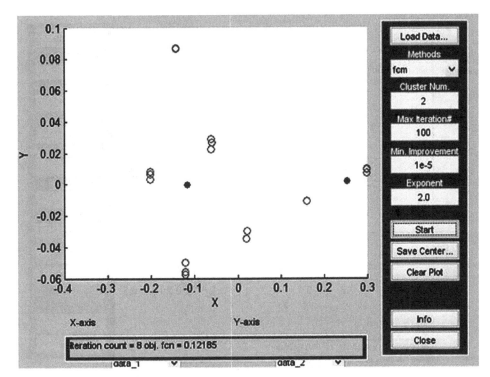

Figure 40. FCM clustering of Servo data when user assign k=3

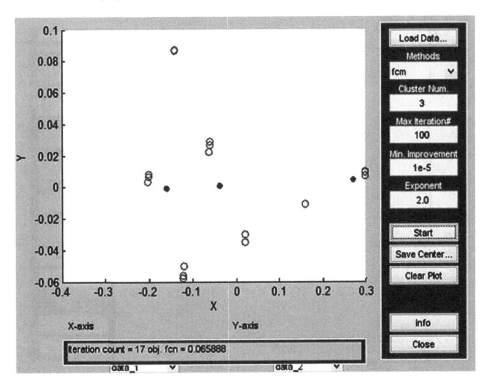

Figure 41. FCM clustering of Servo data when user assign k=4

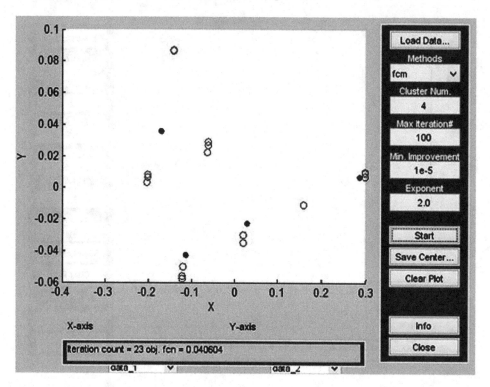

Figure 42. FCM clustering of Servo data when user assign k=5

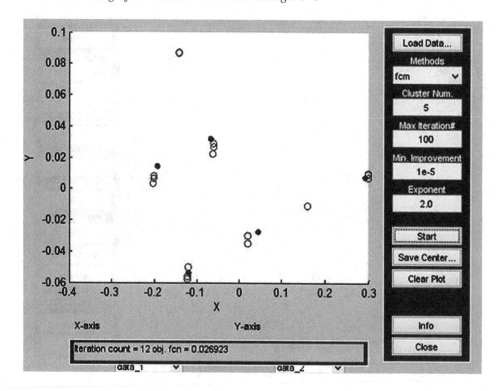

Figure 43. FCM and subtractive clustering of Servo data automatically it assigns clusters k

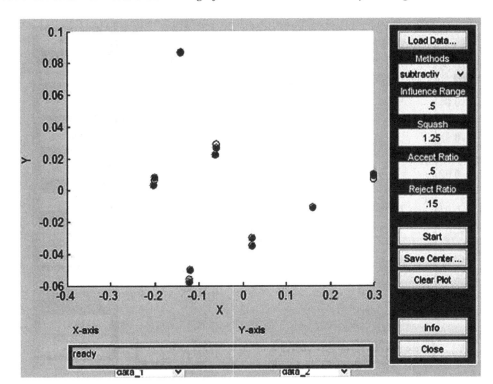

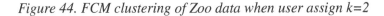

Figure 44. FCM clustering of Zoo data when user assign k=2

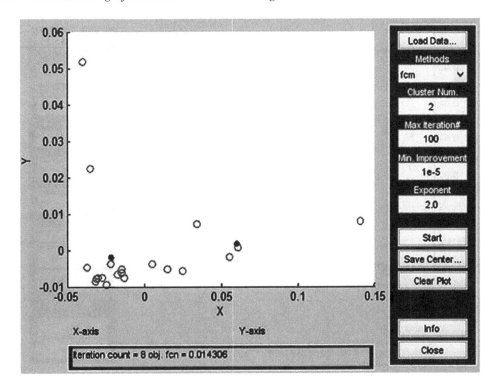

Figure 45. FCM clustering of Zoo data when user assign k=3

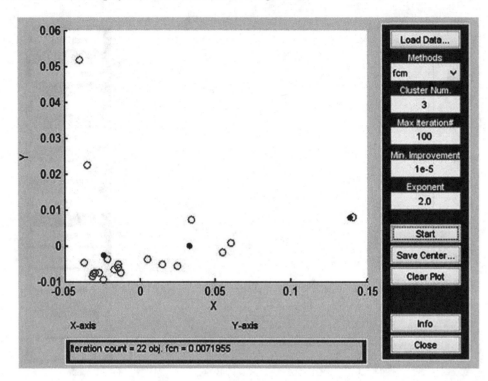

Figure 46. FCM clustering of Zoo data when user assign k=4

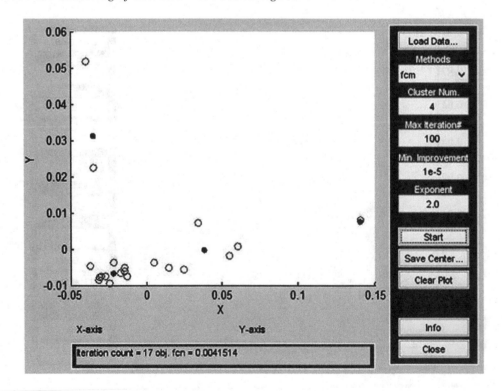

Figure 47. FCM clustering of Zoo data when user assign k=5

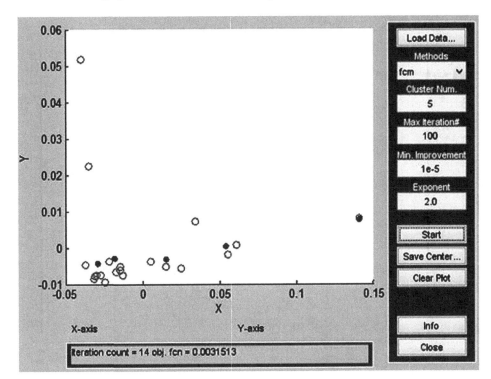

Figure 48. FCM clustering of Zoo data automatically assigns k

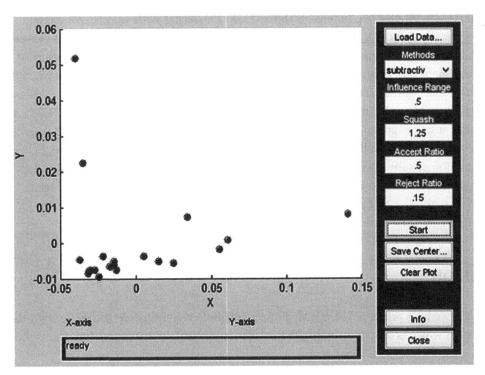

Figure 49. Cluster Evaluation of Abalone data with PCA using k-means

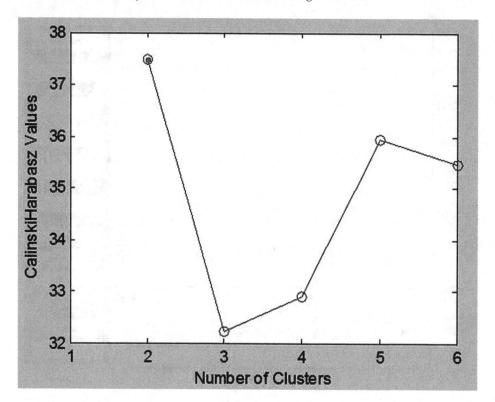

Figure36 shows FCM clustering of CA data when user assign k=4, Figure37 shows FCM clustering of CA data when user assign k=5, Figure 38 shows FCM clustering with subtractive method of CA data which automatically assigns k, Figure 39 shows FCM clustering of Servo data when user assign k=2, Figure40 shows FCM clustering of Servo data when user assign k=3, Figure41 shows FCM clustering of Servo data when user assign k=4, Figure 42 shows FCM clustering of Servo data when user assign k=5, Figure43 shows FCM and subtractive clustering of Servo data automatically it assigns clusters, Figure44 shows FCM clustering of Zoo data when user assign k=2, Figure45 shows FCM clustering of Zoo data when user assign k=3, Figure 46 shows FCM clustering of Zoo data when user assign k=4, Figure 47 shows FCM clustering of Zoo data when user assign k=5, Figure 48 shows FCM clustering of Zoo data automatically assigns k, Figure 49 shows Cluster Evaluation of Abalone data with PCA using k-means, Figure 50 shows Cluster Evaluation of Servo data with PCA using k-means, Figure 51 shows Cluster Evaluation of CA data with PCA using k-means, Figure 52 shows Cluster Evaluation of Zoo data with PCA using k-means.

CONCLUSION

In this chapter, we have presented MWKM, a mixed attribute weighting algorithm for high-dimensional categorical data which is an extension of the k-modes algorithm. In this algorithm, a new weighted dis-

Figure 50. Cluster Evaluation of Servo data with PCA using k-means

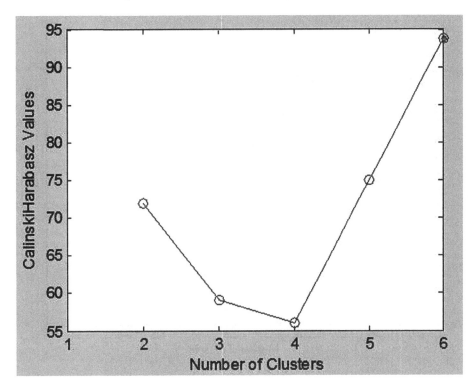

Figure 51. Cluster Evaluation of CA data with PCA using k-means

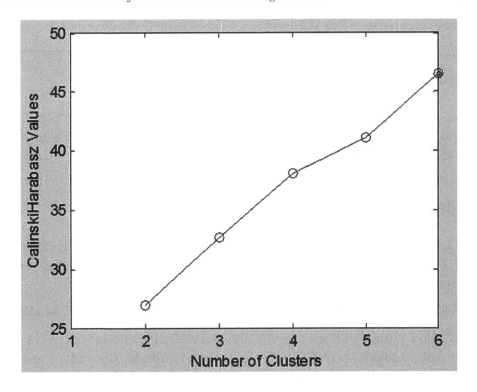

Figure 52. Cluster Evaluation of Zoo data with PCA using k-means

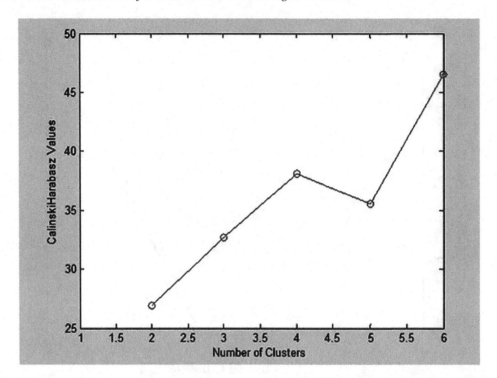

similarity measure has been proposed to eliminate the effect of a problem that the attribute weight does not work while the comparative result of an object and a cluster centre in an attribute is 0. Experimental results show that the analysis is effective and efficient in clustering high-dimensional categorical data sets.

FUTURE WORK

The FCM gives the locally optimal solution. Therefore Genetic algorithm can be used for the global optimal solution. More analysis can be done on feature selection and extraction for more number of attributes of mixed datasets such as Credit approval, Servo Zoo etc.

REFERENCES

Barbará, D., Li, Y., & Couto, J. (2002, November). COOLCAT: an entropy-based algorithm for categorical clustering. In *Proceedings of the eleventh international conference on Information and knowledge management* (pp. 582-589). ACM. doi:10.1145/584792.584888

Blake, C., & Merz, C. J. (1998). *{UCI} Repository of machine learning databases*. Academic Press.

Chatzis, S. P. (2011). A fuzzy c-means-type algorithm for clustering of data with mixed numeric and categorical attributes employing a probabilistic dissimilarity functional. *Expert Systems with Applications*, *38*(7), 8684–8689. doi:10.1016/j.eswa.2011.01.074

Cheeseman, P., Self, M., Kelly, J., Stutz, J., Taylor, W., & Freeman, D. (1996). Bayesian Classification. *AAAI-88 Proceedings*.

Chiu, S. L. (1994). Fuzzy model identification based on cluster estimation. *Journal of Intelligent and Fuzzy Systems, 2*(3), 267-278.

David, G., & Averbuch, A. (2012). SpectralCAT: Categorical spectral clustering of numerical and nominal data. *Pattern Recognition, 45*(1), 416–433. doi:10.1016/j.patcog.2011.07.006

Deng, S., He, Z., & Xu, X. (2010). G-ANMI: A mutual information based genetic clustering algorithm for categorical data. *Knowledge-Based Systems, 23*(2), 144–149. doi:10.1016/j.knosys.2009.11.001

Dutta Baruah, R., & Angelov, P. (2010). Clustering as a tool for self-generation of intelligent systems: A survey. *Evolving Intelligent Systems, EIS, 10*, 34–41.

Fisher, D. H. (1987). Knowledge acquisition via incremental conceptual clustering. *Machine Learning, 2*(2), 139–172. doi:10.1007/BF00114265

Goodall, D. W. (1966). A new similarity index based on probability. *Biometrics, 22*(4), 882–907. doi:10.2307/2528080

Han, J., Kamber, M., & Pei, J. (2001). *Data mining: concepts and techniques*. New York: Elsevier.

He, H., & Tan, Y. (2012). A two-stage genetic algorithm for automatic clustering. *Neurocomputing, 81*, 49–59.

Hsu, C. C. (2006). Generalizing self-organizing map for categorical data. *Neural Networks. IEEE Transactions on, 17*(2), 294–304.

Hsu, C. C., & Huang, Y. P. (2008). Incremental clustering of mixed data based on distance hierarchy. *Expert Systems with Applications, 35*(3), 1177–1185. doi:10.1016/j.eswa.2007.08.049

Hsu, C. C., Lin, S. H., & Tai, W. S. (2011). Apply extended self-organizing map to cluster and classify mixed-type data. *Neurocomputing, 74*(18), 3832–3842. doi:10.1016/j.neucom.2011.07.014

Huang, Z. (1997, May). A Fast Clustering Algorithm to Cluster Very Large Categorical Data Sets in Data Mining. In DMKD.

Huang, Z. (1997, February). Clustering large data sets with mixed numeric and categorical values. In *Proceedings of the 1st Pacific-Asia Conference on Knowledge Discovery and Data Mining,(PAKDD)* (pp. 21-34).

Huang, Z. (1997, February). Clustering large data sets with mixed numeric and categorical values. In *Proceedings of the 1st Pacific-Asia Conference on Knowledge Discovery and Data Mining,(PAKDD)* (pp. 21-34).

Huang, Z., & Ng, M. K. (1999). A fuzzy k-modes algorithm for clustering categorical data. Fuzzy Systems. *IEEE Transactions on, 7*(4), 446–452.

Jain, A. K., Murty, M. N., & Flynn, P. J. (1999). Data clustering: A review. *ACM Computing Surveys, 31*(3), 264–323. doi:10.1145/331499.331504

Ji, J., Pang, W., Zhou, C., Han, X., & Wang, Z. (2012). A fuzzy k-prototype clustering algorithm for mixed numeric and categorical data. *Knowledge-Based Systems, 30*, 129–135. doi:10.1016/j.knosys.2012.01.006

Kaufman, L., & Rousseeuw, P. J. (2009). *Finding groups in data: an introduction to cluster analysis* (Vol. 344). John Wiley & Sons.

Li, C., & Biswas, G. (2002). Unsupervised learning with mixed numeric and nominal data. *Knowledge and Data Engineering. IEEE Transactions on, 14*(4), 673–690.

Lu, Y., Ma, T., Yin, C., Xie, X., Tian, W., & Zhong, S. (2013). Implementation of the Fuzzy C-Means Clustering Algorithm in Meteorological Data. *International Journal of Database Theory and Application, 6*(6), 1–18. doi:10.14257/ijdta.2013.6.6.01

MacQueen, J. (1967, June). Some methods for classification and analysis of multivariate observations. In *Proceedings of the fifth Berkeley symposium on mathematical statistics and probability*.

Manning, C. D., Raghavan, P., & Schütze, H. (2008). *Introduction to information retrieval* (Vol. 1). Cambridge, UK: Cambridge University Press. doi:10.1017/CBO9780511809071

Maulik, U., & Bandyopadhyay, S. (2000). Genetic algorithm-based clustering technique. *Pattern Recognition, 33*(9), 1455–1465. doi:10.1016/S0031-3203(99)00137-5

Rokach, L., & Maimon, O. (2005). Clustering methods. In Data mining and knowledge discovery handbook (pp. 321-352). Springer US. doi:10.1007/0-387-25465-X_15

Sharma, A., & Thakur, R. S. (2012). Challenges in categorical data clustering. In *Proceedings of the International Conference on Intelligent Computing and Information System* (ICICIS).

Sharma, A., & Thakur, R. S. (2014). Cluster Analysis for Categorical Data Using Matlab International Journal of Research in Management. *Science & Technology, 2*(2), 65–68.

Sharma, A., & Thakur, R.S. (2016). Variant of Genetic Algorithm based Categorical data Clustering for Compact Clusters and an Experimental Study on Soybean data for Local and Global Optimal Solution. *International Journal of Advanced Computer Science and Engineering*.

Shih, M. Y., Jheng, J. W., & Lai, L. F. (2010). A two-step method for clustering mixed categroical and numeric data. *Tamkang Journal of Science and Engineering, 13*(1), 11–19.

KEY TERMS AND DEFINITIONS

Clustering: To find out the inherent structure of datasets based on similarity and dissimilarity.

Data Mining: Extraction of hidden and predictive information for large databases.

Fuzzy C-Means: The clustering algorithm for numeric data based on fuzzy concept where the data object has a degree of membership to be in any cluster i.e. any object can be in more than one cluster.

***k*-Means Algorithm:** The basic algorithm for numeric data clustering which became the base for almost all the clustering algorithm.

k-**Modes Algorithm:** The basic algorithm for categorical data clustering which became the base for almost all the categorical clustering algorithm.

k-**Prototypes Algorithm:** This is the basic algorithm for mixed data which is the combination of k-Means and k-Modes algorithm.

Mixed Data: Datasets having both numeric and categorical types attribute values.

Subtractive Method: This method is the enhance version of mountain method to calculate the number of clusters in advance.

Compilation of References

Abdelsamea, M., Gnecco, G., & Medhat Gaber, M. (2015). A SOM-based Chanâ€"Vese model for unsupervised image segmentation. *Soft Computing*. doi:10.1007/s00500-015-1906-z

Abdoh Tabrizi, H., & Jouhare, H. (1996). The Investigation of Efficiency of Stock Price Index of T.S.E. *Journal of Financial Research*, *13*, 11–12.

Abdulsalam Sulaiman Olaniyi, S., Adewole Kayode, S., & Jimoh, R. G. (2011). Stock Trend Prediction Using Regression Analysis – A Data Mining Approach. *ARPN Journal of Systems and Software*, *1*(4), 651–656.

Acharya, U. R., Joseph, K. P., Kannathal, N., Lim, C. M., & Suri, J. S. (2006). Heart rate variability: A review. *Medical & Biological Engineering & Computing*, *44*(12), 1031–1051. doi:10.1007/s11517-006-0119-0 PMID:17111118

Adetunji, , & Aderounmu, , Olusayo, & Adigun. (2013). Forecasting Movement of the Nigerian Stock Exchange All Share Index Using Artificial Neural and Bayesian Networks. *Journal of Finance and Investment Analysis*, *2*(1), 41–59.

Adeyemi, E. O., Desai, K., Towsey, M., & Ghista, D. (1999). Characterization of autonomic dysfunction in patients with irritable bowel syndrome by means of heart rate variability studies. *The American Journal of Gastroenterology*, *94*(3), 816–823. doi:10.1111/j.1572-0241.1999.00861.x PMID:10086672

Adleman, L. (1994). Molecular Computation of Solutions to Combinatorial Problems. *Science*, *266*(5187), 1021–1024. doi:10.1126/science.7973651 PMID:7973651

Agatonovic-Kustrin, S., & Beresford, R. (2000). Basic concepts of artificial neural network (ANN) modeling and its application in pharmaceutical research. *Journal of Pharmaceutical and Biomedical Analysis*, *22*(5), 717–727. doi:10.1016/S0731-7085(99)00272-1 PMID:10815714

Aggarwal, C. C., & Yu, P. S. (2000). Finding Generalized Projected Clusters in High Dimensional Spaces. *ACM SIGMOD Conference.*

Aggarwal, C. C., Gates, S. C., & Yu, P. S. (2004). On Using Partial Supervision for Text Categorization. *IEEE Transactions on Knowledge and Data Engineering*, *16*(2), 245–255. doi:10.1109/TKDE.2004.1269601

Aggarwal, C. C., Procopiuc, C., Wolf, J., Yu, P. S., & Park, J.-S. (1999). Fast Algorithms for Projected Clustering. *ACM SIGMOD Conference.* doi:10.1145/304181.304188

Aggarwal, C. C., & Yu, P. S. (2001). On Effective Conceptual Indexing and Similarity Search in Text. In *ICDM, Proceedings IEEE International Conference.* doi:10.1109/ICDM.2001.989494

Aggarwal, C. C., & Yu, P. S. (2006). A Framework for Clustering Massive Text and Categorical Data Streams. In *SIAM Proceedings, Conference on Data Mining.*

Aggarwal, C. C., Zhao, Y., & Yu, P. S. (2012). Text Clustering with Side Information. In *ICDE Conference*, (pp 894-904).

Agrawal, R., & Srikant, R. (1994). Fast algorithms for mining association rules. In *Proc. 20th Int. Conf. Very Large Data Bases*.

Agrawal, R., Gehrke, J., Raghavan, P., & Gunopulos, D. (1999). Automatic Subspace Clustering of High Dimensional Data for Data Mining Applications. *ACM SIGMOD Conference*.

Agrawal, R., Imielinski, T., & Swami, A. (1993). Mining association rules between sets of items in large databases. In *Proceedings of the ACM SIGMOD Int'l Conf. on Management of data*. doi:10.1145/170035.170072

Agrawal, R., & Shrikanth, R. (1994). Fast Algorithm for Mining Association Rules. In *Proceeding of VLBD Conference*.

Aguado, G., Banon, A., Bateman, J., Bernardos, M. S., Fernandez-Lopez, M., Gomez-Perez, A., … Sanchez, A. (1998). Ontogeneration: Reusing Domain and Linguistic Ontologies for Spanish Text Generation. *Workshop on Applications of Ontologies and Problem Solving Methods*.

Alam, , Napitupulu, & Yohanes Budiman. (2013). Prediction of Stock Price Using Artificial Neural Network: A Case of Indonesia. *Journal of Theoretical and Applied Information Technology*, *54*(1), 104–109.

Ali, H., Badshah, N., Chen, K., & Khan, G. (2016). A variational model with hybrid images data fitting energies for segmentation of images with intensity inhomogeneity. *Pattern Recognition*, *51*, 27–42. doi:10.1016/j.patcog.2015.08.022

Allan, J., Papka, R., & Lavrenko, V. (1998). Online new event detection and tracking. In *ACM SIGIR Proc 21st Int.Conf. On Research and development in information retrieval*.

Alvarcz, G., Li, S., & Hernandez, L. (2007). Analysis of security problems in a medical image encryption system. *Computers in Biology and Medicine*, *37*(3), 424–427. doi:10.1016/j.compbiomed.2006.04.002 PMID:16872592

Amos, M., Paun, G., Rozenberg, G., & Salomaa, A. (2002). Topics in the theory of DNA computing. *Theoretical Computer Science*, *287*(1), 3–38. doi:10.1016/S0304-3975(02)00134-2

Anandhavalli, M., Sudhanshu, S.K., Kumar, A., & Ghose, M.K. (2009). Optimized association rule mining using genetic algorithm. *Advances in Information Mining*, *1*(2).

Ananth, K., & Pannirselvam, S. (2012). A Geodesic Active Contour Level Set Method for Image Segmentation. *International Journal of Image, Graphics, Signal Processing*, *4*(5), 31–37. doi:10.5815/ijigsp.2012.05.04

Anderson. (1980). *Computer Security Threat Monitoring and Surveillance*. Technical Report. James P. Anderson Co.

Andritsos, P., Tsaparas, P., Miller, R., & Sevcik, K. (2004). LIMBO: Scalable Clustering of Categorical Data. In *Proc. 9th international conference EDBT*.

Angelova, R., & Siersdorfer, S. (2006) A neighborhood-based approach for clustering of linked document collections. In *CIKM Proc. Of 15th Int.Conf. On Information and knowledge management*.

Anick, P., & Vaithyanathan, S. (1997). Exploiting Clustering and Phrases for Context-Based Information Retrieval. In *Proc. 20th Int. Conf. ACM SIGIR*.

Anick, P. G., & Tipirneni, S. (1999). The paraphrase search assistant: terminological feedback for iterative information seeking. In *SIGIR '99: Proceedings of the 22nd annual international ACM SIGIR conference on Research and development in information retrieval*. New York, NY:ACM Press. doi:10.1145/312624.312670

Ankerst, M. (2001). *Visual Data Mining with Pixel-Oriented Visualization Techniques.ACM SIGKDD Workshop on Visual Data Mining*, San Francisco, CA.

Appelhans, B. M., & Luecken, L. J. (2006). Heart rate variability as an index of regulated emotional responding. *Review of General Psychology, 10*(3), 229–240. doi:10.1037/1089-2680.10.3.229

Appenzeller, O., & Oribe, E. (1997). *The autonomic nervous system: an introduction to basic and clinical concepts.* Elsevier Health Sciences.

Appleton, B., & Talbot, H. (2005). Globally Optimal Geodesic Active Contours. *Journal of Mathematical Imaging and Vision, 23*(1), 67–86. doi:10.1007/s10851-005-4968-1

Arabshian, K., Danielsen, P., & Afroz, S. (2012). Lexont: Semiautomatic ontology creation tool for programmable web. In *AAAI 2012 Spring Symposium on Intelligent Web Services Meet Social Computing.*

Arabshian, K., Danielsen, P., & Afroz, S. (2012, March). Lexont: Semiautomatic ontology creation tool for programmable web. In *AAAI 2012 Spring Symposium on Intelligent Web Services Meet Social Computing.*

Armstrong Scott, J. (2012). Illusions in Regression Analysis. *Journal of Forecasting, 28*(3), 689-695.

Arpirez, J., G'omez-P'erez, A., Lozano, A., & Pinto, S. (1998). (onto)2agent: An ontology-based www broker to select ontologies. In A. Gomez-Perez, & V. R. Benjamins (Eds.), *Proceedings of the Workshop on Applications of Ontologies and Problem-Solving Methods, held in conjunction with ECAI-98.* Brighton, UK: ECAI.

Arvind, T.S., & Badhe, V. (2014). Comparative Analysis of Fuzzy, Rough, Vague & Soft set Theories in Association Rule Mining. *International Journal Of Scientific Progress And Research, 2*(1).

Arvind, T.S., & Badhe, V. (2015). The Application of Vague Set Theory in Association Rule Mining: A Survey. *International Journal Advanced Research in Computer Science, 6*(1).

Avrma. (2004). Stock Return Predictability and Asset Pricing Models. *The Review of Financial Studies, 17*(3).

Bacharova, L., Selvester, R. H., Engblom, H., & Wagner, G. S. (2005). Where is the central terminal located?: In search of understanding the use of the Wilson central terminal for production of 9 of the standard 12 electrocardiogram leads. *Journal of Electrocardiology, 38*(2), 119–127. doi:10.1016/j.jelectrocard.2005.01.002 PMID:15892021

Baeza-Yates, R. A., & Ribeiro-Neto, B. A. (2011). *Modern Information Retrieval- the concepts and technology behind search* (2nd ed.). Harlow, UK: Pearson Education Ltd.

Bajpayee, Priya, & Kumar. (2015). Big Data: A Brief investigation on NoSQL Databases. *International Journal of Innovations & Advancement in Computer Science, 4*(1).

Baker, L., & McCallum, A. (1998). Distributional Clustering of Words for Text Classification. In *SIGIR Proc. Of 21ˢᵗ Int.ACM Conf. On Research and development in information retrieval.*

Barbara, D., Wu, N., & Jajodia, S. (2001). Detecting novel network intrusions using bayes estimators. In *Proceedings of the First SIAM International Conference on Data Mining* (SDM 2001). doi:10.1137/1.9781611972719.28

Barbara, D., Couto, J., Jajodia, S., & Wu, N. (2001). *Special section on data mining for intrusion detection and threat analysis*, Adam: A testbed for exploring the use of data mining in intrusion detection. *SIGMOD Record, 30*, 15–24. doi:10.1145/604264.604266

Barbará, D., Li, Y., & Couto, J. (2002, November). COOLCAT: an entropy-based algorithm for categorical clustering. In *Proceedings of the eleventh international conference on Information and knowledge management* (pp. 582-589). ACM. doi:10.1145/584792.584888

Barr, R. C., & van Oosterom, A. (2010). *Genesis of the electrocardiogram. In Comprehensive electrocardiology* (pp. 167–190). Springer. doi:10.1007/978-1-84882-046-3_5

Basu, S., Banerjee, A., & Mooney, R. J. (2002). Semi-supervised Clustering by Seeding. In *ICML Proc. Of 19th Int. Conf. On Machine Learning.*

Basu, S., Bilenko, M., & Mooney, R. J. (2004). A probabilistic framework for semi-supervised clustering. In *KDD Proc. Of 10th ACM SIGKDD Int.Conf. On knowledge discovery and data mining.*

Beaver, W. H. (1966). Financial Ratios, as Predictors of Failure. *Journal of Accounting Research, 4,* 71–111. doi:10.2307/2490171

Bechhofer, S., Broekstra, J., Decker, S., Erdmann, M., Fensel, D., Goble, C., … Studer, R. (2002). *An Informal Description of OIL-Core and Standard OIL: A Layered Proposal for DAML-O*. Retrieved from: www.ontoknowledge.org/oil/downl/dialects.pdf.

Beil, F., Ester, M., & Xu, X. (2002). Frequent term-based text clustering. In *Proc. of International conf. ACMKDD.* doi:10.1145/775047.775110

Bekkerman, R., El-Yaniv, R., Winter, Y., & Tishby, N. (2001) On Feature Distributional Clustering for Text Categorization. In *SIGIR Proc. Of 24th Int.ACM Conf. On development in information retrieval.*

Benninghoff, H., & Garcke, H. (2014). Efficient Image Segmentation and Restoration Using Parametric Curve Evolution with Junctions and Topology Changes. *SIAM Journal on Imaging Sciences, 7*(3), 1451–1483. doi:10.1137/130932430

Berbar, M. A., Gahe, S. F., & Ismail, N. A. (2003). *Image Fusion Using Multi Decomposition Levels Of Discrete Wavelet Transform,The Institution of Electrical Engineers*. Stevenage: Michael Faraday House, Six Hills Way.

Bernaras, A., Laresgoiti, I., & Corera, J. (1996). Building and reusing ontologies for electrical network applications. In *Proceedings of the 12th ECAI.*

Bernardi, L., Porta, C., & Sleight, P. (2006). Cardiovascular, cerebrovascular, and respiratory changes induced by different types of music in musicians and non-musicians: The importance of silence. *Heart (British Cardiac Society), 92*(4), 445–452. doi:10.1136/hrt.2005.064600 PMID:16199412

Bhasker, G.V., Shekar, K.C., & Chaitanya, V.L. (2011). Mining Frequent Itemsets for Non Binary Data Set Using Genetic Algorithm. *International Journal of Advanced Engineering Sciences and Technologies, 11*(1), 143-152.

Bhowmick, P.K., Roy, D., Sarkar, S., & Basu, A. (2010). *A Framework For Manual Ontology Engineering For Management Of Learning Material Repository.* Academic Press.

Bhowmick, Roy, Sarkar, & Basu. (2010). *A Framework For Manual Ontology Engineering For Management Of Learning Material Repository.* Academic Press.

Big Data Analytics Advanced Analytics in Oracle Database. (2013). Oracle White Paper.

Bilchick, K. C., & Berger, R. D. (2006). Heart rate variability. *Journal of Cardiovascular Electrophysiology, 17*(6), 691–694. doi:10.1111/j.1540-8167.2006.00501.x PMID:16836727

Blake, C., & Merz, C. J. (1998). *[UCI] Repository of machine learning databases.* Academic Press.

Blake, Keogh, & Merz. (2008). *UCI repository of machine learning databases.* Academic Press.

Blaz, F., Marko, G., & Dunja, M. (2007). OntoGen: Semi-automatic Ontology. In Human Interface, Part II, HCII 2007, (LNCS), (vol. 4558, pp. 309–318). Springer.

Blaz, F., Marko, G., & Dunja, M. (2006). Semi-automatic Data-driven Ontology Construction System. In *Proceedings of the 9th International multi-conference Information Society IS-2006.*

Blei, D., & Lafferty, J. (2006) Dynamic topic models. In *ICML Proc. Of 23ʳᵈ Int.Conf. On Machine Learning*.

Blei, D., Ng, A., & Jordan, M. (2003). Latent Dirichlet allocation, *In Journal of Machine Learning Research. Vole, 3*, 993–1022.

Blum, A. L., & Langley, P. (1997). Selection of Relevant Features and Examples in Machine Learning. *Artificial Intelligence, 97*(1-2), 245–271. doi:10.1016/S0004-3702(97)00063-5

Bolton, S. (1997). Analysis of variance. In *Pharmaceutical statistics: Practical and clinical applications*. Basel: Marcel Dekker.

Borgo, Guarino, & Masolo. (1996). Stratified ontologies: the case of physical objects. In *Proceedings of the Workshop on Ontological Engineering, held in conjunction with ECAI-96*. Budapest: ECAI.

Boso, M., Politi, P., Barale, F., & Enzo, E. (2006). Neurophysiology and neurobiology of the musical experience. *Functional Neurology, 21*(4), 187–191. PMID:17367577

Boston, R. (1998). *A Measure of Uncertainty for Stock Performance.IEEE/IAFE/INFORMS Conference Computational Intelligence for Financial Engineering (CIFEr)*, New York, NY. doi:10.1109/CIFER.1998.690072

Boyce, S., & Pahl, C. (2007). Developing Domain Ontologies for Course Content. *Journal of Educational Technology & Society, 10*(3), 275–288.

Boyett, M. R., Honjo, H., & Kodama, I. (2000). The sinoatrial node, a heterogeneous pacemaker structure. *Cardiovascular Research, 47*(4), 658–687. doi:10.1016/S0008-6363(00)00135-8 PMID:10974216

Bray, T., Paoli, J., Sperberg-McQueen, C. M., & Maler, E. (2000). *Extensible MarkupLanguage (XML) 1.0, Second Edition, W3C Recommendation, 2000*. Retrieved from http://www.w3.org/TR/REC-xml

Bresson, X., & Esedog, Ì. (2007). Fast Global Minimization of the Active Contour/Snake Model. *Journal of Mathematical Imaging and Vision, 28*(2), 151–167. doi:10.1007/s10851-007-0002-0

Brickley, D., & Guha, R. V. (2002). *RDF Vocabulary Description Language 1.0: RDF Schema, W3C Working Draft*. Retrieved from: http://www.w3.org/TR/PR-rdf-schema

Bridges & Rayford. (2000). Fuzzy data mining and genetic algorithms applied to intrusion detection. In *Proceedings of the Twenty-third National Information Systems Security Conference*. National Institute of Standards and Technology.

Brin, S., Motwani, R., Ullman, J. D., & Tsurb, S. (1997). Dynamic itemset counting and implication rules for market basket data. *Proc. ACM SIGMOID Int. Conf. Manage. Data*. doi:10.1145/253260.253325

Brown, P. F., deSouza, P. V., Mercer, R. L., & Della Pietra, V. J. (1992). Class-based n-gram models of natural language. Journal of Computational Linguistics, 18(4).

Brown, D. P., & Jennings, R. H. (1989). On Technical Analysis. *Review of Financial Studies, 2*(4), 527–551. doi:10.1093/rfs/2.4.527

Buitelaar, S., & Olejnik, D. (2004). *A protege plug-in for ontology extraction from text based on linguistic analysis*. Academic Press.

Burns, N. (2013). *Cardiovascular physiology*. Retrieved from School of Medicine, Trinity College, Dublin: http://www.medicine.tcd.ie/physiology/assets/docs12_13/lecturenotes/NBurns/Trinity%20CVS%20lecture

Can, A., Leclercq, L., Lelong, J., & Botteldooren, D. (2010). Traffic noise spectrum analysis: Dynamic modeling vs. experimental observations. *Applied Acoustics, 71*(8), 764–770. doi:10.1016/j.apacoust.2010.04.002

Cardiology, T. F. E. S., & Cardiology, T. F. E. S. (1996). the North American Society of Pacing and Electrophysiology. Heart rate variability: Standards of measurement, physiological interpretation and clinical use. *Circulation, 93*(5), 1043–1065. doi:10.1161/01.CIR.93.5.1043 PMID:8598068

Carney, R. M., Blumenthal, J. A., Stein, P. K., Watkins, L., Catellier, D., Berkman, L. F., & Freedland, K. E. et al. (2001). Depression, heart rate variability, and acute myocardial infarction. *Circulation, 104*(17), 2024–2028. doi:10.1161/hc4201.097834 PMID:11673340

Carney, R. M., Freedland, K. E., & Veith, R. C. (2005). Depression, the autonomic nervous system, and coronary heart disease. *Psychosomatic Medicine, 67*, S29–S33. doi:10.1097/01.psy.0000162254.61556.d5 PMID:15953797

Ceusters, W., & Martens, P. (2001). LinKFactory: an Advanced Formal Ontology Management System.*Proceedings of Interactive Tools for Knowledge Capture Workshop,KCAP 2001.*

Chakrabarti, K., & Mehrotra, S. (2000). Local Dimension reduction: A new Approach to Indexing High Dimensional Spaces. In *VLDB Proc. Of 26th Int. conf. on Very Large Databases.*

Chakrabarti, P., Bhuyan, B., Chowdhuri, A., & Bhunia, C. (2008). A novel approach towards realizing optimum data transfer and Automatic Variable Key (AVK) in cryptography. IJCSNS, 8(5), 241-250.

Chakrabarti. (2007). Application of Automatic Variable Key (AVK) in RSA. *International Journal HIT Transactions on ECCN, 2*(5), 301-305.

Chakraborty, Mondal, Chaudhuri, & Bhunia. (2006). Various new and modified approaches for selective encryption (DES, RSA and AES) with AVK and their comparative study. International Journal HIT Transaction on ECCN, 1(4), 236-244.

Chandrasekaran, B., Josephson, J. R., & Benjamins, V. R. (1999). What are ontologies?Why do we need them? *IEEE Intelligent Systems.*

Chang, J., & Blei, D. (2009). Topic Models for Document Networks. In *Proc. Of 12th Int.Conf. Artificial Intelligence and Statistics.*

Charniak, U. (2001).Unsupervised learning of name structure from conference data. In *Proceedings of the 2nd Meeting of the North American Chapter of the Association for Computational Linguistics.*

Chatzis, S. P. (2011). A fuzzy c-means-type algorithm for clustering of data with mixed numeric and categorical attributes employing a probabilistic dissimilarity functional. *Expert Systems with Applications, 38*(7), 8684–8689. doi:10.1016/j.eswa.2011.01.074

Chaudhri, V. K., Farquhar, A., Fikes, R., Karp, P. D. & Rice, J. P. (1998). *Open Knowledge Base Connectivity 2.0.3.* Technical Report.

Cheeseman, P., Self, M., Kelly, J., Stutz, J., Taylor, W., & Freeman, D. (1996). Bayesian Classification. *AAAI-88 Proceedings.*

Chen, C. L., Tseng, F. S. C., & Liang, T. (2010). Mining fuzzy frequent item sets for hierarchical document clustering. Process Manag, 46(2), 193–211.

Chen, A. S., Leung, M. T., & Daouk, H. (2003). Application of Neural Networks to an Emerging Financial Market: Forecasting and Trading the Taiwan Stock Index. *Computers & Operations Research, 30*(6), 901–923. doi:10.1016/S0305-0548(02)00037-0

Chen, A., Deeley, M., Niermann, K., Moretti, L., & Dawant, B. (2010). Combining registration and active shape models for the automatic segmentation of the lymph node regions in head and neck CT images. *Medical Physics*, *37*(12), 6338. doi:10.1118/1.3515459 PMID:21302791

Chen, C. L. P., & Zhang, C.-Y. (2014). Data-intensive applications, challenges, techniques and technologies: A survey on Big Data. *Information Sciences*, *275*, 314–347. doi:10.1016/j.ins.2014.01.015

Chen, C.-L., Tseng, F. S. C., & Liang, T. (2010, November). An integration of WordNet and Fuzzy association rule mining for multi-label document clustering. *Data & Knowledge Engineering*, *69*(11), 1208–1226. doi:10.1016/j.datak.2010.08.003

Chen, D. (2013). A Novel Image Segmentation Algorithm: Region Merging Using Superpixel-based Local CRF Model. *J. Inf. Comput. Sci.*, *10*(16), 5145–5153. doi:10.12733/jics20103063

Chen, J. (2003) A DNA-based biomolecular cryptography design. *IEEE International Symposium on Circuits and Systems*, (pp. 822–825).

Chen, Y., & Chen, O. (2009). Image Segmentation Method Using Thresholds Automatically Determined from Picture Contents. *EURASIP Journal on Image and Video Processing*, *2009*, 1–15. doi:10.1155/2009/140492

Chih-Fong, T. (2010). Combining Multiple Feature Selection Methods for Stock Prediction: Union, Intersection, and Multi-Intersection Approaches. *Decision Support Systems*, *50*(1), 258–269. doi:10.1016/j.dss.2010.08.028

Chiu, S. L. (1994). Fuzzy model identification based on cluster estimation. *Journal of Intelligent and Fuzzy Systems*, *2*(3), 267-278.

Choudhary J. & Devshri, R. (2012). An Approach to Build Ontology in Semi-Automated way. *Journal of Information and Communication Technologies, 2*(5).

Choudhary, J., & Roy, D. (2012, May). An Approach to Build Ontology in Semi-Automated way. *Journal of Information and Communication Technologies*, *2*(5).

Cowie, J., & Wilks, Y. (2000). *Information extraction*. New York: Academic Press.

Craig, J., & Patterson, V. (2005). Introduction to the practice of Telemedicine. *Journal of Telemedicine and Telecare*, *11*(1), 3–9. doi:10.1258/1357633053430494 PMID:15829036

Cristi, R. (2004). *Modern digital signal processing*. Cl-Engineering.

Croft, W. B. (1977). Clustering large files of documents using the single-link method. *Journal of the American Society for Information Science*, *28*(6), 341–344. doi:10.1002/asi.4630280606

Cui & Potok. (2005). Document Clustering Analysis Based on Hybrid PSO+K-means Algorithm. *Journal of Computer Sciences*, 27-33.

Cui, G. Z., Qin, L. M., Wang, Y. F., & Zhang, X. (2007). Information Security Technology Based on DNA Computing. *IEEE International Workshop on Anti-counterfeiting, Security, Identification*, (pp. 288–291). doi:10.1109/IWASID.2007.373746

Cui, G. Z., Qin, L. M., Wang, Y. F., & Zhang, X. (2008). An Encryption Scheme using DNA Technology. *International Conference on Bio-Inspired Computing: Theories and Applications*, (pp. 37-42).

Cui, Z., Zhang, G., & Wu, J. (2009). Medical Image Fusion Based on Wavelet Transform and Independent Component Analysis. *International Joint Conference on Artificial Intelligence*. IEEE.

Cure, O., Hecht, R., Le Duc, C., & Lamolle, M. (2011). Data Integration over NoSQL Stores Using Access Path Based Mappings. DEXA 2012.

Cutting, D., Karger, D., & Pederson, J. (n.d.). Constant Interaction-time Scatter/Gather Browsing of Large Document Collections. In *SIGIR Proc. Of 16th Int.ACM SIGIR Conf. on Research and Development in information retrieval*.

Cutting, D., Karger, D., Pedersen, J., & Tukey, J. (1992). A Cluster-based Approach to Browsing Large Document Collections. In *SIGIR Proc. Of 15th Int.ACM SIGIR Conf. on Research and Development in information retrieval*.

Daniel, R. M., & Shukla, A. K. (2014). Improving Text Search Process using Text Document Clustering Approach. *International Journal of Science and Research, 3*(5), 14-24.

Danielsen, P. J., & Arabshian, K. (2013). User Interface Design in Semi-Automated Ontology Construction. *IEEE 20th International Conference on Web Services*.

Dardzinska, A. (2013). *Action Rules Mining, Studies in Computational Intelligence* (Vol. 468). Springer. doi:10.1007/978-3-642-35650-6

Dardzinska, A., & Ras, Z. (2006). *Extracting rules from incomplete decision systems. In Foundations and Novel Approaches in Data Mining, Studies in Computational Intelligence* (pp. 143–154). Springer.

Das, A. P. (2008). *Security Analysis and Portfolio Management* (3rd ed.). New Delhi, India: I.K. International Publication.

Dash, M., & Liu, H. (1997). Feature Selection for Clustering. In *Proc. of Int. Conf. PAKDD*. doi:10.1007/3-540-45571-X_13

Davenport, T. H., & Patil, D. J. (2012). Data Scientist: The Sexiest Job of the 21st Century. *Harvard Business Review, 90*(10), 70–76. PMID:23074866

David, G., & Averbuch, A. (2012). SpectralCAT: Categorical spectral clustering of numerical and nominal data. *Pattern Recognition, 45*(1), 416–433. doi:10.1016/j.patcog.2011.07.006

Davis, W. B., Gfeller, K. E., & Thaut, M. H. (2008). *An introduction to music therapy: Theory and practice*. ERIC.

Dawoud, A., & Netchaev, A. (2012). Fusion of visual cues of intensity and texture in Markov random fields image segmentation. *IET Computer Vision, 6*(6), 603–609. doi:10.1049/iet-cvi.2011.0233

Dean & Ghemawat. (2004). *MapReduce: Simplified Data Processing on Large Clusters*. Academic Press.

Dean & Ghemawat. (2015). *Map Reduce: Simplified Data Processing on Large Clusters*. Google, Inc.

Dean, M., Connolly, D., van Harmelen, F., Hendler, J., Horrocks, I., McGuinness, D. L., . . . Stein, L. A. (2002). *OWL Web Ontology Language 1.0Reference, W3C Working Draft*. Retrieved from: http://www.w3.org/TR/owl-ref/

DeCandia, G. (2007). Dynamo: Amazon's Highly Available Key-Value Store. *Proc. 21st ACM SIGOPS Symp. Operating Systems Principles (SOSP 07)*. doi:10.1145/1294261.1294281

Deerwester, S., Dumais, S., Landauer, T., Furnas, G., & Harshman, R. (1990). Indexing by Latent Semantic Analysis. *JASIS, 41*(6), 391–407. doi:10.1002/(SICI)1097-4571(199009)41:6<391::AID-ASI1>3.0.CO;2-9

Deng, S., He, Z., & Xu, X. (2010). G-ANMI: A mutual information based genetic clustering algorithm for categorical data. *Knowledge-Based Systems, 23*(2), 144–149. doi:10.1016/j.knosys.2009.11.001

Denning. (1987). An Intrusion Detection Model. *IEEE Transactions on Software Engineering, 13*(2), 222–232.

Dhillon, I. (2001). Co-clustering Documents and Words using bipartitespectral graph partitioning. In *KDD Proc. Of 7th Int.ACM SIGKDD Conf. on Knowledge discovery and data mining*.

Dhillon, I., & Modha, D. (2001). Concept Decompositions for Large Sparse Data using Clustering. Springer.

Dilaveris, P. E., & Gialafos, J. E. (2001). P-wave dispersion: A novel predictor of paroxysmal atrial fibrillation. *Annals of Noninvasive Electrocardiology*, 6(2), 159–165. doi:10.1111/j.1542-474X.2001.tb00101.x PMID:11333174

Ding, C., He, X., Zha, H., & Simon, H. D. (2002). Adaptive Dimension Reduction for Clustering High Dimensional Data. In *ICDM Proc. Of 24th Int Conf. on Machine Learning*.

Diop, E., & Burdin, V. (2013). Bi-planar image segmentation based on variational geometrical active contours with shape priors. *Medical Image Analysis*, 17(2), 165–181. doi:10.1016/j.media.2012.09.006 PMID:23168322

Dorow, B., & Widdows, D. (2003). Discovering corpus-specific word senses. In *Proceedings of the tenth conference on European chapter of the Association for Computational Linguistics*.

Drapikowski, P., & Domaga, Å. (2014). Semi-Automatic Segmentation of Ct/Mri Images Based on Active Contour Method for 3D Reconstruction of Abdominal Aortic Aneurysms. *Image Processing & Communications*, 19(1). doi:10.1515/ipc-2015-0002

Dutta Baruah, R., & Angelov, P. (2010). Clustering as a tool for self-generation of intelligent systems: A survey. *Evolving Intelligent Systems, EIS*, 10, 34–41.

Dutta, A. (2001). Investors Reaction to the Good and Bad News in Secondary Market. A Study Relating to Investors Behavior. *Finance India*, 15(2), 567–576.

Dzeroski, S., & Zenko, B. (2002). Is Combining Classifiers Better than Selecting the Best One. *Proc. 19th Int'l Conf. Machine Learning (ICML '02)*.

Eiben, A.E., & Smith, J.E. (2001). *Introduction to Evolutionary Computing*. Springer.

Ekanayake, J., Pallickara, S., & Fox, G. (2008). Mapreduce for data intensive scientific analyses. *Proceedings of IEEE Fourth International Conference on eScience*.

Elith, J., Leathwick, J. R., & Hastie, T. (2008). A working guide to boosted regression trees. *Journal of Animal Ecology*, 77(4), 802–813. doi:10.1111/j.1365-2656.2008.01390.x PMID:18397250

Elminaam, Kader, & Hadhoud. (2008). Performance Evaluation of Symmetric Encryption Algorithms. *International Journal of Computer Science and Network Security, 8*(12), 280–286.

Esler, M., & Kaye, D. (2000). Sympathetic nervous system activation in essential hypertension, cardiac failure and psychosomatic heart disease. *Journal of Cardiovascular Pharmacology*, 35, S1–S7. doi:10.1097/00005344-200000004-00001 PMID:11346214

Esler, P. D. M., & Kaye, P. D. D. (2000). Measurement of sympathetic nervous system activity in heart failure: The role of norepinephrine kinetics. *Heart Failure Reviews*, 5(1), 17–25. doi:10.1023/A:1009889922985 PMID:16228913

Everitt, B. S., Landau, S., & Leese, M. (2001). *Cluster Analysis* (4th ed.). London: Arnold.

Fadai Nejad, M. I. (1994). Stock Market Efficiency: Some Misconceptions. *Journal of Financial Research, 1*(2), 227–236.

Fama Eugene, F. (1965). The Behavior of Stock Market Prices. *The Journal of Business*, 38(1), 34–105. doi:10.1086/294743

Fang, H., Tao, T., & Zhai, C. (2004). A formal study of information retrieval heuristics. *Proceedings of ACM SIGIR Int. conf. On research and development in Information retrieval*. doi:10.1145/1008992.1009004

Farquhar, A., Fikes, R., & Rice, J. (1996). The Ontolingua Server: a Tool for Collaborative Ontology Construction. In *Proceedings of the 10th Bank Knowledge Acquisition for Knowledge Based System Workshop* (KAW95). doi:10.1006/ijhc.1996.0121

Faure, D., & Poibeau, T. (2000). First experiments of using semantic knowledge learned by ASIUM for information extraction task using INTEX. In S. Staab, A.Maedche, C. Nedellec, & P. Wiemer-Hastings (Eds.), *Proceedings of the Workshop on Ontology Learning,14th European Conference on Artificial Intelligence ECAI'00.*

Fayyad, U. M., Piatetsky, Shapiro, G., Smith, P., & Uthurusamy, R. (Eds.). (1996). Advances in Knowledge Discovery and Data Mining. AAAI Press/MIT Press.

Feierabend, R., & Shahram, M. (2009). Hoarseness in adults. *American Family Physician, 80*(4), 363–370.

Feigenbaum, E.A. (1977). The art of artificial intelligence – Themes and case studies of knowledge engineering. *Proc. of 5th IJCAI.*

Fernandez Lopez, M. (1999). Overview of Methodologies for Building Ontologies. In *Proceedings of the IJCAI99 Workshop on Ontologies and Problem-Solving Methods:Lessons Learned and Future Trends.*

Fisher, D. (1979). Knowledge Acquisition via incremental conceptual clustering.Machine Learning, 2, 139–172.

Fisher, D. H. (1987). Knowledge acquisition via incremental conceptual clustering. *Machine Learning, 2*(2), 139–172. doi:10.1007/BF00114265

Floras, J. S. (2009). Sympathetic nervous system activation in human heart failure: Clinical implications of an updated model. *Journal of the American College of Cardiology, 54*(5), 375–385. doi:10.1016/j.jacc.2009.03.061 PMID:19628111

Frank, L. (2011). Countermeasures against consistency anomalies in distributed integrated databases with relaxed ACID properties. *Innovations in Information Technology (IIT),International Conference.*

Franz, M., Ward, T., McCarley, J., & Zhu, W.-J. (2001). Unsupervised and supervised clustering for topic tracking.*Proceedings of ACM SIGIR 24th Int. conf. On research and development in Information retrieval.* doi:10.1145/383952.384013

Freedman David, A. (2005). *Statistical Models: Theory and Practice.* Cambridge University Press. doi:10.1017/CBO9781139165495

Friedman, B. H., & Thayer, J. F. (1998). Autonomic balance revisited: Panic anxiety and heart rate variability. *Journal of Psychosomatic Research, 44*(1), 133–151. doi:10.1016/S0022-3999(97)00202-X PMID:9483470

Frohlich, H. (2003). Feature selection for support vector machines by means of genetic algorithm. In *15th IEEE International Conf. on Tools with Artificial Intelligence.* doi:10.1109/TAI.2003.1250182

Fugate, M., & Gattiker, J. R. (2002). Anomaly Detection Enhanced Classification in Computer Intrusion Detection. In *Pattern Recognition with Support Vector Machines, First International Workshop* (LNCS), (vol. 2388, pp. 186-197). Springer. doi:10.1007/3-540-45665-1_15

Fung, G. P. C., Yu, J. X., Yu, P., & Lu, H. (2005). Parameter Free Bursty Events Detection in Text Streams. In *Proceeding of 31st int. conf. VLDB.*

Fung, B., Wang, K., & Ester, M. (2003). Hierarchical Document Clustering using Frequent Itemsets. In *Proc. of SIAM Intl. Conf. on Data Mining.*

Fussenegger, M., Roth, P., Bischof, H., Deriche, R., & Pinz, A. (2009). A level set framework using a new incremental, robust Active Shape Model for object segmentation and tracking. *Image and Vision Computing, 27*(8), 1157–1168. doi:10.1016/j.imavis.2008.10.014

Gaizauskas, R., Wakao, T., Humphreys, K., Cunningham, H., & Wilks, Y. (1996).Description of the lasie system as used for muc-6. In *Proceedings of the Sixth Message Understanding Conference* (MUC-6).

Gao, Y., Kikinis, R., Bouix, S., Shenton, M., & Tannenbaum, A. (2012). A 3D interactive multi-object segmentation tool using local robust statistics driven active contours. *Medical Image Analysis*, *6*(6), 1216–1227. doi:10.1016/j.media.2012.06.002 PMID:22831773

Gau, W.-L., & Buehrer, D. J. (1993). *Vague Sets*. IEEE.

Gehan, A., LaBean, T., & Reif, J. (2000). DNA Based Cryptography. *DIMACS Series in Discrete Mathematics and Theoretical Computer Science.*, *54*, 233–249.

Genesereth, M. (1991). Knowledge Interchange Format. *Proceedings of the Second International Conference on the Principles of Knowledge Representation and Reasoning* (KR-91). Morgan Kaufman Publishers.

Gennari, J. H., Langley, P., & Fisher, D. (1989). Models of incremental concept formation. Journal of Artificial Intelligence, 40, 11–61.

Gennari, J. H., Musen, M. A., Fergerson, R. W., Grosso, W. E., Crubzy, M., Eriksson, H., & Tu, S. W. et al. (2002). The evolution of Protege: An Environment for Knowledgebased Systems Development. *International Journal of Human-Computer Studies*, *58*(1), 89–123. doi:10.1016/S1071-5819(02)00127-1

Gervais, R., Leclercq, C., Shankar, A., Jacobs, S., Eiskjaer, H., Johannessen, A., & Daubert, C. et al. (2009). Surface electrocardiogram to predict outcome in candidates for cardiac resynchronization therapy: A sub-analysis of the CARE-HF trial. *European Journal of Heart Failure*, *11*(7), 699–705. doi:10.1093/eurjhf/hfp074 PMID:19505883

Ghezelbash. (2012). Predicting Changes in Stock Index and Gold Prices to Neural Network Approach. *The Journal of Mathematics and Computer Science, 4*(2), 227 – 236.

Ghosh, S., Biswas, S., Sarkar, D., & Sarkar, P. P. (2010). Mining Frequent Itemsets Using Genetic Algorithm. *International Journal of Artificial Intelligence & Applications*, *1*(4).

Gibson, D., Kleinberg, J., & Raghavan, P. (1998). Clustering Categorical Data. An Approach Based on Dynamical Systems. In *Proc. of 24th Int. conf.VLDB Conference.*

Gilbert & Lynch. (2002). *Brewer's conjecture and the feasibility of consistent, available, partition-tolerant web services.* SigAct News.

Girolami, M., & Kaban, A. (2003). On the Equivalence between PLSI and LDA. *SIGIR Conference.* doi:10.1145/860435.860537

Goerge, M. A. (1995). Wordnet: A Lexical Database for English. *Communications of the ACM*, *38*(11), 39–41. doi:10.1145/219717.219748

Goldberger, J. J. (1999). Sympathovagal balance: How should we measure it? *American Journal of Physiology. Heart and Circulatory Physiology*, *276*(4), H1273–H1280. PMID:10199852

Goodall, D. W. (1966). A new similarity index based on probability. *Biometrics*, *22*(4), 882–907. doi:10.2307/2528080

Good, M., Anderson, G. C., Ahn, S., Cong, X., & Stanton-Hicks, M. (2005). Relaxation and music reduce pain following intestinal surgery. *Research in Nursing & Health*, *28*(3), 240–251. doi:10.1002/nur.20076 PMID:15884029

Gottfrid, D. (2007). *Self-service, Prorated Super Computing Fun!* Retrieved from: http://open.blogs.nytimes.com/2007/11/01/self-service-prorated-super-computing-fun/

Grobelnik, M., & Mladenic, D. (2002). Efficient visualization of large text corpora. In *Proceedings of the 17th TELRI seminar.*

Gruber T. R. (1993). A Translation Approach to Portable Ontology Specifications. *Knowledge Acquisition, 5*, 199–220.

Gruber, T. R. (1993). A Translation Approach to Portable Ontology Specifications. *Knowledge Acquisition, 5*, 199–220.

Gruber, T. R. (1995). Towards principles for the design of ontologies used for knowledge sharing. *International Journal of Human-Computer Studies, 43*(5-6), 907–928. doi:10.1006/ijhc.1995.1081

Guha, S., Rastogi, R., & Shim, K. (1998). CURE: An Efficient Clustering Algorithm for Large Databases. *ACM SIGMOD Conference*. doi:10.1145/276304.276312

Guha, S., Rastogi, R., & Shim, K. (1999). ROCK a robust clustering algorithm for categorical attributes. In *15th International Conference on Data Engineering*. doi:10.1109/ICDE.1999.754967

Gupta, & Nath. (2010). Layered Approach Using Conditional Random Fields for Intrusion Detection. *IEEE Transactions on Dependable and Secure Computing, 7*(1).

Gupta, K. K., Nath, B., & Kotagiri, R. (2007). Conditional Random Fields for Intrusion Detection. *Proc. 21st Int'l Conf. Advanced Information Networking and Applications Workshops (AINAW '07)*. doi:10.1109/AINAW.2007.126

Gupta, S. C., & Kapoor, V. K. (2000). *Fundamentals of Mathematical Statistics* (10th ed.). New Delhi, India: Sultan Chand and Sons.

Hadavandi, E., Shavandi, H., & Ghanbari, A. (2010). Integration of Genetic Fuzzy Systems and Artificial Neural Networks for Stock Price Forecasting. *Knowledge-Based Systems, 23*(8), 800–808. doi:10.1016/j.knosys.2010.05.004

Hahn, U., & Schulz, S. (2000). Towards Very Large Terminological Knowledge Bases: A Case Study from Medicine. In *Canadian Conference on AI 2000*. doi:10.1007/3-540-45486-1_15

Haldulakar & Agrawal. (2011). Optimization of Association Rule Mining through Genetic Algorithm. *International Journal on Computer Science and Engineering, 3*(3), 1252–1259.

Hale, R. (2005). Text mining: Getting more value from literature resources. *Drug Discovery Today, 10*(6), 377–379. doi:10.1016/S1359-6446(05)03409-4 PMID:15808812

Hall, J. E. (2010). *Guyton and Hall textbook of medical physiology*. Elsevier Health Sciences.

Han & Kamber. (2001). *Data Mining: Concepts and techniques*. Morgan Kaufmann Publishers.

Han, J., Haihong, E., Le, G., & Du, J. (2011). Survey on NoSQL database. *Pervasive Computing and Applications (ICPCA). 2011 6th International Conference*.

Han, J., & Kamber, M. (2006). *Data Mining: Concepts and Techniques* (2nd ed.). San Francisco, CA: Morgan Kaufmann.

Han, J., Kamber, M., & Pei, J. (2001). *Data mining: concepts and techniques*. New York: Elsevier.

Han, J., Pei, I., Yin, Y., & Mao, R. (2004). Mining frequent patterns without candidate generation: A frequent pattern tree approach. *Data Mining and Knowledge Discovery, 8*(1), 53–87. doi:10.1023/B:DAMI.0000005258.31418.83

Harland, C., Clark, T., Peters, N., Everitt, M. J., & Stiffell, P. (2005). A compact electric potential sensor array for the acquisition and reconstruction of the 7-lead electrocardiogram without electrical charge contact with the skin. *Physiological Measurement, 26*(6), 939–950. doi:10.1088/0967-3334/26/6/005 PMID:16311443

Harrell, F. E. (2013). *Regression modeling strategies: with applications to linear models, logistic regression, and survival analysis*. Springer Science & Business Media.

Haun, M., Mainous, R. O., & Looney, S. W. (2001). Effect of music on anxiety of women awaiting breast biopsy. *Behavioral Medicine (Washington, D.C.), 27*(3), 127–132. doi:10.1080/08964280109595779 PMID:11985186

Hearst, M. A. (1998, May). Automated discovery of wordnet relations. In WordNet: An Electronic Lexical Database. MIT Press.

Hebb, D. O. (1949). *The Organization of Behavior: A Neuropsychological Theory*. New York: Wiley.

He, H., & Tan, Y. (2012). A two-stage genetic algorithm for automatic clustering. *Neurocomputing, 81*, 49–59.

Hejjel, L., & Gal, I. (2001). Heart rate variability analysis. *Acta Physiologica Hungarica, 88*(3-4), 219–230. doi:10.1556/APhysiol.88.2001.3-4.4 PMID:12162580

Hellman. (2002). An Overview of Public Key Cryptography. IEEE Communication Magazine, 16(6), 24-32.

He, Q., Chang, K., Lim, E.-P., & Zhang, J. (2007). Bursty feature representation for clustering text streams.*SDM Conference*. doi:10.1137/1.9781611972771.50

Herodotou, H., Lim, H., Luo, G., Borisov, N., & Dong, L. (2014). Starfish: a self-tuning system for big data analytics. *The Biennial Conference on Innovative Data Systems Research*.

Hill, P., Canagarajah, N., & Bull, D. (2002). *Image Fusion using Complex Wavelets*. BMVC-2002.

Hill, P., Canagarajah, N., & Bull, D. (2005). Image Fusion Using A New Framework For Complex Wavelet Transform. IEEE.

Hinal, M. M., & Chavan, P. V. (2015). Fuzzy Logic Based Image Encryption For Confidential Data Transfer Using (2, 2) Secret Sharing Scheme. *International Conference on Advances in Computer Engineering and Applications*. ICACEA.

Hirji, K. K. (2001). Exploring Data Mining Implementation. *Communications of the ACM, 44*(7), 87–93. doi:10.1145/379300.379323

Hobbs, R., Appelt, D., Bear, J., Israel, D., Kameyama, M., Stickel, M., & Tyson, M. (1997). *FASTUS: A cascaded finite-state transducer for extraction information from natural language text.*In E. Roche & Y. Schabes (Eds.), *Finite States Devices for Natural Language Processing* (pp. 383–406).

Hofmann, T. (1999). Probabilistic Latent Semantic Indexing. In *Proc. of 22nd Int. conf. On Research development in information retrieval ACM SIGIR Conference*.

Hong, T.-P., Horng, C.-Y., Wu, C.-H., & Wang, S.-L. (2009). An Improved Data Mining Approach Using Predictive Item sets. *Expert Systems with Applications, 36*(1), 72–80. doi:10.1016/j.eswa.2007.09.009

Horrocks, I., & van Harmelen, F. (2001). *Reference Description of the DAMLOIL Ontology Markup Language*. Technical report. Retrieved from http://www.daml.org/2001/03/reference.html

Horrocks, I., Fensel, D., Harmelen, F., Decker, S., Erdmann, M., & Klein, M. (2000). OIL in a Nutshell. In *ECAI'00 Workshop on Application of Ontologies and PSMs*.

Hotho, A., Staab, S., & Stumme, G. (2003). Wordnet improves text document clustering. In SIGIR international conference on Semantic Web Workshop.

Hsu, C. C. (2006). Generalizing self-organizing map for categorical data. *Neural Networks. IEEE Transactions on, 17*(2), 294–304.

Hsu, C. C., & Huang, Y. P. (2008). Incremental clustering of mixed data based on distance hierarchy. *Expert Systems with Applications, 35*(3), 1177–1185. doi:10.1016/j.eswa.2007.08.049

Hsu, C. C., Lin, S. H., & Tai, W. S. (2011). Apply extended self-organizing map to cluster and classify mixed-type data. *Neurocomputing, 74*(18), 3832–3842. doi:10.1016/j.neucom.2011.07.014

Hu, C., Yu, Q., Li, Y., & Ma, S. (2000). *Extraction of Parametric Human model for posture recognition using Genetic Algorithm*. 4th IEEE international conference on automatic face and gesture recognition, Grenoble, France.

Huang, G., & Pun, C. (2015). Robust Interactive Segmentation Using Color Histogram and Contourlet Transform. *IJCTE, 7*(6), 489–494. doi:10.7763/IJCTE.2015.V7.1007

Huang, Z. (1997, February). Clustering large data sets with mixed numeric and categorical values. In *Proceedings of the 1st Pacific-Asia Conference on Knowledge Discovery and Data Mining,(PAKDD)* (pp. 21-34).

Huang, Z. (1997, May). A Fast Clustering Algorithm to Cluster Very Large Categorical Data Sets in Data Mining. In DMKD.

Huang, Z., & Ng, M. K. (1999). A fuzzy k-modes algorithm for clustering categorical data. Fuzzy Systems. *IEEE Transactions on, 7*(4), 446–452.

Hurst, J. W. (1998). Naming of the waves in the ECG, with a brief account of their genesis. *Circulation, 98*(18), 1937–1942. doi:10.1161/01.CIR.98.18.1937 PMID:9799216

Hu, W., Liao, Y., & Rao Vemuri, V. (2003). Robust Support Vector Machines for Anomaly Detection in Computer Security. In *Proceedings of 2003 International Conference on Machine Learning and Applications*.

Indira, K., & Kanmani, S. (2012). Performance Analysis of Genetic Algorithm for Mining Association Rules. *International Journal of Computer Science Issues, 9*(2).

Irbil, A. M., Moh'd, A., & Khan, Z. (2011). *A Semi-Automated Approach To Transforming Database Schemas Into Ontology Language*. IEEE.

Jain, A. K., Mao, J., & Mohiuddin, K. (1996). Artificial neural networks: A tutorial. *Computer, 29*(3), 31–44. doi:10.1109/2.485891

Jain, A. K., Murty, M. N., & Flynn, P. J. (1999). Data Clustering: A Review. *ACM Computing Surveys, 31*(3), 264–323. doi:10.1145/331499.331504

Jajoo, P. (2008). *Document Clustering*. (Masters' Thesis). IIT Kharagpur.

Jardine, N., & van Rijsbergen, C. J. (1971). The use of hierarchical clustering in information retrieval. *Information Storage and Retrieval, 7*(5), 217–240. doi:10.1016/0020-0271(71)90051-9

Ji, X., & Xu, W. (2006). Document clustering with prior knowledge. In *Proc. of ACM SIGIR 29th int. conf. On research development on information retrieval*.

Jia, M., Yang, B., Zheng, D., Sun, W., Liu, L., & Yang, J. (2009). Automatic Ontology Construction Approaches and Its Application on Military Intelligence. *Asia-Pacific Conference on Information Processing* (APCIP).

Jiang, G., & Lin, Y. (2010). Skin color segmentation algorithm combining adaptive model and fixed model. *Journal Of Computer Applications, 30*(10), 2698–2701. doi:10.3724/SP.J.1087.2010.02698

Jiang, X., & Tan, A. H. (2005). Mining Ontological Knowledge from Domain-Specific Text Documents. *Proceedings of the Fifth IEEE International Conference on Data Mining*. IEEE. doi:10.1109/ICDM.2005.97

Ji, C., & Ma, S. (1997). Combinations of Weak Classifiers. *IEEE Transactions on Neural Networks, 8*(1), 32–42. doi:10.1109/72.554189 PMID:18255608

Jie, S., & Hui, L. (2008). Data Mining Method for Listed Companies Financial Distress Prediction. *Knowledge-Based-SystemsJournal, 21*(1), 1–5.

Ji, J., Pang, W., Zhou, C., Han, X., & Wang, Z. (2012). A fuzzy k-prototype clustering algorithm for mixed numeric and categorical data. *Knowledge-Based Systems, 30*, 129–135. doi:10.1016/j.knosys.2012.01.006

Jones, R., Ghani, R., Mitchell, T., & Riloff, E. (2003).Active learning for information extraction with multiple view feature sets. *Conference on Machine Learning (ICML 2003).*

Joseph, A. A., Lehmanny, C. U., Green, M. D., Pagano, M. W., Zachary, N. J. P., & Rubin, A. D. (2010). *Self-Protecting Electronic Medical Records Using Attribute-Based Encryption.* Retrieved from: https://eprint.iacr.org/2010/565.pdf

Josh, B., Melissa, C., Horvitz, E., & Lauter, K. (n.d.). *Patient Controlled Encryption: Ensuring Privacy of Electronic Medical Records.* Microsoft Research.

Jung, Y., Kang, M., & Heo, J. (2014). Clustering performance comparison using K -means and expectation maximization algorithms. *Biotechnology & Biotechnological Equipment, 28*(sup1), S44-S48.10.1080/13102818.2014.949045

Juslin, P. N., & Sloboda, J. A. (2001). *Music and emotion: Theory and research.* Oxford University Press.

Kaisler, S., & Armour, F., Espinosa, & Money. (2013). Big data: issues and challenges moving forward. *IEEE,46th Hawaii International Conference on System Sciences.*

Kambatla, K., Kollias, G., Kumar, V., & Grama, A. (2014). Trends in big data analytics. *Journal of Parallel and Distributed Computing, 74*(7), 2561–2573. doi:10.1016/j.jpdc.2014.01.003

Kamley, S., & Jaloree, S. (2014). Stock Market Behavior Prediction Using NN based Model. *British Journal of Mathematics and Computer Science, 4*(17), 2502–2515. doi:10.9734/BJMCS/2014/9819

Kamley, S., & Jaloree, S., & Thakur, R.S. (2015). Rule Based Approach for Stock Selection: An Expert System. *International Journal of Computing Algorithm, 4*(Special Issue), 1142–1146.

Kanhaiya & Mohanti. (2011). Role of soft computing as a tool in data mining. *International Journal of Computer Science and Information Technologies, 2*(1), 526–537.

Karanikas, H., Tjortjis, C., & Theodoulidis, B. (2000). An approach to text mining using information extraction. In *Proceedings of Workshop of Knowledge Management: Theory and Applications in Principles of Data Mining and Knowledge Discovery 4th European Conference.*

Karasulu, B. (2013). An approach based on simulated annealing to optimize the performance of extraction of the flower region using mean-shift segmentation. *Applied Soft Computing, 13*(12), 4763–4785. doi:10.1016/j.asoc.2013.07.019

Karp, R., Chaudhri, V., & Thomere, J. (1999). *XOL: An XML-Based Ontology Exchange Language.* Technical Report. Retrieved from http://www.ai.sri.com/pkarp/xol/xol.html

Kashyap, S. K. (2015). *IR and Color Image Fusion Using Interval Type 2 Fuzzy Logic System.* IEEE. doi:10.1109/CCIP.2015.7100732

Kass, M., Witkin, A., & Terzopoulos, D. (1988). Snakes: Active contour models. *International Journal of Computer Vision, 1*(4), 321–331. doi:10.1007/BF00133570

Katal, A., Wazid, M., & Goudar, R. H. (2013). Big data: issues, challenges, tools and good practices. *Contemporary Computing (IC3), 2013 Sixth International Conference.*

Kaufman, L., & Rousseeuw, P. J. (1990). *Finding Groups in Data: An Introduction to Cluster Analysis*. Wiley Interscience. doi:10.1002/9780470316801

Kaufman, L., & Rousseeuw, P. J. (2009). *Finding groups in data: an introduction to cluster analysis* (Vol. 344). John Wiley & Sons.

Kavitha, C. T., & Chellamuthu, C. (2010). *Multimodal Medical Image Fusion Based on Integer Wavelet Transform and Neuro-Fuzzy*. IEEE.

Kawashima, T. (2005). The autonomic nervous system of the human heart with special reference to its origin, course, and peripheral distribution. *Anatomy and Embryology*, *209*(6), 425–438. doi:10.1007/s00429-005-0462-1 PMID:15887046

Ke, W., Sugimoto, C., & Mostafa, J. (2009) Dynamicity vs. effectiveness: studying online clustering for scatter/gather. *ACM SIGIR Conference, 2009.A Survey of Text Clustering Algorithms 125*. doi:10.1145/1571941.1571947

Kiernan, J., & Rajakumar, R. (2013). *Barr's the human nervous system: an anatomical viewpoint*. Lippincott Williams & Wilkins.

Kietz, J. U., Maedche, A., & Volz, R. (2000). A Method for Semi-Automatic Ontology Acquisition from a Corporate Intranet. In N. Aussenac-Gilles, B. Biebow, & S. Szulman (Eds.), *EKAW'00 Workshop on Ontologies and Texts*. Juan-Les-Pins, France: CEUR. Available: http://CEURWS.org/Vol-51

Kietz, J. U., Maedche, A., & Volz, R. (2001). A Method for Semi-Automatic Ontology Acquisition from a Corporate Intranet. In N. Aussenac-Gilles, B. Biebow, & S. Szulman (Eds.), *EKAW'00 Workshop on Ontologies and Texts*. Juan-Les-Pins, France: CEUR. Available: http://CEURWS.org/Vol-51

Kifer, M., Lausen, G., & Wu, J. (1995). Logical foundations of object-oriented and frame-based languages. *Journal of the ACM*, *42*(4), 741–843. doi:10.1145/210332.210335

Kim, D. S., & Park, J. S. (2003). Network-based Intrusion Detectio with Support Vector Machines. In *Information Networking, Networking Technologies for Enhanced Internet Services International Conference* (ICOIN 2003), (LNCS), (vol. 2662, pp. 747-756). Springer.

Kim, D., & Park, J. (2005). Connectivity-based local adaptive thresholding for carotid artery segmentation using MRA images. *Image and Vision Computing*, *23*(14), 1277–1287. doi:10.1016/j.imavis.2005.09.005

Kim, H., & Lee, S. (2000). A Semi-supervised document clustering technique for information organization. *CIKM Conference*. doi:10.1145/354756.354777

Kleiger, R. E., Stein, P. K., & Bigger, J. T. (2005). Heart rate variability: Measurement and clinical utility. *Annals of Noninvasive Electrocardiology*, *10*(1), 88–101. doi:10.1111/j.1542-474X.2005.10101.x PMID:15649244

Kleinberg, J. (2002).Bursty and hierarchical structure in streams. In *Proc. of Int conf.ACMKDD Conference*.

Knight, K., & Luk, S. K. (1994). Building a Large Knowledge Base for Machine Translation. *Proceedings of the American Association of Artificial Intelligence Conference*.

Kocher, M., & Leonardi, R. (1986). Adaptive region growing technique using polynomial functions for image approximation. *Signal Processing*, *11*(1), 47–60. doi:10.1016/0165-1684(86)90094-0

Koelsch, S. (2009). A neuroscientific perspective on music therapy. *Annals of the New York Academy of Sciences*, *1169*(1), 374–384. doi:10.1111/j.1749-6632.2009.04592.x PMID:19673812

Kong, H., Hwang, M., & Kim, P. (2006). Design of the automatic ontology building system about the specific domain knowledge. *8th International Conference on Advanced Com-munication Technology (ICACT)*.

Kosztyła-Hojna B., Moskal, D., Kuryliszyn-Moskal, A., & Rutkowski, R. (2013). The innovative method of visualization of vocal folds vibrations in the chosen cases of occupational dysphonia. *Otorynolaryngologia - Przegląd Kliniczny*, 23-28.

Kosztyła-Hojna, B. (2013). Ocena przydatności metody szybkiego filmu highspeed imaging (HSI) w diagnostyce zaburzeń jakości głosu. *Annals of the Rheumatic Diseases*, *72*(suppl. 3), 837–840. doi:10.1136/annrheumdis-2013-eular.2491

Kosztyła-Hojna, B. et al.. (2007). Usefulness of some diagnostic methods in differential diagnosis of occupational voice disorders. *Polish Journal of Environmental Studies*, *16*(no 1A), 23–29.

Labbé, E., Schmidt, N., Babin, J., & Pharr, M. (2007). Coping with stress: The effectiveness of different types of music. *Applied Psychophysiology and Biofeedback*, *32*(3-4), 163–168. doi:10.1007/s10484-007-9043-9 PMID:17965934

Lakhina, Joseph, & Verma. (2010). Feature Reduction using Principal Component Analysis for Effective Anomaly-Based Intrusion Detection on NSL-KDD. *International Journal of Engineering Science and Technology, 2*(6), 1790-1799.

Langley. (1994). Selection of Relevant Features in Machine Learning. *Proc. AAAI Fall Symp. Relevance.*

Lankton, S., & Tannenbaum, A. (2008). Localizing Region-Based Active Contours. *IEEE Transactions on Image Processing*, *17*(11), 2029–2039. doi:10.1109/TIP.2008.2004611 PMID:18854247

Larson, M. G. (2008). Analysis of variance. *Circulation*, *117*(1), 115–121. doi:10.1161/CIRCULATIONAHA.107.654335 PMID:18172051

Lassila, O., & Swick, R. (1999). *Resource description framework (RDF) model and syntax specification, W3C Recommendation*. Retrieved from: http://www.w3.org/TR/REC-rdf-syntax/

Lee, W., & Stolfo, S. J. (1998). Data Mining Approaches for Intrusion Detection. In *Proc. of the 7th USENIX Security Symp.*

Lee, W., Stolfo, & Mok. (1998). Mining audit data to build intrusion detection models. In *Proceedings of the Fourth International Conference on Knowledge Discovery and Data Mining* (KDD '98).

Lee, D. D., & Seung, H. S. (1999). Learning the parts of objects by non negative matrix factorization. *Nature*, *401*(6755), 788–791. doi:10.1038/44565 PMID:10548103

Lee, P.-C., Chen, S.-A., & Hwang, B. (2009). Atrioventricular node anatomy and physiology: Implications for ablation of atrioventricular nodal reentrant tachycardia. *Current Opinion in Cardiology*, *24*(2), 105–112. doi:10.1097/HCO.0b013e328323d83f PMID:19225293

Lee, W., & Stolfo, S. J. (1998). Data Mining Approaches for Intrusion Detection. In *Proc. of the 7th USENIX Security Symp.*

Lee, W., Stolfo, S., & Mok, K. W. (2000). Adaptive Intrusion Detection: A Data Mining Approach. *Artificial Intelligence Review, Kluwer Academic Publishers*, *14*(6), 533–567. doi:10.1023/A:1006624031083

Legendre, P., & Legendre, L. (1998). *Numerical Ecology* (2nd ed.). Academic Press.

Lemon, S. C., Roy, J., Clark, M. A., Friedmann, P. D., & Rakowski, W. (2003). Classification and regression tree analysis in public health: Methodological review and comparison with logistic regression. *Annals of Behavioral Medicine*, *26*(3), 172–181. doi:10.1207/S15324796ABM2603_02 PMID:14644693

Lenat, D. B., & Guha, R. V. (1990). *Building Large Knowledge-Based Systems: Representation and Inference in the Cyc Project*. Boston: Addison-Wesley.

Levene, M., & Poulovassilis, A. (2004). *Adapting to Change in Content,Size, Topology and Use* (W. Dynamics, Ed.). Springer.

Lewis, R. J. (2000). *An introduction to classification and regression tree (CART) analysis.* Paper presented at the Annual Meeting of the Society for Academic Emergency Medicine, San Francisco, CA.

Li, Guan, & Zan. (2003). Network intrusion detection based on support vector machine. *Journal of Computer Research and Development, 6,* 800-807.

Li, T., Ma, S., & Ogihara, M. (2004). Document Clustering via Adaptive Subspace Iteration. In *Proc. Of 27th Int. conf. ACM SIGIR Conference.*

Li, C., & Biswas, G. (2002). Unsupervised learning with mixed numeric and nominal data. *Knowledge and Data Engineering. IEEE Transactions on, 14*(4), 673–690.

Licai, Y., Xin, L., & Yucui, Y. (2008). *Medical Image Fusion Based on Wavelet Packet Transform and Self-adaptive Operator.* IEEE.

Ligia, C., & Vaida, M. F. (2009). Medical Image Fusion Based on Discrete Wavelet Transform Using Java Technology. *Proceedings of the ITI 2009 31st Int.Conf. on Information Technology Interfaces.*

Liritano, S., & Ruffolo, M. (2001). Managing the Knowledge Contained in Electronic Documents: a Clustering Method for Text Mining. IEEE.

Li, T., Ding, C., & Zhang, Y. (2008). Knowledge transformation from word space to document space.*ACM SIGIR Conference.*

Liu, F., Liu, J., & Gao, Y. (2007). Image Fusion Based On Wedgelet And Wavelet.*Proceedings of 2007 International Symposium on Intelligent Signal Processing and Communication Systems.* IEEE.

Liu, H., & Motoda, H. (Eds.). (2001). *Feature Extraction, Construction and Selection a Data Mining Perspective.* Kluwer Academic.

Liu, S., & Peng, Y. (2012). A local region-based Chanâ€"Vese model for image segmentation. *Pattern Recognition, 45*(7), 2769–2779. doi:10.1016/j.patcog.2011.11.019

Liu, T., Lin, S., Chen, Z., & Ma, W.-Y. (2003). An Evaluation on Feature Selection for Text Clustering. *ICML Conference.*

Liu, Y.-B., Cai, J.-R., Yin, J., & Fu, A. W.-C. (2008). Clustering Text Data Streams. *Journal of Computer Science and Technology, 23*(1), 112–128. doi:10.1007/s11390-008-9115-1

Liu, Y., & Yang, J. (2010). *PET/CT Medical Image Fusion Algorithm Based on Multiwavelet Transform.* IEEE.

Li, Y., Luo, S., & Zou, Q. (2010). Active Contour Model Based on Salient Boundary Point Image for Object Contour Detection in Natural Image. *IEICE Transactions on Information and Systems, E93-D*(11), 3136–3139. doi:10.1587/transinf.E93.D.3136

Li, Z., & Weng, G. (2011). Segmentation of cDNA Microarray Image Using Fuzzy c-Mean Algorithm and Mathematical Morphology. *KEM, 464,* 159–162. doi:10.4028/www.scientific.net/KEM.464.159

Lu, A., Ke, Y., Cheng, J., & Ng, W. (2007). Mining Hesitation Information by Vague Association Rules. In ER 2007 (LNCS), (vol. 4801, pp. 39–55). Springer-Verlag Berlin Heidelberg.

Lu, A., Ke, Y., Cheng, J., & Ng, W. (2007). *Mining Vague Association Rules.* Springer. doi:10.1007/978-3-540-71703-4_75

Lu, A., & Ng, W. (2004). *Managing Merged Data by Vague Functional Dependencies.* Springer. doi:10.1007/978-3-540-30464-7_21

Lu, A., & Ng, W. (2005). *Vague Sets or Intuitionistic Fuzzy Sets for Handling Vague Data- Which One Is Better?* Springer. doi:10.1007/11568322_26

Lu, A., & Ng, W. (2007). *Handling Inconsistency of Vague Relations with Functional Dependencies. In Conceptual Modeling - ER 2007 (LNCS),* (Vol. 4801, pp. 229–244). Springer.

Lu, Y., Ma, T., Yin, C., Xie, X., Tian, W., & Zhong, S. (2013). Implementation of the Fuzzy C-Means Clustering Algorithm in Meteorological Data. *International Journal of Database Theory and Application, 6*(6), 1–18. doi:10.14257/ijdta.2013.6.6.01

Lu, Y., Mei, Q., & Zhai, C. (2011). Investigating task performance of probabilistic topic models: An empirical study of PLSA and LDA. *Information Retrieval, 14*(2), 178–203. doi:10.1007/s10791-010-9141-9

MacGregor, R. (1991). Inside the LOOM classifier. *SIGART Bulletin, 2*(3), 70-76.

Maciejewski, M., Surtel, W., Maciejewska, B., & Małecka-Massalska, T. (2015). Level-set image processing methods in medical image segmentation. *Bio-Algorithms And Med-Systems, 11*(1). doi:10.1515/bams-2014-0017

MacQueen, J. (1967, June). Some methods for classification and analysis of multivariate observations. In *Proceedings of the fifth Berkeley symposium on mathematical statistics and probability.*

Maedche, A. & Staab, S. (2001). *Ontology Learning for the Semantic Web.* IEEE.

Maedche, A., & Staab, S. (2001). *Ontology Learning for the Semantic Web.* IEEE.

Maedche, A., & Staab, S. S. (2000). Semi-automatic engineering of ontologies from text. In *12th International Conference on Software Engineering and Knowledge Engineering.*

Majewski, J., & Rosenblatt, D. (2012). Exome and whole-genome sequencing for gene discovery: The future is now! *Human Mutation, 33*(4), 591–592. doi:10.1002/humu.22055 PMID:22411407

Malik, H. H., & Kender, J. R. (2006). High Quality, Efficient Hierarchical Document Clustering Using Closed Interesting Itemsets. In *Proc. of IEEE Intl. Conf. on Data Mining.*

Manning, C. D., Raghavan, P., & Schütze, H. (2008). *Introduction to information retrieval* (Vol. 1). Cambridge, UK: Cambridge University Press. doi:10.1017/CBO9780511809071

Manyika, J., Chui, M., Brown, B., Bughin, J., Dobbs, R., Roxburgh, C., & Byers, A. H. (2011). *Big data: The next frontier for innovation, competition, and productivity.* McKinsey Global Institute. Retrieved from: http://www.mckinsey.com/insights/business_technology/big_data_the_next_frontier_for_innovation

Martínez-Lavín, M., & Hermosillo, A. G. (2000). *Autonomic nervous system dysfunction may explain the multisystem features of fibromyalgia.* Paper presented at the Seminars in arthritis and rheumatism. doi:10.1016/S0049-0172(00)80008-6

Martínez-Lavín, M., Hermosillo, A. G., Rosas, M., & Soto, M. E. (1998). Circadian studies of autonomic nervous balance in patients with fibromyalgia: A heart rate variability analysis. *Arthritis and Rheumatism, 41*(11), 1966–1971. doi:10.1002/1529-0131(199811)41:11<1966::AID-ART11>3.3.CO;2-F PMID:9811051

Martini, F. (2005). *Human anatomy.* San Francisco, CA: Pearson/Benjamin Cummings.

Masudianpour, A. (2013). *An Introduction to Redis Server, an Advanced Key Value Database.* SlideShare. Retrieved from: www.slideshare.net/masudianpour/redis-25088079

Maulik, U., & Bandyopadhyay, S. (2000). Genetic algorithm-based clustering technique. *Pattern Recognition, 33*(9), 1455–1465. doi:10.1016/S0031-3203(99)00137-5

Mau, T. (2010). Diagnostic evaluation and management of hoarseness. *The Medical Clinics of North America*, *94*(5), 945–960. doi:10.1016/j.mcna.2010.05.010

McCreadie, R., Macdonald, C., & Ounis, I. (2012). MapReduce indexing strategies: Studying scalability and efficiency. *Journal of Information Processing and Management: An International Journal, 48*(5), 873-888.

Mcculloch, W. S., & Pitts, W. H. (1943). A Logical Calculus of the Ideas Immanent in Nervous Activity. *Bull. Math. Biopsy, 5*(4), 115–133. doi:10.1007/BF02478259

McGuinness, D. L., Fikes, R., Hendler, J., & Stein, L. A. (2002). DAML + OIL: An Ontology Language for the Semantic Web. *IEEE Intelligent Systems, 17*(5), 72–80. doi:10.1109/MIS.2002.1039835

Mei, Q., Cai, D., Zhang, D., & Zhai, C.-X. (2008). Topic Modeling with Network Regularization. In *Proc. of 17th international conf.On WWW Conference.*

Metzger, L. K. (2004). Assessment of use of music by patients participating in cardiac rehabilitation. *Journal of Music Therapy, 41*(1), 55–69. doi:10.1093/jmt/41.1.55 PMID:15157124

Metzler, D., Dumais, S. T., & Meek, C. (2007). Similarity Measures for Short Segments of Text. *Proceedings of ECIR*. doi:10.1007/978-3-540-71496-5_5

Millan, M. J., Agid, Y., Brüne, M., Bullmore, E. T., Carter, C. S., Clayton, N. S., & Young, L. J. et al. (2012). Cognitive dysfunction in psychiatric disorders: Characteristics, causes and the quest for improved therapy. *Nature Reviews. Drug Discovery, 11*(2), 141–168. doi:10.1038/nrd3628 PMID:22293568

Ming, Z., Wang, K., & Chua, T.-S. (2010). Prototype hierarchy-based clustering for the categorization and navigation of web collections.*ACMSIGIR Conference*. doi:10.1145/1835449.1835453

Mitchell, M. (1996). *An Introduction to Genetic Algorithms*. PHI.

Mitchell, T. M. (1999). The role of unlabeled data in supervised learning.*Proceedings of the Sixth International Colloquium on Cognitive Science.*

Mizoguchi, R. (1995). *Tutorial on ontological engineering*. Academic Press.

Monfredi, O., Dobrzynski, H., Mondal, T., Boyett, M. R., & Morris, G. M. (2010). The anatomy and physiology of the sinoatrial node—a contemporary review. *Pacing and Clinical Electrophysiology, 33*(11), 1392–1406. doi:10.1111/j.1540-8159.2010.02838.x PMID:20946278

Motro, A. (1995). *Management of Uncertainty in Database Systems*. New York, NY: ACM Press/Addison-Wesley Publishing Co.

Mukkamala, S., Janoski, G., & Sung, A. H. (2002). Intrusion Detection Using Neural Networks and Support Vector Machines. In *Proceedings of IEEE International Joint Conference on Neural Networks*. IEEE Computer Society Press. doi:10.1109/IJCNN.2002.1007774

Murtagh, F. (1983). A Survey of Recent Advances in Hierarchical Clustering Algorithms. *The Computer Journal, 26*(4), 354–359. doi:10.1093/comjnl/26.4.354

Murtagh, F. (1984). Complexities of Hierarchical Clustering Algorithms: State of the Art. *Computational Statistics Quarterly, 1*(2), 101–113.

Muschold, M. (1996). Ontologies: principle, methods and application. *The Knowledge Engineering Review, 1*(2), 93-136.

Nadeem, A., & Javed, M. Y. (2005, Aug). A Performance comparison of data encryption algorithms. *IEEE-International Conference of Information and Communication Technologies.* doi:10.1109/ICICT.2005.1598556

Nahm, U., & Mooney, R. (2002). Text mining with information extraction. In *Proceedings of the AAAI 2002 Spring Symposium on Mining Answers from Texts and Knowledge Bases.*

Nandagopal, S., Arunachalam, V. P., & Karthik, S. (2012). A Novel Approach for Mining Inter-Transaction Itemsets. *European Scientific Journal, 8*, 14–22.

Narnaware, S., & Khedgaonkar, R. (2005). Image Enhancement using Artificial Neural Network and Fuzzy Logic. *IEEE Sponsored 2nd International Conference on Innovations in Information Embedded and Communication Systems ICIIECS'15.* IEEE. doi:10.1109/ICIIECS.2015.7193203

Navigli, R., Gangemi, A. & Velardi, P. (2003). *Ontology learning and its application.* Academic Press.

Navigli, R., Gangemi, A., & Velardi, P. (2003). *Ontology learning and its application.* Academic Press.

Nedellec, C., & Nazarenko, A. (2005). *Ontologies and information extraction: A necessary symbiosis. In Ontology Learning from Text: Methods, Evaluation and Applications.* IOS Press Publication.

Nguyen, H., Franke, K., & Petrovic, S. (2010). Improving Effectiveness of Intrusion Detection by Correlation Feature Selection. *2010 International Conference on Availability, Reliability and Security.* IEEE. doi:10.1109/ARES.2010.70

Nikolov, S. G., Bull, D. R., Canagarajah, C. N., Halliwell, M., & Wells, P. N. T. (1999). *Image Fusion Using A 3-D Wavelet Transform. Image Processing And Its Applications.* IEEE.

Niles, I., & Pease, A. (2001). Towards a Standard Upper Ontology.*Proceedings of the International Conference on Formal Ontology in Information Systems.*

Ning, K. (2009). A pseudo DNA cryptography Method. *CoRR.* Retrieved from http://arxiv.org/abs/0903.2693

Norcen, R., Podesser, M., Pommer, A., Schmidt, H. P., & Uhl, A. (2003). Confidential storage and transmission of medical image data. *Computers in Biology and Medicine, 33*(3), 273–292. doi:10.1016/S0010-4825(02)00094-X PMID:12726806

Noy, N.F., & McGuinness, D.L. (2000). *Ontology Development 101: A Guide to Creating Your First Ontology.* Academic Press.

NSL KDD Dataset. (n.d.). Available at http://nsl.cs.unb.ca/NSL-KDD/

Okin, P. M., Devereux, R. B., Howard, B. V., Fabsitz, R. R., Lee, E. T., & Welty, T. K. (2000). Assessment of QT interval and QT dispersion for prediction of all-cause and cardiovascular mortality in American Indians the Strong Heart Study. *Circulation, 101*(1), 61–66. doi:10.1161/01.CIR.101.1.61 PMID:10618305

Olatunji, S. O. (2013). Forecasting the Saudi Arabia Stock Prices based on Artificial Neural Networks Model. *International Journal of Intelligent Information Systems, 2*(5), 77–86. doi:10.11648/j.ijiis.20130205.12

Olshansky, B., Sabbah, H. N., Hauptman, P. J., & Colucci, W. S. (2008). Parasympathetic nervous system and heart failure pathophysiology and potential implications for therapy. *Circulation, 118*(8), 863–871. doi:10.1161/CIRCULA-TIONAHA.107.760405 PMID:18711023

Omelayenko, B. (2001). Learning of Ontologies for the web: the analysis of existent Approaches. In *Proceedings of the international Workshop on web Dynamics, held in conj. withthe 8th International Conference on Database theory* (ICDT'01).

Opthof, T., Coronel, R., Wilms-Schopman, F. J., Plotnikov, A. N., Shlapakova, I. N., Danilo, P. Jr, & Janse, M. J. et al. (2007). Dispersion of repolarization in canine ventricle and the electrocardiographic T wave: T pe interval does not reflect transmural dispersion. *Heart Rhythm*, *4*(3), 341–348. doi:10.1016/j.hrthm.2006.11.022 PMID:17341400

Oracle NoSQL Database. (2012). Oracle White Paper.

Ortiz, A., Gorriz, J., Ramirez, J., & Salas-Gonzalez, D. (2012). Unsupervised Neural Techniques Applied to MR Brain Image Segmentation. *Advances in Artificial Neural Systems*, *2012*, 1–7. doi:10.1155/2012/457590

Overview of Attack Trends. (2002). Retrieved from http://www.cert.org/archive/pdf/attack_trends.pdf

Palit, I., & Reddy, C. K. (2012). Scalable and parallel boosting with MapReduce. *IEEE Transactions on Knowledge and Data Engineering*, *24*(10), 1904–1916. doi:10.1109/TKDE.2011.208

Pandey, A., & Pardasani. (2012). A Model for Mining Course Information using Vague Association Rule. *International Journal of Computer Applications*, *58*(20).

Pantel, P., & Lin, D. (2002). Document Clustering with Committees. In *Proc. of 25th int. conf.ACMSIGIR Conference*.

Parati, G., Saul, J. P., Di Rienzo, M., & Mancia, G. (1995). Spectral analysis of blood pressure and heart rate variability in evaluating cardiovascular regulation a critical appraisal. *Hypertension*, *25*(6), 1276–1286. doi:10.1161/01.HYP.25.6.1276 PMID:7768574

Park, J. S., Lee, J., Kim, D. S., & Chi, S.-D. (2002). Using Support Vector Ma-chine to Detect the Host based Intrusion. In *IRC International Conference on Internet Information Retrieval*.

Patel, D. K., & More, S. A. (2013). Edge Detection Technique by Fuzzy Logic and Cellular Learning Automata using Fuzzy Image Processing. *International Conference on Computer Communication and Informatics*. ICCCI. doi:10.1109/ICCCI.2013.6466130

Pawlak, Z. (1982). *Rough sets*. Elsevier Inc.

Pawlak, Z. (1991). Information systems - theoretical foundations. *Information Systems Journal*, *6*(3), 205–218. doi:10.1016/0306-4379(81)90023-5

Pawlak, Z., & Skowron, A. (2006). Rudiments of rough sets. *Information Sciences*, *177*.

Paxinos, G., & Mai, J. K. (2004). *The human nervous system*. Academic Press.

Peng, S.-M., Koo, M., & Yu, Z.-R. (2009). Effects of music and essential oil inhalation on cardiac autonomic balance in healthy individuals. *Journal of Alternative and Complementary Medicine (New York, N.Y.)*, *15*(1), 53–57. doi:10.1089/acm.2008.0243 PMID:19769477

Peter, I., Osakwe, C., Kayode, A.A., & Adagunodo, E.R. (2012). Prediction of Stock Market in Nigeria Using Artificial Neural Network. *International Journal of Intelligent Systems and Applications*, *11*, 68–74.

Petitjean, C., & Dacher, J. (2011). A review of segmentation methods in short axis cardiac MR images. *Medical Image Analysis*, *15*(2), 169–184. doi:10.1016/j.media.2010.12.004 PMID:21216179

Philip, M. T., Paul, K., Choy, S. O., Reggie, K., Ng, S. C., Mak, J., & Tak-Lam, W. et al. (2007). Design and Implementation of NN5 for Hong Stock Price Forecasting. *Journal of Engineering Applications of Artificial Intelligence*, *20*(4), 453–461. doi:10.1016/j.engappai.2006.10.002

Pillar Global. (n.d.). Retrieved from: http://www.3pillarglobal.com/insights/exploring-the-different-types-of-nosql-databases

Polikar, R. (1996). *The Wavelet Transform* (2nd ed.). Part I, Fundamental Concepts and An Overview of the Wavelet Theory.

Prajapat et al. (2012). A Novel Approach For Information Security With Automatic Variable Key Using Fibonacci Q-Matrix. *International Journal of Computer & Communication Technology, 3*(3).

Prajapat, & Thakur. (2013, Sep). *Recurrence relation approach for key prediction.* 18th International Conference of Gwalior Academy of Mathematical Science (GAMS), MANIT, Bhopal, India.

Prajapat, & Thakur. (2014a, Mar). Time variant key using exact differential equation model. *National Conference in Emerging Trends in cloud Computing and Digital Communication* (ETCDC-2014).

Prajapat, & Thakur. (2014b, Jun). *Sparse approach for realizing AVK for Symmetric Key Encryption.* Presented on second days, International Research Conference on Engineering, Science and Management (IRCESM 2014), Dubai, UAE.

Prajapat, & Thakur. (2014c, Oct). *Time variant key using Fuzzy differential equation model.* Oriental Bhopal, India.

Prajapat, & Thakur. (2014d, Oct). Association Rule Extraction in AVK based cryptosystem. *International Conferences on Intelligent Computing and Information System* (ICICIS-2014).

Prajapat, & Thakur. (2015a). Towards Optimum size of key for AVK based cryptosystem. Covenant Journal of Informatics and Communication Technology, 3(2).

Prajapat, & Thakur. (2015b, Jun). Markov Analysis of AVK Approach of Symmetric Key Based Cryptosystem. *LNCS, 9159*, 164-176.

Prajapat, Parmar, & Thakur. (2015). Investigation of Efficient Cryptosystem Using SGcrypter. *IJAER,* 853-858.

Prajapat, Rajput, & Thakur. (2013, Oct). Time variant approach towards Symmetric Key. *IEEE- Science and Information Conference 2013.*

Prajapat, S., & Thakur. (2015a). Optimal Key Size of the AVK for Symmetric Key Encryption. *Covenant Journal of Information & Communication Technology, 71.*

Prajapat, S., & Thakur. (2015b). Various Approaches towards Crypt-analysis. *International Journal of Computer Applications, 127*(14), 15-24.

Prajapat, S., & Thakur. (2016b). Realization of information exchange with Fibo-Q based Symmetric Cryptosystem. *International Journal of Computer Science and Information Security.*

Prajapat, S., & Thakur. (2016c). Cryptic Mining: Apriori Analysis of Parameterized Automatic Variable Key based Symmetric Cryptosystem. *International Journal of Computer Science and Information Security.*

Prajapat, Swami, Singroli, Thakur, Sharma, & Rajput. (2014). Sparse approach for realizing AVK for Symmetric Key Encryption. *International Journal of Recent Development in Engineering and Technology, 2*(4), 13-18.

Prajapat, S., & Thakur, R. S. (2016a). Cryptic Mining for Automatic Variable Key Based Cryptosystem. *Elsevier Procedia Computer Science, 78*(78C), 199–209. doi:10.1016/j.procs.2016.02.034

PratimAcharjya, P., & Ghoshal, D. (2012). A Modified Watershed Segmentation Algorithm using Distances Transform for Image Segmentation. *International Journal of Computers and Applications, 52*(12), 46–50. doi:10.5120/8258-1791

Pratondo, A., Chui, C., & Ong, S. (2016). Robust Edge-Stop Functions for Edge-Based Active Contour Models in Medical Image Segmentation. *IEEE Signal Processing Letters, 23*(2), 222–226. doi:10.1109/LSP.2015.2508039

Pujari, A. K. (2006). Data Mining Techniques (10th ed.). Hyderabad, India: Universites (India) Press Private Limited.

Pujari, A. K. (2001). *Data Mining Techniques*. University Press.

Qiang, Z., Xue, X., & Wei, X. (2012). A Novel Image Encryption Algorithm based on DNA Subsequence Operation. *TheScientificWorldJournal*.

Qi, G., Aggarwal, C., & Huang, T. (2012). Community Detection with Edge Content in Social Media works. *ICDE Conference*.

Qin, L., Rueda, L., Ali, A., & Ngom, A. (2005). Spot Detection and Image Segmentation in DNA??Microarray Data. *Applied Bioinformatics*, *4*(1), 1–11. doi:10.2165/00822942-200504010-00001 PMID:16000008

Racker, D. K., & Kadish, A. H. (2000). Proximal atrioventricular bundle, atrioventricular node, and distal atrioventricular bundle are distinct anatomic structures with unique histological characteristics and innervation. *Circulation*, *101*(9), 1049–1059. doi:10.1161/01.CIR.101.9.1049 PMID:10704174

Rahman, M. (2012). Unsupervised Natural Image Segmentation Using Mean Histogram Features. *Journal Of Multimedia*, *7*(5). doi:10.4304/jmm.7.5.332-340

Rajesh, , & Sulabha. (2012). Fragment Based Approach to Forecast Association Rules from Indian IT Stock Transaction Data. *International Journal of Computer Science and Information Technologies*, *3*(2), 3493–349.

Ramesh Kumar & Iyakutti. (2011). Genetic algorithms for the prioritization of Association Rules. *IJCA*, 35-38.

Ranamuka, N. G., Gayan, R., & Meegama, N. (2013). Detection of hard exudates from diabetic retinopathy images using fuzzy logic. IET.

Rao, R. (2003). From unstructured data to actionable intelligence. In *Proceedings of the IEEE Computer Society*.

Ras, Z., & Dardzinska, A. (2006). Action rules discovery, a new simplified strategy. *Foundations of Intelligent Systems, Proceedings of ISMIS'06 Symposium* (LNAI) (vol. 4203, pp. 445-453). Springer.

Ras, Z., & Dardzinska, A. (2008). Action rules discovery without pre-existing classification rules. *Proceedings of the International Conference on Rough Sets and Current Trends in Computing* (LNAI), (vol. 5306, pp. 181-190). Springer.

Ras, Z., & Wieczorkowska, A. (2000). Action-Rules: How to increase profit of a company. *Proceedings of PKDD 2000* (LNAI), (vol. 1910, pp. 587-592). Springer.

Ravits, J. M. (1997). AAEM minimonograph# 48: Autonomic nervous system testing. *Muscle & Nerve*, *20*(8), 919–937. doi:10.1002/(SICI)1097-4598(199708)20:8<919::AID-MUS1>3.0.CO;2-9 PMID:9236782

Ray, M., Sharma, H. S., & Choudhary, S. (2006). A Reference book on Mathematical Statistics (4th ed.). Agra, India: Ram Prakash and Sons.

Reddy, G., Ramudu, K., Srinivas, A., & Rao, R. (2011). Fast Level Set Evolution of Region Based Segmentation of Satellite and Medical Imagery on Noisy Images. *International Journal Of Applied Physics And Mathematics*, *78-81*. doi:10.7763/ijapm.2011.v1.15

Rege, M., Dong, M., & Fotouhi, F. (2006). Co-clustering Documents and Words Using Bipartite Isoperimetric Graph Partitioning.*ICDM Conference*. doi:10.1109/ICDM.2006.36

Reif, J. (1997). Local Parallel Biomolecular Computation.*3rd DIMACS workshop on DNA based computers*, (pp. 243-258).

Renka, R. (2009). Image segmentation with a Sobolev gradient method. *Nonlinear Analysis: Theory. Methods & Applications*, *71*(12), e774–e780. doi:10.1016/j.na.2008.11.070

Rentschler, S., Vaidya, D. M., Tamaddon, H., Degenhardt, K., Sassoon, D., & Morley, G. E. (2001). Visualization and functional characterization of the developing murine cardiac conduction system. *Development, 128*(10), 1785–1792. PMID:11311159

Richa, H. R., & Phulpagar, B. D. (2013). Review on Multi-Cloud DNA Encryption Model for Cloud Security. *Int. Journal of Engineering Research and Applications, 3*(6), 1625–1628.

Richter, C., Leier, A., Banzhaf, W., & Rauhe, H. (2000). Private and Public Key DNA steganography.*6th DIMACS Workshop on DNA Based Computers*, (pp. 1-10).

Risca, V. I. (2001). DNA-based Steganography. *Cryptologia, Taylor and Francis, 25*(1), 37–49. doi:10.1080/0161-110191889761

Robertson, S. E., & Walker, S. (1994). Some simple effective approximations to the 2-poisson model for probabilistic weighted retrieval. In SIGIR.

Rokach, L., & Maimon, O. (2005). Clustering methods. In Data mining and knowledge discovery handbook (pp. 321-352). Springer US. doi:10.1007/0-387-25465-X_15

Roque, A. L., Valenti, V. E., Guida, H. L., Campos, M. F., Knap, A., Vanderlei, L. C. M., & Abreu, L. C. et al. (2013). The effects of auditory stimulation with music on heart rate variability in healthy women. *Clinics (Sao Paulo), 68*(7), 960–967. doi:10.6061/clinics/2013(07)12 PMID:23917660

Rosenblatt, F. (1958). The Perceptron: A Probabilistic Model for Information Storage and Organization in the Brain. *Psychological Review, 65*(6), 386–408. doi:10.1037/h0042519 PMID:13602029

Ross. (2010). Introduction to Probability models (10th ed.). Academic Press.

Rothemund P W K. (1996). A DNA and restriction enzyme implementation of Turing machines. *DNA Based Computers, 6*, 75-120.

Rothemund, P. W. K., Papadakis, N., & Winfree, E. (2004). Algorithmic self-assembly of DNA Sierpinski triangles. *PLoS Biology, 2*(12), e424. doi:10.1371/journal.pbio.0020424 PMID:15583715

Rozenberg, G., & Salomaa, A. (2006). DNA computing: New ideas and paradigms. Lecture Notes in Computer Science, 7, 188-200.

Rozenberg, G., Bäck, T., & Kok, J. (2012). *Handbook of Natural Computing*. Springer. doi:10.1007/978-3-540-92910-9

Rubin J., Sataloff, R.T., & Korovin, G.S. (2006). *Diagnosis and treatment of voice disorders*. Plural Publishing Inc.

Ruud, E. (2010). *Music therapy: A perspective from the humanities*. Barcelona Publishers.

Sadeg, S. (2010). An Encryption algorithm inspired from DNA.*IEEE International Conference on Machine and Web Intelligence*, (pp. 344 – 349).

Saecker, M., & Markl, V. (2013). Big Data Analytics on Modern Hardware Architectures: A Technology Survey. *Springer Lecture Notes in Business Information Processing, 138*, 125–149. doi:10.1007/978-3-642-36318-4_6

Saeedmanesh, M., Izadi, T., & Ahvar, E. (2002). *A Hybrid Data Mining Technique for Stock Exchange Prediction*. International Multi Conference, China.

Saggar, M., Agarwal, A. K., & Lad, A. (2004). *Optimization of Association Rule Mining using Improved Genetic Algorithms*. IEEE. doi:10.1109/ICSMC.2004.1400923

Sagiroglu, S., & Sinanc, D. (2013). Big Data: A review. *Collaboration Technologies and Systems (CTS), 2013 International Conference.*

Sahami, M., & Heilman, T. D. (2006). A web-based kernel function for measuring the similarity of short text snippets. *Proceedings of WWW2006*, 377–386.

Sahoo, N., Callan, J., Krishnan, R., Duncan, G., & Padman, R. (2006). Incremental Hierarchical Clustering of Text Documents. In *Proc. of Int. conf.ACM CIKM Conference.*

Sakakibara, Y. (2005). Development of a bacteria computer: From in silico finite automata to *in vitro* and *invivo*. *Bulletin of EATCS*, *87*, 165–178.

Salahuddin, L., Cho, J., Jeong, M. G., & Kim, D. (2007). *Ultra short term analysis of heart rate variability for monitoring mental stress in mobile settings.* Paper presented at the Engineering in Medicine and Biology Society, 2007. EMBS 2007. 29th Annual International Conference of the IEEE. doi:10.1109/IEMBS.2007.4353378

Salton, G. (1983). *An Introduction to Modern Information Retrieval.* McGraw Hill.

Salton, G., & Buckley, C. (1988). Term Weighting Approaches in Automatic Text Retrieval. *Information Processing & Management*, *24*(5), 513–523. doi:10.1016/0306-4573(88)90021-0

Sánchez, R., Grau, R., & Morgado, E. (2006). A Novel Lie Algebra of the Genetic Code over the Galois Field of Four DNA Bases. *Mathematical Biosciences*, *202*(1), 156–174. doi:10.1016/j.mbs.2006.03.017 PMID:16780898

Sandhu, Dhaliwal, Panda, & Bisht. (2010). An Improvement in Apriori algorithm Using Profit And Quantity. *Second International Conference on Computer and Network Technology.* IEEE. DOI doi:10.1109/ICCNT.2010.46

Savasere, A., Omieccinski, E., & Navathe, S. (1995). An efficient algorithm for mining association rules in Large databases. *Proceedings of the 21st international Conference on Very Large Databases.*

Sawah, A. E. (2007). A framework for 3D hand tracking and gesture recognition using elements of genetic programming. *4th Canadian conference on Computer and robot vision*, Montreal, Canada. doi:10.1109/CRV.2007.3

Scheufele, P. M. (2000). Effects of progressive relaxation and classical music on measurements of attention, relaxation, and stress responses. *Journal of Behavioral Medicine*, *23*(2), 207–228. doi:10.1023/A:1005542121935 PMID:10833680

Schijvenaars, B. J., Kors, J. A., van Herpen, G., Kornreich, F., & van Bemmel, J. H. (1997). Effect of electrode positioning on ECG interpretation by computer. *Journal of Electrocardiology*, *30*(3), 247–256. doi:10.1016/S0022-0736(97)80010-6 PMID:9261733

Schneier. (1996). *Applied cryptography: Protocols, Algorithms, and Source Code in C.* Wiley.

Schutze, H., & Silverstein, C. (1997). Projections for Efficient Document Clustering. In *Proc. of 20th Int. conf.ACM SIGIR Conference.*

Schwartz, S. R., Cohen, S. M., Dailey, S. H., Rosenfield, R. M., Deutsch, E. S., Gillepsie, M. B., & Patel, M. M. et al. (2009). Clinical practice guideline: Hoarseness (dysphonia). *Otolaryngology - Head and Neck Surgery*, *141*(3Suppl 2), S1–S31. doi:10.1016/j.otohns.2009.06.744

Sedding, J., & Kazakov, D. (2004). WordNet-based text document clustering. In COLING-2004 workshop on robust methods in analysis of natural language data. doi:10.3115/1621445.1621458

Segev, A., Jung, & Jung. (2013). Analysis of technology trends based on big data. *Big Data (BigData Congress), 2013 IEEE International Congress.*

Se, H. (2001). Advances in Predictive Models for Data Mining. *Pattern Recognition Letters*, *22*(1), 55–61. doi:10.1016/S0167-8655(00)00099-4

Shahid, M., & Gupta, S. (2006). Novel Masks for Multimodality Image Fusion using DTCWT. IEEE International Conference on Image Fusion.

Shang, S. (2010). *DNA microarray analysis of the gene expression profile of kidney tissue in a type 2 diabetic rat model.* Mol Med Rep. doi:10.3892/mmr.2010.367

Shan, H., He, C., & Wang, N. (2014). MCA aided geodesic active contours for image segmentation with textures. *Pattern Recognition Letters*, *45*, 235–243. doi:10.1016/j.patrec.2014.04.018

Shannon, C. E. (1949). Communication theory of secrecy system. *Journal of Bell System Technology*, *28*(4), 656–715. doi:10.1002/j.1538-7305.1949.tb00928.x

Shao, G., Li, T., Zuo, W., Wu, S., & Liu, T. (2015). A Combinational Clustering Based Method for cDNA Microarray Image Segmentation. *PLoS ONE*, *10*(8), e0133025. doi:10.1371/journal.pone.0133025 PMID:26241767

Sharma, A., & Thakur, R. S. (2012). Challenges in categorical data clustering. In *Proceedings of theInternational Conference on Intelligent Computing and Information System* (ICICIS).

Sharma, A., & Thakur, R.S. (2016). Variant of Genetic Algorithm based Categorical data Clustering for Compact Clusters and an Experimental Study on Soybean data for Local and Global Optimal Solution. *International Journal of Advanced Computer Science and Engineering*.

Sharma, A., & Thakur, R. S. (2014). Cluster Analysis for Categorical Data Using Matlab International Journal of Research in Management. *Science & Technology*, *2*(2), 65–68.

Sherif, T. A., Magdy, S., & El-Gindi, S. (2006). A DNA based Implementation of YAEA Encryption Algorithm.*IASTED International Conference on Computational Intelligence*.

Sheth & Amit. (2014). Transforming big data into smart data: deriving value via harnessing volume, variety, and velocity using semantic techniques and technologies. *Data Engineering (ICDE). IEEE 30th International Conference*.

Shi, C. (2006). A Parametric Active Contour Model for Medical Image Segmentation Using Priori Shape Force Field. *Journal Of Computer Research And Development*, *43*(), 2131. doi:10.1360/crad20061215

Shih, M. Y., Jheng, J. W., & Lai, L. F. (2010). A two-step method for clustering mixed categroical and numeric data. *Tamkang Journal of Science and Engineering*, *13*(1), 11–19.

Shi, J., & Malik, J. (2000). Normalized cuts and image segmentation. *IEEE Transactions on Pattern Analysis and Machine Intelligence*, 888–905.

Shi, S., Ying, S. Y., & Li, W. Y. (2014). *Medical Ultrasound Image Denoising based on Fuzzy Logic*. IEEE. doi:10.1109/ISDEA.2014.143

Shon, T., Seo, J., & Moon, J. (2005). SVM approach with a genetic algorithm for network intrusion detection. In *Proc. of 20th International Symposium on Computer and Information Sciences (ISCIS 2005)*. Berlin: Springer-Verlag. doi:10.1007/11569596_25

Shukla, Pandey, & Kumar. (2015). Big Data Framework: At a Glance. *International Journal of Innovations & Advancement in Computer Science, 4*.

Silverstein, C., & Pedersen, J. (1997). Almost-constant time clustering of arbitrary corpus subsets.*ACM SIGIR Conference*.

Sim, K., Gopalkrishnan, V., Phua, C., & Cong, G. (2012). 3D Subspace Clustering for Value Investing. *IEEE Intelligent Systems, 99*(1), 1–8.

Singh, N. (2004). *The use of syntactic structure in relationship extraction.* (Master's thesis). MIT.

Singhal, A., Buckley, C., & Mitra, M. (1996). Pivoted Document Length Normalization. *ACM SIGIR Conference.*

Singh, S., & Singh, N. (2012). Big data analytics. *IEEE, International Conference on Communication, Information & Computing Technology (ICCICT).*

Siromoney, R., & Bireswar, D. (2003). DNA algorithm for breaking a propositional logic based cryptosystem. *Bulletin of the European Association for Theoretical Computer Science, 79*, 170–177.

Sivanandam, S. N., & Deepa, S. N. (2007). *Principles of soft computing.* New Delhi: Wiley India.

Sivanandam, S. N., Sumathi, S., & Deepa, S. N. (2006). *Introduction to Neural Networks Using Matlab 6.0* (7th ed.). New Delhi, India: Tata McGraw Hill Publishing Company Limited.

Skrodzka D., et al. (2006). Powikłania laryngologiczne choroby refluksowej przełyku. *Prz. Lek. 2006, 63*(9), 752-755. (in Polish)

Slonim, N., Friedman, N., & Tishby, N. (2002). Unsupervised document classification using sequential information maximization.*ACM SIGIR Conference.* doi:10.1145/564376.564401

Slonim, N., & Tishby, N. (2000). Document Clustering using word clusters via the information bottleneck method. *ACM SIGIR Conference.* doi:10.1145/345508.345578

Smith, D. (2002). Detecting and browsing events in unstructured text. In *Proceedings of ACM SIGIR Conference on Research and Development in Information Retrieval.* doi:10.1145/564376.564391

Sneddon, I. N. (1995). *Fourier transforms.* Courier Corporation.

Soderland, S. (1999). Learning information extraction rules for semi-structured and free text. *Machine Learning, 34*(1/3), 233–272. doi:10.1023/A:1007562322031

Solin, P., Kaye, D. M., Little, P. J., Bergin, P., Richardson, M., & Naughton, M. T. (2003). Impact of sleep apnea on sympathetic nervous system activity in heart failure. *CHEST Journal, 123*(4), 1119–1126. doi:10.1378/chest.123.4.1119 PMID:12684302

Sorensen, T. (1948). A method of establishing groups of equal amplitude in plant sociology based on similarity of species and its application to analyses of the vegetation on Danish commons. *Biologiske Skrifter, 5*, 1–34.

Soria, D., Garibaldi, J., Ambrogi, F., Biganzoli, E., & Ellis, I. (2011). A 'non-parametric' version of the naive Bayes classifier. *Knowledge-Based Systems, 24*(6), 775–784. doi:10.1016/j.knosys.2011.02.014

Sowa, J. F. (1995). Top-level Ontological Categories. *International Journal of Human-Computer Studies, 43*(5-6), 669–685. doi:10.1006/ijhc.1995.1068

Sowa, J. F. (2000). *Knowledge Representation – Logical, Philosophical, and Computational Foundations.* Pacific Grove, CA: Brooks/Cole.

Srinivasulu, Satya Prasad, & Ramesh Babu. (2010). Intelligent Network Intrusion Detection Using DT and BN Classification Techniques. *Int. J. Advance. Soft Compute. Appl., 2*(1).

Srisawat. (2011). An Application of Association Rule Mining Based on Stock Market. *3rd International Conference on Data Mining and Intelligent Information Technology Applications* (ICMIA).

Srivastava & Divesh. (2014). Data quality: the other face of big data. *Data Engineering (ICDE). IEEE 30th International Conference.*

Stakhov, A. P. (2006). Fibonacci matrices, a generalization of the 'Cassini formula', and a new coding theory. Chaos, Solutions & Fractals, 30(1), 56–66.

Stallings W. (n.d.). *Cryptography and Network Security – Principles and Practice* (5th ed.). Prentice Hall.

Stauss, H. M. (2003). Heart rate variability. *American Journal of Physiology. Regulatory, Integrative and Comparative Physiology, 285*(5), R927–R931. doi:10.1152/ajpregu.00452.2003 PMID:14557228

Steinbach, M., Karypis, G., & Kumar, V. (2000). A comparison of document clustering techniques. In *Proceedings of KDD Workshop on Text Mining,6th ACM SIGKDD International Conference on Knowledge Discovery and Data Mining* (KDD).

Steinbach, M., Karypis, G., & Kumar, V. (2000). A Comparison of Document Clustering Techniques. *KDD Workshop on text mining.*

Stewart, J. M. (2000). Autonomic nervous system dysfunction in adolescents with postural orthostatic tachycardia syndrome and chronic fatigue syndrome is characterized by attenuated vagal baroreflex and potentiated sympathetic vasomotion. *Pediatric Research, 48*(2), 218–226. doi:10.1203/00006450-200008000-00016 PMID:10926298

Stock Market Data Source. (n.d.). Retrieved from http://www.bseindia.com

Stonebraker, M. (2010). Sql databases vs. nosql databases. *Communications of the ACM, 53*(4), 10–11. doi:10.1145/1721654.1721659

Strobl, C., Malley, J., & Tutz, G. (2009). An introduction to recursive partitioning: Rationale, application, and characteristics of classification and regression trees, bagging, and random forests. *Psychological Methods, 14*(4), 323–348. doi:10.1037/a0016973 PMID:19968396

Strozzi & Carlo. (2010). *NoSQ L – A relational database management system.* Retrieved from: http://www.strozzi.it/cgibin/CSA/tw7/I/en_US/nosql/Home%20Page

Studer, R., Benjamins, V. R., & Fensel, D. (1998). Knowledge engineering, principles and methods. *Data & Knowledge Engineering, 25*(1-2), 161–197. doi:10.1016/S0169-023X(97)00056-6

Sung, A. H., & Mukkamala, S. (2004). The Feature Selection and Intrusion Detection Problems. In *Proceedings of the 9th Asian Computing Science Conference*, (LNCS) (vol. 3029). Springer. doi:10.1007/978-3-540-30502-6_34

Sun, S. (2013). High Precision Infrared Image Data Rendering Algorithm Based on Probability Sequence. *J. Inf. Comput. Sci., 10*(16), 5293–5299. doi:10.12733/jics20102304

Sun, Y., Han, J., Gao, J., & Yu, Y. (2009). iTopicModel: Information Network Integrated Topic Modeling. *ICDM Conference.*

SUO. (n.d.). *Standard Upper Ontology.* Retrieved from: http://suo.ieee.org/

Sure, Y., Angele, J., & Staab, S. (2002). OntoEdit: Guiding Ontology Development by Methodology and Inferencing. *Proceedings of the 1st International Conference on Ontologies, Databases and Applications of Semantics for Large Scale Information Systems.* doi:10.1007/3-540-36124-3_76

Susan, K. L., & Hellman, M. E. (1994). Differential-Linear Cryptanalysis. *LNCS, 839*, 17–25.

Sutheebanjard, P., & Premchaiswadi, W. (2010). Stock Exchange of Thailand Index Prediction Using Back Propagation Neural Networks. *2nd International Conference on Computer and Network Technology (IEEE).* doi:10.1109/ICCNT.2010.21

Sutherland et al. (2010). *Cracking Codes and Cryptograms for Dummies.* Wiley.

Su, X., Lan, Y., Wan, R., & Qin, Y. (2009). A Fast Incremental Clustering Algorithm. *Proceedings of the 2009 International Symposium on Information Processing (ISIP'09).*

Svetnik, V., Liaw, A., Tong, C., Culberson, J. C., Sheridan, R. P., & Feuston, B. P. (2003). Random forest: A classification and regression tool for compound classification and QSAR modeling. *Journal of Chemical Information and Computer Sciences, 43*(6), 1947–1958. doi:10.1021/ci034160g PMID:14632445

Sztajzel, J. (2004). Heart rate variability: A noninvasive electrocardiographic method to measure the autonomic nervous system. *Swiss Medical Weekly, 134,* 514–522. PMID:15517504

Tan, P., Kumar, V., & Shrivastava, J. (2004). Selecting the Right Interesting Measure for Association Patterns. *Information Systems, 29*(4), 293–331. doi:10.1016/S0306-4379(03)00072-3

Tao, W., & Tai, X. (2011). Multiple piecewise constant with geodesic active contours (MPC-GAC) framework for interactive image segmentation using graph cut optimization. *Image and Vision Computing, 29*(8), 499–508. doi:10.1016/j.imavis.2011.03.002

Tausif, A., Sanchita, P., & Kumar, S. (2014). Message Transmission Based on DNA Cryptography[Review]. *International Journal of Bio-Science and Bio-Technology, 6*(5), 215–222. doi:10.14257/ijbsbt.2014.6.5.22

Tavallaee, M., Bagheri, E., Lu, W., & Ghorbani, A. A. (2009). A Detailed Analysis of the KDDCUP 99 Data Set. *Proceedings of the 2009 IEEE Symposium on Computational Intelligence in Security and Defense Application (CISDA 2009).* IEEE. doi:10.1109/CISDA.2009.5356528

Tawara, S., Suma, K., & Shimada, M. (2000). *The conduction system of the mammalian heart: an anatomico-histological study of the atrioventricular bundle and the Purkinje fibers.* Imperial College Press.

Taylor, C., Risca, V., & Bancroft, C. (1999). Hiding messages in DNA Microdots. *Nature, 399*(6736), 533–534. doi:10.1038/21092 PMID:10376592

Terec, R. (2011). DNA Security using Symmetric and Asymmetric Cryptography. *International Journal of New Computer Architectures and Their Applications,* 34-51.

Tew, C., Giraud-Carrier, C., Tanner, K., & Burton, S. (2014). Behaviour based clustering and analysis of interesting measures for association rule mining: Vol. 28. *Issue 4* (pp. 1004–1045). Springer.

Thayer, J. F., Yamamoto, S. S., & Brosschot, J. F. (2010). The relationship of autonomic imbalance, heart rate variability and cardiovascular disease risk factors. *International Journal of Cardiology, 141*(2), 122–131. doi:10.1016/j.ijcard.2009.09.543 PMID:19910061

Tiwari, V., & Thakur, R. S. (2012). A level wise Tree Based Approach for Ontology-Driven Association Rules Mining. *CiiT International Journal of Data Mining and Knowledge Engineering, 4*(5).

Tiwari, V., & Thakur, R. S. (2015). Contextual Snowflake Modeling for Pattern Warehouse Logical Design. Sadhana - Academy Proceedings in Engineering Science, 40(1), 15-33.

Tiwari, A., Gupta, R. K., & Agrawal, D. P. (2010). A survey on Frequent Pattern Mining: Current Status and Challenging issues. *Information Technology Journal, 9*(7), 1278–1293. doi:10.3923/itj.2010.1278.1293

Tiwari, V., Tiwari, V., Gupta, S., & Mishra, R. (2010). Association Rule Mining- A Graph based approach for mining Frequent Itemsets.*IEEE International Conference on Networking and Information Technology (ICNIT).* doi:10.1109/ICNIT.2010.5508505

Toivonen, H. (1996). Sampling Large Databases for Association Rules. In *Proc. 22nd VLDB*.

Toivonen, H. (1996). Sampling large databases for association rules. *Proceedings of 22th International Conference on Very Large Databases*.

Tombini, E., Debar, H., Me, L., & Ducasse, M. (2004). A Serial Combination of Anomaly and Misuse IDSes Applied to HTTP Traffic. *Proc. 20th Ann. Computer Security Applications Conf. (ACSAC '04)*. doi:10.1109/CSAC.2004.4

Torrent-Guasp, F., Ballester, M., Buckberg, G. D., Carreras, F., Flotats, A., Carrió, I., & Narula, J. et al. (2001). Spatial orientation of the ventricular muscle band: Physiologic contribution and surgical implications. *The Journal of Thoracic and Cardiovascular Surgery*, *122*(2), 389–392. doi:10.1067/mtc.2001.113745 PMID:11479518

Traister, R. S., Fajt, M. L., Landsittl, D., & Petrov, A. A. (2014). A novel scoring system to distinguish vocal cord dysfunction from asthma. *Journal of Allergy Clinical Immunology Practice*, *2*(10), 65–69. doi:10.1016/j.jaip.2013.09.002

Trappe, H.-J. (2010). The effects of music on the cardiovascular system and cardiovascular health. *Heart (British Cardiac Society)*, *96*(23), 1868–1871. doi:10.1136/hrt.2010.209858 PMID:21062776

Triposkiadis, F., Karayannis, G., Giamouzis, G., Skoularigis, J., Louridas, G., & Butler, J. (2009). The sympathetic nervous system in heart failure: Physiology, pathophysiology, and clinical implications. *Journal of the American College of Cardiology*, *54*(19), 1747–1762. doi:10.1016/j.jacc.2009.05.015 PMID:19874988

Tsatsanis, M. K., & Giannakis, G. B. (1995). Principal component filter banks for optimal multiresolution analysis. *Signal Processing. IEEE Transactions on*, *43*(8), 1766–1777. doi:10.1109/78.403336

Tuzhilin, A., & Silberschatz, A. (1996). What Makes Patterns Interesting in Knowledge Discovery Systems. *IEEE Transactions on Knowledge and Data Engineering*, *8*(6), 970–974. doi:10.1109/69.553165

Tzung-Pei, H., Kuei-Ying, L., & Shyue-Liang, W. (2003). Fuzzy Data Mining for Interesting Generalized Association Rules. *Fuzzy Sets and Systems*, *138*(2), 255–269. doi:10.1016/S0165-0114(02)00272-5

Udo, F., Saghaf, S., Wolfgang, B., & Rauhe, H. (2002). DNA Sequence Generator: A program for the construction of DNA sequences. *DNA Computing*, 23-32.

Ugwu, C., & Onwuachu, C. (2014). Machine Learning Application for Stock Market Price Prediction. *The Pacefic Journal of Science and Technology*, *15*(2), 155–166.

Umemura, M., & Honda, K. (1998). Influence of Music on Heart Rate Variability and Comfort. A Consideration Through Comparison of Music and Noise. *Journal of Human Ergology*, *27*(1/2), 30–38. PMID:11579697

Umetani, K., Singer, D. H., McCraty, R., & Atkinson, M. (1998). Twenty-four hour time domain heart rate variability and heart rate: Relations to age and gender over nine decades. *Journal of the American College of Cardiology*, *31*(3), 593–601. doi:10.1016/S0735-1097(97)00554-8 PMID:9502641

Upendra & Kumar. (2012). An Efficient Intrusion detection based on Decision Tree Classifier Using Feature Reduction. *International Journal of Scientific and Research*, *2*(1).

Vaisla, , & Bhatt, . (2010). An Analysis of the Performance of Artificial Neural Network Technique for Stock Market Forecasting. *International Journal on Computer Science and Engineering*, *2*(6), 2104–2109.

van Rijsbergen, C. J., & Croft. Document Clustering, W. B. (1975). An Evaluation of some experiments with the Cranfield 1400 collection. *Information Processing & Management*, *11*(5-7), 171–182. doi:10.1016/0306-4573(75)90006-0

Vard, A., Jamshidi, K., & Movahhedinia, N. (2012). An automated approach for segmentation of intravascular ultrasound images based on parametric active contour models. *Australasian Physical & Engineering Sciences in Medicine*, *35*(2), 135–150. doi:10.1007/s13246-012-0131-7 PMID:22415899

Vard, A., Monadjemi, A., Jamshidi, K., & Movahhedinia, N. (2011). Fast texture energy based image segmentation using Directional Walshâ€"Hadamard Transform and parametric active contour models. *Expert Systems with Applications*, *38*(9), 11722–11729. doi:10.1016/j.eswa.2011.03.058

Vazirani, V. (2004). *Approximation Algorithms*. Berlin: Springer.

Vega, J. C. A. (2000). *WebODE 1.0: User's Manual.* Laboratory of Artificial Intelligence, Technical University of Madrid.

Vlachos, M., & Dermatas, E. (2013). Finger vein segmentation in infrared images using supervised and unsupervised clustering algorithms. *Pattern Recognition and Image Analysis*, *23*(2), 328–334. doi:10.1134/S1054661813020168

Volos, C. K., Kyprianidis, I., & Stouboulos, I. (2013). Image encryption process based on chaotic synchronization phenomena. *Signal Processing*, *93*(5), 1328–1340. doi:10.1016/j.sigpro.2012.11.008

Voorhees, E. M. (1986). *Implementing Agglomerative Hierarchical Clustering for use in Information Retrieval*. Technical Report TR86-765. Cornell University.

Wakabi-Waiswa & Baryamureeba. (2008). Extraction of Interesting Association Rules Using Genetic Algorithms. *International Journal of Computing and ICT Research, 2*(1).

Wang, K., Zhou, S., & Han, J. (2002). Profit Mining: From Patterns to Actions. In EDBT 2002 (LNCS) (vol. 2287, pp. 70–87). Springer-VerlagBerlin Heidelberg.

Wang, F., & Zhang, C. (2007) T. Li. Regularized clustering for documents. *ACM SIGIR Conference.*

Wang, H., & Liu, M. (2012). Medical Images Segmentation Using Active Contours Driven By Global And Local Image Fitting Energy. *International Journal of Image and Graphics*, *12*(02), 1250015. doi:10.1142/S0219467812500155

Wang, H., Zhang, H., & Ray, N. (2013). Adaptive shape prior in graph cut image segmentation. *Pattern Recognition*, *46*(5), 1409–1414. doi:10.1016/j.patcog.2012.11.002

Wang, J., Wang, C., Liu, J., & Wu, C. (2006). Information Extraction forlearning of Ontology Instances. *IEEE International Conference on Industrial Informatics.*

Wang, L., Li, C., Sun, Q., Xia, D., & Kao, C. (2009). Active contours driven by local and global intensity fitting energy with application to brain MR image segmentation. *Computerized Medical Imaging and Graphics*, *33*(7), 520–531. doi:10.1016/j.compmedimag.2009.04.010 PMID:19482457

Wang, P., Hu, J., Zeng, H.-J., & Chen, Z. (2009). Wikipedia knowledge to improve text classification. *Knowledge and Information Systems*, *19*(3), 265–281. doi:10.1007/s10115-008-0152-4

Wang, X., & Wang, Q. (2014). A novel Image Encryption Algorithm based on Dynamic S-Boxes constructed by chaos. *Nonlinear Dynamics*, *75*(3), 567–576. doi:10.1007/s11071-013-1086-2

Wang, Y., & Sun, Y. (2011). Adaptive Mean Shift Based Image Smoothing and Segmentation. *Acta Automatica Sinica*, *36*(12), 1637–1644. doi:10.3724/SP.J.1004.2010.01637

Wang, Z., & Yu, Z. (2011). Index-based symmetric DNA encryption algorithm. *Fourth International Congress on Image and Signal Processing*, (pp. 15-17).

Warner, B., & Misra, M. (1996). Understanding Neural Networks as Statistical Tools. *The American Statistician, 50*, 284–293.

Watkins, G. R. (1997). Music therapy: Proposed physiological mechanisms and clinical implications. *Clinical Nurse Specialist CNS, 11*(2), 43–50. doi:10.1097/00002800-199703000-00003 PMID:9233140

Watson. (2014). Big Data Tutorial: Concepts, Technologies and Applications. *Communications of the Association for Information Systems, 34*.

Watson, J. D., & Crick, F. H. C. (1953). Molecular structure of nucleic acids: A structure for De-oxy ribose nucleic acid. *Nature, 25*(4356), 737–738. doi:10.1038/171737a0 PMID:13054692

Wee-Chung Liew, A., Yan, H., & Yang, M. (2003). Robust adaptive spot segmentation of DNA microarray images. *Pattern Recognition, 36*(5), 1251–1254. doi:10.1016/S0031-3203(02)00170-X

Weichang, C., & Zhihua, C. (2000). Digital Coding of the Genetic Codons and DNA Sequences in High Dimension Space. *Acta Biophysica Sinica, 16*(4), 760–768.

Wellens, H. J., Bär, F. W., & Lie, K. (2000). *The value of the electrocardiogram in the differential diagnosis of a tachycardia with a widened QRS complex*. Springer.

Westlund, B. H. (2002). NIST reports measurable success of Advanced Encryption Standard. *Journal of Research of the National Institute of Standards and Technology*.

White. (2010). *Hadoop: The Definitive Guide* (3rd ed.). O'Reilly Media.

White, H. (1988). Economic Prediction Using Neural Networks: The Case of IBM Daily Stock Returns. In *Proc. of the IEEE International Conference on Neural Networks*. doi:10.1109/ICNN.1988.23959

Wielki, J. (2013). Implementation of the big data concept in organizations - possibilities, impediments and challenges. *Computer Science and Information Systems (FedCSIS), 2013 Federated Conference*.

Wierman, M. J. (2010). *An Introduction to the Mathematics of Uncertainty*. Center for the Mathematics of Uncerteainty, Creighton University.

Wilbur, J., & Sirotkin, K. (1992). The automatic identification of stop words. *Information Sciences, 18*, 45–55.

Willett, P. (1980). Document Clustering using an inverted file approach. *Journal of Information Science, 2*(5), 223–231. doi:10.1177/016555158000200503

Willett, P. (1988). Recent Trends in Hierarchical Document Clustering: A Critical Review. *Information Processing & Management, 24*(5), 577–597. doi:10.1016/0306-4573(88)90027-1

Windeatt, T., & Ardeshir, G. (2002). *Boosted tree ensembles for solving multiclass problems. In Multiple Classifier Systems* (pp. 42–51). Springer.

Winfree, A. (1980). *The Geometry of Biological Time*. Academic Press.

Winfree, E. (1996) On the Computational Power of DNA Annealing and Ligation.*1st DIMACS Workshop on DNA Based Computers*.

Wootton, R., & Craig, J. (1999). *History of Telemedicine. Introduction to telemedicine*. London: Royal Society of Medical Press.

World Health Organization. (1997). *Health-for-all Policy for the 21st Century, HQ (document EB101/8)*. Geneva: WHO.

Wu, Y., Noonan, J. P., & Agaian, S. (2011). NPCR and UACI Randomness Tests for Image Encryption. *Journal of Selected Areas in Telecommunications, 4*, 31–38.

Wu, Y., Zhou, Y., Noonan, J. P., & Agaian, S. (2013). Design of Image Cipher Using Latin Squares. *Information Sciences, 00*, 1–30.

Xiang, P., Hou, R., & Zhou, Z. (2010). Cache and consistency in nosql. *Computer Science and Information Technology (ICCSIT).3rd IEEE International Conference.*

Xiangwei, L. (2012). Based on BP Neural Network Stock Prediction. *Journal of Curriculum and Teaching, 1*(1), 45–50.

Xiao, G., Lu, M., Qin, L., & Lai, X. (2006). New field of cryptography: DNA cryptography. *Chinese Science Bulletin, 51*, 1139–1144.

Xiao, J. H., Zhang, X. Y., & Xu, J. (2012). A membrane evolutionary algorithm for DNA sequence design in DNA computing. *Chinese Science Bulletin, 57*(2), 698–706. doi:10.1007/s11434-011-4928-7

Xu, W., Liu, X., & Gong, Y. (2003). Document Clustering based on negative matrix factorization. In *Proc. of ACM SIGIR 26th International Conference.*

Xu, C., & Zhang, Y. (2014). Cell Contour Irregularity Feature Extraction Methods based on Linear Geometric Heat Flow Curve Evolution. *International Journal Of Signal Processing, Image Processing. Pattern Recognition, 7*(3), 181–192. doi:10.14257/ijsip.2014.7.3.15

XueJia, L., MingXin, L., Lei, Q., JunSong, H., & XiWen, F. (2010). Asymmetric Encryption and signature method with DNA technology. *Information Sciences, 53*, 506–514.

Xu, X., & He, C. (2013). Implicit Active Contour Model with Local and Global Intensity Fitting Energies. *Mathematical Problems in Engineering, 2013*, 1–13. doi:10.1155/2013/367086

Yahoo Launches World's Largest Hadoop Production Application. (2008). Retrieved from http://developer .yahoo.net/blogs/hadoop/2008/02/yahoo-worlds-largest-production-hadoop.html

Yamashita, S., Iwai, K., Akimoto, T., Sugawara, J., & Kono, I. (2006). Effects of music during exercise on RPE, heart rate and the autonomic nervous system. *The Journal of Sports Medicine and Physical Fitness, 46*(3), 425. PMID:16998447

Yang, T., Jin, R., Chi, Y., & Zhu, S. (2009). Combining link and content for community detection: a discriminative approach. In *Proc. of Int. conf.ACM KDD Conference.*

Yang, Y. (1995). Noise Reduction in a Statistical Approach to Text Categorization. In *Proc. Of 18th Int. conf. ACM SIGIR.*

Yang, Y., & Pederson, J. O. (1995). A comparative study on feature selection in text categorization. In *Proc. of Int. conf. ACM SIGIR Conference.*

Yang, Y., Park, D.S., Huang, S., Fang, Z., & Wang, Z. (2009). Wavelet based Approach for Fusing Computed Tomography and Magnetic Resonance Images. IEEE.

Yangarber, R., Grishman, R., Tapanainen, P., & Huttunen, S. (2000). Automatic acquisition of domain knowledge for information extraction. In *Proceedings of the 18th International Conference on Computational Linguistics.* doi:10.3115/992730.992782

Yang, B., & Chen, E. (2009). *Image Fusion Using an Improved Max-lifting Scheme.* IEEE.

Yang, H., Zhao, L., & Tang, S. (2014). Brain Tumor Segmentation Using Geodesic Region-based Level Set without Re-initialization. *International Journal Of Signal Processing, Image Processing. Pattern Recognition*, 7(1), 213–224. doi:10.14257/ijsip.2014.7.1.20

Yang, Q., Kai-min, C., Jun-li, S., & Li, Y. (2010). Design Analysis and Implementation for Ontology Learning Model. *2nd International Conference on Computer Engineering and Technology*.

Yan, X., Zhang, C., & Zhang, S. (2009). Genetic algorithmbased strategy for identifying association rules without specifying actual minimum support. *Elsevier, Expert Systems with Application*, 36(2), 3066–3077. doi:10.1016/j.eswa.2008.01.028

Yao, L., & Mimno, D. (2009). Efficient methods for topic model inference on streaming document collections. In *Proc. of 15th Int. conf.ACM KDD Conference*.

Yao, , Teng, , Poh, , & Tan, . (1998). Forecasting and Analysis of Marketing Data Using Neural Networks. *J. Inf. Sci. Eng.*, 14(4), 843–862.

Ye, K., & Zhan, Y. (2009). Image segmentation algorithm based on mathematical morphology and active edgeless contour model without edges. *Journal Of Computer Applications*, 29(9), 2398–2401. doi:10.3724/SP.J.1087.2009.02398

Yin, F. Mickan, & Abbott. (2007). Terahertz Computed Tomographic Reconstruction and its Wavelet-based Segmentation by Fusion. IEEE.

Yin, X., Ferguson, H., Mickan, S. P., & Fischer, B. M. (2006). Information Fusion and Wavelet Based Segment Detection with Applications to the Identification of 3D Target T-ray CT Imaging. *Biomedical Image Fusion Using Wavelet Transform and SOFM Neural Network*, 1, 1189–1194.

Youssef, M. I., Emam, A. E., Saafan, S. M., & Abd Elghany, M. (2013). Secured Image Encryption Scheme Using both Residue Number System and DNA Sequence. *The Online Journal on Electronics and Electrical Engineering*, 6(3), 656–664.

Yuan, J. (2012). Active contour driven by region-scalable fitting and local Bhattacharyya distance energies for ultrasound image segmentation. *IET Image Processing*, 6(8), 1075–1083. doi:10.1049/iet-ipr.2012.0120

Yuasa, M., Watanabe, M., Nishiura, M., Yamaguchi, K., Kondo, T., Anno, H., & Muto, K. (2003). Automatic heart wall contour extraction from MR images using active contour models: Initial contour setting based on principal component analysis. *Systems and Computers in Japan*, 34(4), 72–82. doi:10.1002/scj.1202

Yuhuang, W., & Yuhuang, L. (2009). *Design and realization for ontology learning model based on web*. IEEE. doi:10.1109/ITCS.2009.234

Yunpeng, Z. (2012). *Research on DNA Cryptography*. InTech Press.

Yunpeng, Z., Fu, B., & Zhang, X. (2012). DNA cryptography based on DNA Fragment assembly.*IEEE International Conference Information Science and Digital Content Technology*.

Zadeh, L. (1965). *Fuzzy Sets*. Elsevier Inc.

Zaki, M. (2000). Scalable algorithms for association mining. *IEEE Transactions on Knowledge and Data Engineering*, 12(3), 372–390. doi:10.1109/69.846291

Zaki, M., Parthasarathy, S., Ogihara, M., & Li, W. (1997). Parallel algorithm for discovery of association rules. *Data Mining and Knowledge Discovery*, 1(4), 343–374. doi:10.1023/A:1009773317876

Zaman, S., & Karray, F. (2009). Features selection for intrusion detection systems based on support vector machines. In *Proceedings of the 6th IEEE Conference on Consumer Communications and Networking Conference*.

Zamir, O., & Etzioni, O. (1998). Web Document Clustering: A Feasibility Demonstration. *ACM SIGIR Conference.*

Zamir, O., Etzioni, O., Madani, O., & Karp, R. M. (1997). Fast and Intuitive Clustering of Web Documents. *ACM KDD Conference.*

Zesiewicz, T. A., Baker, M. J., Wahba, M., & Hauser, R. A. (2003). Autonomic nervous system dysfunction in Parkinson's disease. *Current Treatment Options in Neurology, 5*(2), 149–160. doi:10.1007/s11940-003-0005-0 PMID:12628063

Zhang, H., Liu, L., & Nan Lin, N. (2007). A Novel Wavelet Medical Image Fusion Method. *International Conference on Multimedia and Ubiquitous Engineering.*

Zhang, J., Ghahramani, Z., & Yang, Y. (2005). A probabilistic model for online document clustering with application to novelty detection. Advances in Neural Information Processing Letters, 17.

Zhang, C., Pan, H., & Zhou, K. (2015). Comparision of Back Propagation Neural Networks and EMD-Base Neural Networks in Forecasting the Three Asian Stock Markets. *Journal of Applied Sciences, 15*(1), 90–99. doi:10.3923/jas.2015.90.99

Zhang, D., Wang, J., & Si, L. (2011). Document clustering with universum. In *Proc. of Int. conf. On ACM SIGIR Conference.*

Zhang, J., Zhou, Z., Jionghua, T., & Ting, L. (2009). *Miao Zhiping Fusion Algorithm of Functional Images and Anatomical Images Based on Wavelet Transform.* IEEE.

Zhang, T., Ramakrishnan, R., & Livny, M. (1996). BIRCH: An Efficient Data Clustering Method for Very Large Databases. In *Proc. Of International conference on Management of Data ACM SIGMOD.* doi:10.1145/233269.233324

Zhang, X., Hu, X., & Zhou, X. (2008). A comparative evaluation of different link types on enhancing document clustering. In *Proc. Of 31st international ACM SIGIR Conference.* doi:10.1145/1390334.1390429

Zhao, M., Wang, J., & Fan, G. (2008). Research on Application of Improved Text Cluster Algorithm in intelligent QA system. *Proceedings of the Second International Conference on Genetic and Evolutionary Computing.* IEEE Computer Society. doi:10.1109/WGEC.2008.49

Zhao, Y., & Karypis, G. (2002). Evaluation of hierarchical clustering algorithms for document data set. *CIKM Conference.*

Zhao, Y., & Karypis, G. (2004). Empirical and Theoretical comparisons of selected criterion functions for document clustering. *Machine Learning, 55*(3), 311–331. doi:10.1023/B:MACH.0000027785.44527.d6

Zheng, Q. (2012). New local segmentation model for images with intensity inhomogeneity. *Optical Engineering (Redondo Beach, Calif.), 51*(3), 037006. doi:10.1117/1.OE.51.3.037006

Zhong, S. (2005). Efficient Streaming Text Clustering. *Neural Networks, 18*(5–6), 2005. PMID:16085385

Zhou, Y., Cheng, H., & Yu, J. X. (2009). Graph Clustering based on Structural/Attribute Similarities. In *Proceeding of VLDB Conference.*

Zhou, W., Liu, Z., Zhao, Y., Xu, L., Chen, G., Wu, Q., & Qiang, Y. et al. (2006). *A Semi-automatic Ontology Learning Based on WordNet and Event-based Natural Language Processing.* ICIA. doi:10.1109/ICINFA.2006.374119

Zou, X. (2013). Improved Dcut and its application in image segmentation. *Journal Of Computer Applications, 32*(8), 2291–2295. doi:10.3724/SP.J.1087.2012.02291

Zuo, Y., & Kita, E. (2012). Stock Price Forecasting Using Bayesian Network. *Expert Systems with Applications, 39*(8), 6729–6737. doi:10.1016/j.eswa.2011.12.035

About the Contributors

Vivek Tiwari is from India. He is the recipient of Young scientist award by Govt. by the MPCST, Govt. of M.P., India. He has published more than 25 research papers and book chapters in the areas of data mining, data warehousing, pattern warehousing, distributed computing and cloud computing in leading international journals (Springer, Inderscience, Elsevier, ACM and IGI-Global) indexed by Science Citation Index (SCI) and conferences (IEEE and ACM). He is Editors-in-chief of book "Handbook of Research on Pattern and Data Analysis in Healthcare Settings" under the series of Advances in Data Mining & Database Management (ADMDM), published by IGI-Global, USA. A research project "Aakash for Education" of cost 5 lac funded by MHRD, India is in his credit. He has been invited from various universities of India as keynote speaker/expert/visiting/guest faculty. He has given their services for various conferences under the umbrella of Springer, ACM, IEEE. He is an active member of the CSI, IAENG and IACSIT and regular reviewer of various international journals including Inderscience and IGI-Global.

Ramjeevan Singh Thakur is an Associate Professor in the Department of Computer Applications at Maulana Azad National Institute of Technology, Bhopal, India. He had a long carrier in teaching and research, including Three Year Teaching in the Department of Computer Applications at National Institute of Technology, Tiruchirapalli, Tamilnadu, India. At Present he is guiding several Ph.D. Research Scholars and handling Government Research Projects of about Rs. One Crore. He has published more than 75 Research Paper in National, International, Journals and Conferences. He has visited several Universities in USA, Hong Kong, Iran, Thailand, Malaysia, and Singapore.

* * *

Murugan Annamalai received his MSc Degree (Gold Medalist) from Manon-Maniam Sundaranar University, Tirunelveli, India in 1994 and Ph.D from University of Madras, Chennai, India in 2005. He is working as Associate Professor in the Department of Computer Science, Dr. Ambedkar Government College, Vyasarpadi, Chennai, India. He has published four papers in the International Journal of Computer Mathematics. His research interests include Molecular Computation, Graph Theory, Data Structure, Analysis of Algorithms and Theoretical Computer Science.He has authored two books. He is a member of the Editorial Board of International Journal of Advanced Computer Science and Technology (IJACST) and International Journal of Statistics and Analysis (IJSA) – Research India Publications.

Vivek Badhe received his M.Tech. in 2006 from School of Information Technology, RGPV Bhopal, The State Technical University of Madhya Pradesh. Currently He is working towards his Ph.D. degree in application of soft computing in Data Mining, from MANIT Bhopal India. His areas of interest are Data Mining, Data Science and Soft Computing.

Agnieszka Dardzinska is a professor of computer science at the Bialystok University of Technology, Poland.Her areas of specialization include Knowledge Discovery and Data Mining, Recommender Systems, Medical Information Retrieval, Flexible Query Answering, and Soft Computing. She is the author of more than 100 publications. Degree: D.Sc. (Habilitation) Computer Science.

Pratima Gautam is Professor at AISECT University, India.

Grasha Jacob received her MCA Degree from Avinashilingam Uni-versity, Coimbatore, India in 1994 and M.Phil Degree in Computer Science from Manonmaniam Sundaranar University in 2003. She is working as an Associate Professor of Computer Science in Rani Anna Government College, Tirunelveli, India. Her research interests include Information Security, Image Processing, Molecular Compu-ting. She is pursing research in Bharathiar University, Coimbatore.

Shailesh Jaloree is an Associate Professor in the Department of Applied Math's and Computer Science at Samrat Ashok Technological Institute (S.A.T.I.), Vidisha, India. He earned his Master Degree from Devi Ahiliya University Indore (M.P.) in 1991 and Ph.D. Degree (Applied Maths) From Barkatullah University, Bhopal (M.P.) in 2002. At Present he is guiding several Ph.D. Research Scholars in Mathematics and Computer Science field. He has published more than 35 Research Paper in National, International, Journals and Conferences. His areas of interest include Special Function, Data Mining, Data Warehousing and Web Mining.

Sachin Kamley did his Masters from S.A.T.I., Computer Applications Department, Rajiv Gandhi Technological University, Bhopal (M.P.) in 2006. He is working at Samrat Ashok Technological Institute (S.A.T.I), Vidisha as a Lecturer from May 2007 to Department of Computer Applications and recently completed Ph.D. from Barkatullah University, Bhopal in the year 2015. He has attended many workshops and conferences of National repute.

Ramgopal Kashyap is Research scholar at AISECT Univerity, India.

Vinod Kumar is a PhD Research Scholar in the Department of Computer Applications, Maulana Azad National Institute of Technology, Bhopal (M.P.), India. He is doing research in the field of Big Data Technology and Techniques.

Biswajit Mohapatra is practicing surgeon at Vesaj Patel Hospital, Rorurkela, India.

Suraj Kumar Nayak received his B. Tech in Electrical Engineering from Government College of Engineering Keonjhar, Odisha, India (formerly known as OSME Keonjhar) and M. Tech in Biomedical Engineering from National Institute of Technology Rourkela, Odisha, India. Currently, he is pursuing his PhD degree in Biotechnology and Medical Engineering from National Institute of Technology Rourkela, Odisha, India. His research interest includes Biomedical Instrumentation, Biomedical Signal & Image Processing, Artificial Neural Network and Trans-dermal Drug Delivery.

Aditi Nema is Assistant Professor in Bansal Institute of Research and Technology, Bhopal under the faculty of Computer Science and Engineering.

Kunal Pal is an Assistant Professor in Biomedical Engineering at NIT Rourkela.

Abha Sharma is a research scholar at the Department of Mathematics and Computer Applications, Maulana Azad National Institute of Technology, Bhopal. She received her M.C.A Degree from Rajeev Gandhi Technical University,Bhopal, India in 2007. Presently she is trying to solve issues in mixed categorical data clustering.

Utkarsh Srivastava is a student in Biomedical Engineering at NIT Rourkela.

Goutam Thakur is an Associate Professor in Biomedical Engineering at Manipal Institute of Technology (Manipal), India.

D. N. Tibarewala is a Professor of Biomedical Engineering at Jadavpur University.

Index

A

B

C

D

E

F

G

H

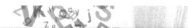
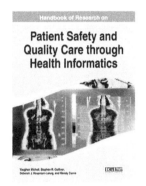
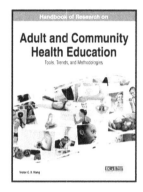
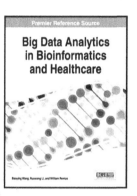
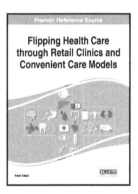
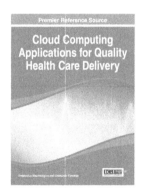
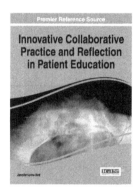
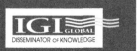
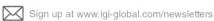

Printed in the United States
By Bookmasters